2013
YEAR BOOK OF
PULMONARY DISEASE®

The 2013 Year Book Series

Year Book of Critical Care Medicine®: Drs Dries, Zanotti-Cavazzoni, Latenser, Martinez, Rincon, and Zwank

Year Book of Emergency Medicine®: Drs Hamilton, Bruno, Handly, Minczak, Quintana, and Ramoska

Year Book of Endocrinology®: Drs Schott, Apovian, Clarke, Eugster, Meikle, Oetgen, Ovalle, Schteingart, and Toth

Year Book of Hand and Upper Limb Surgery®: Drs Yao, Adams, Isaacs, Lee, and Rizzo

Year Book of Medicine®: Drs Barker, Garrick, Gersh, Khardori, LeRoith, Panush, Talley, and Thigpen

Year Book of Neonatal and Perinatal Medicine®: Drs Fanaroff, Benitz, Donn, Neu, Papile, and Van Marter

Year Book of Neurology and Neurosurgery®: Drs Klimo, Minagar, Gandhi, House, Kevill, Liu, Mazia, Panagariya, Ragel, Riesenburger, Robottom, Schwendimann, Shafazand, Uhm, and Yang

Year Book of Obstetrics, Gynecology, and Women's Health®: Drs Dungan and Shulman

Year Book of Oncology®: Drs Arceci, Bauer, Chiorean, Gordon, Lawton, Murphy, Thigpen, and Tsao

Year Book of Ophthalmology®: Drs Rapuano, Cohen, Flanders, Hammersmith, Milman, Myers, Nagra, Nelson, Penne, Pyfer, Sergott, Shields, Talekar, and Vander

Year Book of Orthopedics®: Drs Morrey, Huddleston, Rose, Swiontkowski, and Trigg

Year Book of Otolaryngology-Head and Neck Surgery®: Drs Sindwani, Balough, Franco, Gapany, and Mitchell

Year Book of Pathology and Laboratory Medicine®: Drs Raab and Bissell

Year Book of Pediatrics®: Dr Stockman

Year Book of Plastic and Aesthetic Surgery™: Drs Miller, Boehmler, Gosman, Gutowski, Ruberg, Salisbury, and Smith

Year Book of Psychiatry and Applied Mental Health®: Drs Talbott, Ballenger, Buckley, Frances, Krupnick, and Mack

Year Book of Pulmonary Disease®: Drs Barker, Jones, Maurer, Spradley, Tanoue, and Willsie

Year Book of Sports Medicine®: Drs Shephard, Cantu, Feldman, Galea, Jankowski, Janssen, Lebrun, and Nieman

Year Book of Surgery®: Drs Copeland, Behrns, Daly, Eberlein, Fahey, Huber, Klodell, Mozingo, and Pruett

Year Book of Urology®: Drs Andriole and Coplen

Year Book of Vascular Surgery®: Drs Moneta, Gillespie, Starnes, and Watkins

2013

The Year Book of PULMONARY DISEASE®

Editor-in-Chief

James A. Barker, MD, CPE, FACP, FCCP, FAASM

Chief, Pulmonary, Critical Care Medicine, and Sleep Internal Medicine, Scott & White Health System; Professor of Medicine, Texas A&M Health Science Center, Temple, Texas

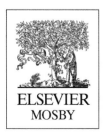

ELSEVIER
MOSBY

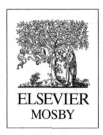

ELSEVIER
MOSBY

Vice President, Continuity: Kimberly Murphy
Developmental Editor: Patrick Manley
Production Supervisor, Electronic Year Books: Donna M. Skelton
Electronic Article Manager: Mike Sheets
Illustrations and Permissions Coordinator: Dawn A. Vohsen

2013 EDITION

Composition by TNQ Books and Journals Pvt Ltd, India

Printed and bound by CPI Group (UK) Ltd, Croydon, CR0 4YY

Transferred to digital print 2012

Editorial Office:
Elsevier, Inc.
Suite 1800
1600 John F. Kennedy Blvd
Philadelphia, PA 19103-2899

International Standard Serial Number: 8756-3452
International Standard Book Number: 978-1-4557-7289-6

Associate Editors

Shirley F. Jones, MD, FCCP, DABSM

Assistant Professor of Internal Medicine, Division of Pulmonary, Critical Care, and Sleep Medicine, Scott & White Memorial Hospital/Texas A&M Health Science Center, Temple, Texas

Janet R. Maurer, MD, MBA

Vice President, Medical Director, Health Dialog Services Corp, Scottsdale, Arizona

Christopher D. Spradley, MD, FCCP

Director, Medical Intensive Care Unit, Pulmonary Hypertension Clinic, Sleep Medicine, Scott & White Memorial Hospital, Temple, Texas

Lynn T. Tanoue, MD

Professor of Medicine, Section of Pulmonary and Critical Care Medicine, Yale School of Medicine, Yale University, New Haven, Connecticut

Sandra K. Willsie, DO, MA

Kansas City Free Clinic, Kansas City, Missouri; Medical Director, PRA International, Lenexa, Kansas

Table of Contents

Journals Represented

Journals represented in this YEAR BOOK are listed below.

Acta Anaesthesiologica Scandinavica
American Journal of Cardiology
American Journal of Emergency Medicine
American Journal of Hypertension
American Journal of Infection Control
American Journal of Medicine
American Journal of Obstetrics and Gynecology
American Journal of Pathology
American Journal of Respiratory and Critical Care Medicine
American Journal of Transplantation
Anesthesiology
Annals of Allergy, Asthma & Immunology
Annals of Emergency Medicine
Annals of Internal Medicine
Annals of Oncology
Annals of the Rheumatic Diseases
Annals of Thoracic Surgery
Archives of Internal Medicine
Archives of Pediatrics & Adolescent Medicine
British Journal of Anaesthesia
British Medical Journal
CA: A Cancer Journal for Clinicians
Chest
Clinical Infectious Diseases
Critical Care Medicine
European Respiratory Journal
Intensive Care Medicine
International Journal of Gynecology & Obstetrics
Journal of Acquired Immune Deficiency Syndromes
Journal of Cardiothoracic and Vascular Anesthesia
Journal of Clinical Anesthesia
Journal of Clinical Investigation
Journal of Clinical Neuroscience
Journal of Clinical Oncology
Journal of Clinical Rheumatology
Journal of Emergency Medicine
Journal of Heart and Lung Transplantation
Journal of Infectious Diseases
Journal of Pediatrics
Journal of the American College of Cardiology
Journal of the American Geriatrics Society
Journal of the American Medical Association
Journal of the National Cancer Institute
Journal of the National Comprehensive Cancer Network
Journal of Thoracic Oncology
Journal of Trauma and Acute Care Surgery
Lancet

Mayo Clinic Proceedings
New England Journal of Medicine
Pediatrics
Pharmacotherapy
Respiratory Medicine
Sleep
Thorax
Tobacco Control
Transplantation

STANDARD ABBREVIATIONS

The following terms are abbreviated in this edition: acquired immunodeficiency syndrome (AIDS), cardiopulmonary resuscitation (CPR), central nervous system (CNS), cerebrospinal fluid (CSF), computed tomography (CT), deoxyribonucleic acid (DNA), electrocardiography (ECG), health maintenance organization (HMO), human immunodeficiency virus (HIV), intensive care unit (ICU), intramuscular (IM), intravenous (IV), magnetic resonance (MR) imaging (MRI), ribonucleic acid (RNA), and ultrasound (US).

NOTE

The YEAR BOOK OF PULMONARY DISEASE is a literature survey service providing abstracts of articles published in the professional literature. Every effort is made to assure the accuracy of the information presented in these pages. Neither the editors nor the publisher of the YEAR BOOK OF PULMONARY DISEASE can be responsible for errors in the original materials. The editors' comments are their own opinions. Mention of specific products within this publication does not constitute endorsement.

To facilitate the use of the YEAR BOOK OF PULMONARY DISEASE as a reference tool, all illustrations and tables included in this publication are now identified as they appear in the original article. This change is meant to help the reader recognize that any illustration or table appearing in the YEAR BOOK OF PULMONARY DISEASE may be only one of many in the original article. For this reason, figure and table numbers will often appear to be out of sequence within the YEAR BOOK OF PULMONARY DISEASE.

1 Asthma, Allergy, and Cystic Fibrosis

Introduction

This year's highlighted publications on asthma and Cystic Fibrosis (CF) were chosen from scores of articles, and those appearing in this chapter reflect what we believe to be the most important investigations of particular significance to the practicing clinician.

Despite minor adjustments in evidence-based guidelines, the same basic therapies exist, and for chronic uncontrolled asthma, inhaled corticosteroids (ICS) play a front-and-center role. Several articles highlighted this year focus on new, 24-hour duration agents.[1,2] As important and attractive as these new, longer half-life agents may be, an investigation by Jentzsch et al[3] demonstrated that even with noncompliance for a bid regimen, as long as patients were using their beclomethasone diproprionate ICS in a dose of 300 mcg daily, control of mild to moderate asthma was preserved. Tiotropium (T), not just for COPD anymore? A study published this year[4] indicates that in poorly controlled asthma, despite appropriate use of ICS and long-acting beta agonists (LABA), addition of T provided modest and sustained bronchodilatation and significantly increased the time to severe exacerbation. And finally, work remains in convincing the global emergency medicine community to provide asthmatics being discharged from the emergency department following an exacerbation with asthma controller therapy.

Several CF articles were chosen to be highlighted this year, including a review of the era of personalized medicine in CF. As most practitioners know, CF is an amalgamation of a variety of mutations, all leading to varied expression of symptoms, disease, and longevity. The article by Clancy et al from Am Rev Resp Crit Care Med is worth reading. Vitamin D deficiency in Puerto Rican children is common[5] and must be addressed as it is associated with asthma exacerbations, and children with CF may require increased supplementation with Vitamin D in order to achieve therapeutic efficacy. Finally, new therapeutic regimens are on the market for CF, but providers must evaluate the genotype when determining whether a particular treatment will provide efficacy. Exciting news about new therapies, but treatment must be tailored for the patient, as always!

Finally, we hope that you enjoy reviewing this selection of publications as much as we enjoyed selecting them for you.

Sandra K. Willsie, DO, MA

References

1. Bleecker ER, Bateman ED, Busse WW, et al. Once-daily fluticasone furoate is efficacious in patients with symptomatic asthma on low-dose inhaled corticosteroids. *Ann Allergy Asthma Immunol.* 2012;109:353-358.e4.
2. Lötvall J, Bateman ED, Bleecker ER, et al. 24-h duration of the novel LABA vilanterol trifenatate in asthma patients treated with inhaled corticosteroids. *Eur Respir J.* 2012;40:570-579.
3. Jentzsch NS, Camargos P, Sarinho ES, Bousquet J. Adherence rate to beclomethasone dipropionate and the level of asthma control. *Respir Med.* 2012;106:338-343.
4. Kerstjens HA, Engel M, Dahl R, et al. Tiotropium in asthma poorly controlled with standard combination therapy. *N Engl J Med.* 2012;367:1198-1207.
5. Brehm JM, Acosta-Pérez E, Klei L, et al. Vitamin D insufficiency and severe asthma exacerbations in Puerto Rican children. *Am J Respir Crit Care Med.* 2012;186: 140-146.

Asthma

Vitamin D Insufficiency and Severe Asthma Exacerbations in Puerto Rican Children

Brehm JM, Acosta-Pérez E, Klei L, et al (Children's Hosp of Pittsburgh of UPMC, PA; Univ of Puerto Rico, San Juan; Univ of Pittsburgh, PA; et al)
Am J Respir Crit Care Med 186:140-146, 2012

Rationale.—Vitamin D insufficiency (a serum 25(OH)D < 30 ng/ml) has been associated with severe asthma exacerbations, but this could be explained by underlying racial ancestry or disease severity. Little is known about vitamin D and asthma in Puerto Ricans.

Objectives.—To examine whether vitamin D insufficiency is associated with severe asthma exacerbations in Puerto Rican children, independently of racial ancestry, atopy, and time outdoors.

Methods.—A cross-sectional study was conducted of 560 children ages 6—14 years with (n = 287) and without (n = 273) asthma in San Juan, Puerto Rico. We measured plasma vitamin D and estimated the percentage of African racial ancestry among participants using genome wide genotypic data. We tested whether vitamin D insufficiency is associated with severe asthma exacerbations, lung function, or atopy (greater than or equal to one positive IgE to allergens) using logistic or linear regression. Multivariate models were adjusted for African ancestry, time outdoors, atopy, and other covariates.

Measurements and Main Results.—Vitamin D insufficiency was common in children with (44%) and without (47%) asthma. In multivariate analyses, vitamin D insufficiency was associated with higher odds of greater than or equal to one severe asthma exacerbation in the prior year (odds ratio [OR], 2.6; 95% confidence interval [CI], 1.5—4.9; $P = 0.001$) and atopy, and a lower FEV_1/FVC in cases. After stratification by atopy, the magnitude of the association between vitamin D insufficiency and severe exacerbations was greater in nonatopic (OR, 6.2; 95% CI, 2−21.6; $P = 0.002$) than in atopic (OR, 2; 95% CI, 1−4.1; $P = 0.04$) cases.

Conclusions.—Vitamin D insufficiency is associated with severe asthma exacerbations in Puerto Rican children, independently of racial ancestry, atopy, or markers of disease severity or control.

▶ Vitamin D deficiency has been considered a fad by some, worrisome and demanding of treatment by others, and pinpointed as causative of a number of diseases by many in the scientific community. More recently, vitamin D deficiency has been studied in many diverse populations, including those with racial and ethnic variances. This provocative study evaluated Puerto Rican children, both nonasthmatics and asthmatics, to evaluate the role of vitamin D in children in general and specifically in asthmatic children. Percentage of African ancestry, time spent out of doors, vitamin D levels, and hospitalizations or acute severe exacerbations in the past year were evaluated. Vitamin D deficiency was common in controls (nonasthmatics). After analyzing for covariates, vitamin D deficiency was associated with more severe asthma; in addition, vitamin D deficiency was more common in older and female children, who are more likely to have had a severe exacerbation within the past year. This increase in the severity of asthma was independent of African ancestry, time spent out of doors, and atopy. This shows us that there continues to be elucidated inflammatory processes at work with asthma and vitamin D deficiency.

S. K. Willsie, DO, MA

Adherence rate to beclomethasone dipropionate and the level of asthma control

Jentzsch NS, Camargos P, Sarinho ESC, et al (Med Sciences School, Brazil; Universidade Federal de São João del-Rei, Brazil; Federal Univ of Pernambuco, Brazil; et al)
Respir Med 106.338-343, 2012

There are only a few studies assessing the relationship between adherence rate to ICS, as assessed by electronic monitoring, and the level of asthma control in childhood. The present study was carried out to examine the relationship between adherence to beclomethasone diprorionate (BDP) as well as other factors related to poor asthma control. In this prospective cohort study, 102 steroid naïve randomly selected subjects with persistent asthma, aged 5−14 years were prescribed 500−750 µg daily of BDP-CFC and followed during one year. Adherence to BDP was measured electronically in the 4th, 8th and 12th months of study. The level of asthma control was classified as either controlled or uncontrolled instead of the current three categories recommended by the Global Initiative for Asthma (GINA). Mean adherence rate was higher in patients with controlled asthma during

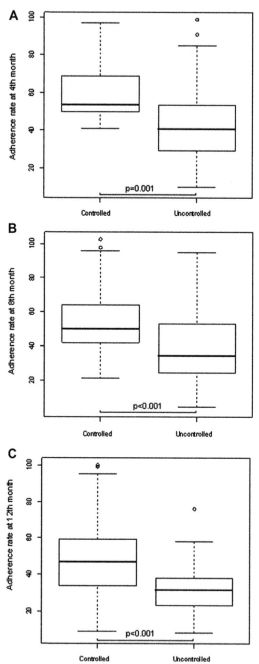

FIGURE 1.—Adherence rate to BDP (%) and the corresponding level of asthma control during the follow-up appointments (A = 4th month; B = 8th month; and C = 12th month). (Reprinted from Respiratory Medicine. Jentzsch NS, Camargos P, Sarinho ESC, et al. Adherence rate to beclomethasone dipropionate and the level of asthma control. *Respir Med.* 2012;106:338-343, Copyright 2012, with permission from Elsevier.)

TABLE 2.—Adherence Rate (%) Stratified by Level of Asthma Control in the 4th, 8th, and 12th Month (N = 102)

Level of asthma control	Mean (SD)	Adherence Min	1st. Q	Median	3rd. Q	Max
4th month						
Controlled	60.4 (17.3)	41.0	49.5	54.0	69.5	97.0
Uncontrolled	43.8 (21.5)	10.0	29.3	41.0	53.8	99.0
8th month						
Controlled	56.2 (22.1)	21.0	42.0	50.0	70.0	100.0
Uncontrolled	39.0 (21.0)	4.0	24.0	34.5	54.0	95.0
12th month						
Controlled	49.8 (20.8)	9.0	24.5	47.0	55.0	100.0
Uncontrolled	31.2 (12.6)	8.0	22.5	31.5	38.0	76.0

follow-up, but went down from 60.4% in the 4th month to 49.8% in the 12th month ($p = 0.038$). Conversely, among patients with uncontrolled asthma, the mean adherence rate decreased from 43.8% to 31.2% ($p = 0.001$). Multivariate analysis showed that the level of asthma control was independently associated to the adherence rate in all follow-up visits (p-values equal or lower than 0.005). The level of asthma control was directly proportional to adherence rate. Our results suggest that a BDP daily dose by 300 μg seems to be enough to attain control over mild and moderate persistent asthma, including exercise induced asthma (Fig 1, Table 2).

▶ Bolstering the literature with regard to efficacy and adherence to the use of inhaled corticosteroid (ICS) therapy in steroid-naive patients, this investigation dispensed 500 (puff morning and evening) or 750 micrograms (250 micrograms administered 3 times daily, once in the morning and 2 puffs at bedtime) of beclomethasone dipropionate and followed the asthma control and medication adherence for 1 year. Doser Clinical Trials (MedTrack Products, USA) was used to record adherence. Adherence rates at the 4th, 8th, and 12th month are depicted, comparing the number of asthma controlled with asthma uncontrolled patients (Table 2). Fig 1 depicts controlled asthma versus uncontrolled asthma as compared with adherence at the 4th, 8th, and 12th month of treatment. The level of asthma control was consistently and independently related to adherence rate at all 3 visits ($P \le .005$). Interestingly and provocatively, adherence rates with ICS of 40% to 50% were enough to maintain control. The question remains, shall we tell our patients to only take half of their ICS dose and hope they'll comply all the time… *or* shall we keep telling patients to continue to take the recommended doses and be happy with controlled asthma as the marker of success, regardless of their actual adherence?

S. K. Willsie, DO, MA

Once-daily fluticasone furoate is efficacious in patients with symptomatic asthma on low-dose inhaled corticosteroids

Bleecker ER, Bateman ED, Busse WW, et al (Wake Forest Univ Health Sciences, Winston-Salem, NC; Univ of Cape Town, South Africa; Univ of Wisconsin, Madison; et al)
Ann Allergy Asthma Immunol 109:353-358.e4, 2012

Background.—Fluticasone furoate (FF) is an inhaled corticosteroid (ICS) with 24-hour activity in development as a once-daily treatment for the long-term management of asthma.

Objective.—To assess the efficacy and safety of 4 doses of once-daily FF administered using a dry powder inhaler in patients ($\geq$12 years) with moderate asthma, uncontrolled on low-dose ICS (fluticasone propionate [FP] 200 μg/day or equivalent).

Methods.—This double-blind, placebo-controlled, dose-ranging study randomized 622 patients to 1 of 6 treatments: FF (100, 200, 300, or 400 μg) once daily in the evening, FP 250 μg twice daily (active control), or placebo for 8 weeks. The primary endpoint was the change from baseline in predose evening forced expiratory colume in 1 second (FEV$_1$) at week 8.

Results.—At week 8, relative to placebo, all doses of FF once daily and FP twice daily demonstrated significantly ($P < .001$) greater increases from baseline and greater than 200-mL increases in predose FEV$_1$. There was no evidence of a dose-response relationship between FF doses. Improvement with once-daily FF was similar to or greater than that for twice-daily FP. Secondary efficacy endpoint findings generally supported the efficacy of FF 100 to 400 μg once daily, although statistically significant improvements versus placebo in symptom-free 24-hour periods were only reported for FF 400 μg. There were few withdrawals due to lack of efficacy. Oral candidiasis was reported in 0 to 4% of patients; 24-hour urinary cortisol excretion ratios were similar across active treatment groups and not significantly different from placebo.

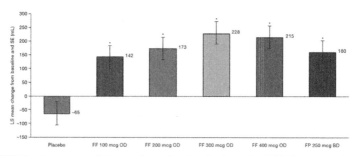

FIGURE 2.—Least squares (LS) mean change from baseline in pre dose FEV$_1$ (last observation carried forward) at week 8 (ITT population). *$P < .001$ relative to placebo. BD, twice daily; FF, fluticasone furoate; FP, fluticasone propionate; ITT, intent-to-treat; OD, once daily; SE, standard error. (Reprinted from Annals of Allergy, Asthma and Immunology. Bleecker ER, Bateman ED, Busse WW, et al. Once-daily fluticasone furoate is efficacious in patients with symptomatic asthma on low-dose inhaled corticosteroids. *Ann Allergy Asthma Immunol.* 2012;109:353-358.e4, Copyright 2012, with permission from American College of Annals of Allergy, Asthma & Immunology.)

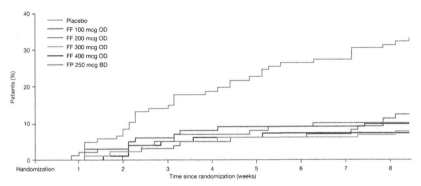

FIGURE 3.—Withdrawals due to lack of efficacy (cumulative incidence) (ITT population). BD, twice daily; FF, fluticasone furoate; FP, fluticasone propionate; ITT, intent to treat; OD, once daily. (Reprinted from Annals of Allergy, Asthma and Immunology. Bleecker ER, Bateman ED, Busse WW, et al. Once-daily fluticasone furoate is efficacious in patients with symptomatic asthma on low-dose inhaled corticosteroids. *Ann Allergy Asthma Immunol.* 2012;109:353-358.e4, Copyright 2012, with permission from American College of Annals of Allergy, Asthma & Immunology.)

Conclusion.—FF 100 to 400 μg once daily in the evening is effective and well tolerated in patients with asthma uncontrolled on low-dose ICS, with 100 μg and 200 μg, considered the most applicable doses in this asthma population.

Trial Registration.—clinicaltrials.gov Identifier: NCT00603278 (Figs 2 and 3).

▶ Fluticasone furoate (FF) is an inhaled corticosteroid (ICS) currently undergoing development for once-daily use in long-term asthma. Moderate asthmatics with uncontrolled asthma who were taking low-dose fluticasone propionate (FP) 200 μg/d or equivalent were randomly assigned to 6 different treatment arms: FF at 100, 200, 300, or 400 μg/d in the evening; or FP 250 μg/d twice daily (active control); or placebo for 8 weeks. Fig 2 shows least-squares mean change from baseline in predose forced expiratory volume in 1 second (FEV_1) at 8 weeks in the intent-to-treat population. All treatment groups had statistically significant improvements in FEV_1 compared with the placebo group. Fig 3 depicts withdrawals caused by lack of efficacy compared with that of placebo. FF doses greater than 200 μg/d did not show superior performance to the 300- and 400-μg/d dose. All FF doses had similar FEV_1 or greater response than the FP group. Adverse events (AE) were considered clinically insignificant, and AEs related to FF 300 μg/d were equivalent to the AE profile for FP. Four serious AEs occurred, none related to the FF. Longer-term studies with comparative doses of other ICS are in order, but clearly the early data show that FF has promise as a once-daily ICS.

S. K. Willsie, DO, MA

Tiotropium in Asthma Poorly Controlled with Standard Combination Therapy

Kerstjens HAM, Engel M, Dahl R, et al (Univ Med Ctr Groningen, the Netherlands; Boehringer Ingelheim Pharma, Germany; Aarhus Univ Hosp, Denmark; et al)

N Engl J Med 367:1198-1207, 2012

Background.—Some patients with asthma have frequent exacerbations and persistent airflow obstruction despite treatment with inhaled glucocorticoids and long-acting beta-agonists (LABAs).

Methods.—In two replicate, randomized, controlled trials involving 912 patients with asthma who were receiving inhaled glucocorticoids and LABAs, we compared the effect on lung function and exacerbations of adding tiotropium (a total dose of 5 μg) or placebo, both delivered by a soft-mist inhaler once daily for 48 weeks. All the patients were symptomatic, had a post-bronchodilator forced expiratory volume in 1 second (FEV₁) of 80% or less of the predicted value, and had a history of at least one severe exacerbation in the previous year.

TABLE 2.—Mean Difference between Tiotropium and Placebo in the Change from Baseline to Week 24 and Week 48 in the Two Trials*

| | | Trial 1 | | Trial 2 |
| | | Difference in Change | | Difference in Change |
Measure and Week	No. of Patients	Mean (95% CI)	No. of Patients	Mean (95% CI)
Forced expiratory volume in 1 sec				
Peak at 0–3 hr (ml)				
24 wk[†]	428	86 (20 to 152)[‡]	423	154 (91 to 217)[§]
48 wk	417	73 (5 to 140)[‡]	403	152 (87 to 217)[§]
Trough (ml)				
24 wk[†]	428	88 (27 to 149)[¶]	422	111 (53 to 169)[§]
48 wk	417	42 (−21 to 104)	402	92 (32 to 151)[¶]
Forced vital capacity				
Peak (ml)				
24 wk	428	89 (6 to 173)[‡]	423	94 (10 to 177)[‡]
48 wk	417	125 (40 to 210)[¶]	403	114 (29 to 200)[¶]
Trough (ml)				
24 wk	428	136 (58 to 214)[§]	422	106 (25 to 186)[¶]
48 wk	417	111 (31 to 190)[¶]	402	71 (−12 to 153)
Peak expiratory flow[‖]				
Morning (liters/min)				
24 wk	414	21.5 (12.7 to 30.4)[§]	407	23.3 (14.5 to 32.1)[§]
48 wk	369	20.3 (11.3 to 29.4)[§]	378	14.0 (5.1 to 22.9)[¶]
Evening (liters/min)				
24 wk	413	22.0 (13.0 to 30.9)[§]	405	29.9 (20.7 to 39.1)[§]
48 wk	369	22.6 (13.5 to 31.7)[§]	377	24.5 (15.1 to 33.8)[§]

*All differences are calculated as the adjusted mean change from baseline, as measured at randomization (visit 2), for tiotropium minus placebo. Baseline was defined as the measurement obtained before any study or maintenance medication was administered. Values for forced expiratory volume in 1 second and forced vital capacity have been adjusted for treatment, center, visit, baseline value, and interactions between treatment and visit and between baseline value and visit.
[†]This category was a coprimary end point in the two trials.
[‡]P<0.05.
[§]P<0.001.
[¶]P<0.01.
[‖]All values are means of weekly measurements of peak expiratory flow.

Results.—The patients had a mean baseline FEV_1 of 62% of the predicted value; the mean age was 53 years. At 24 weeks, the mean ($\pm SE$) change in the peak FEV_1 from baseline was greater with tiotropium than with placebo in the two trials: a difference of 86 ± 34 ml in trial 1 ($P = 0.01$) and 154 ± 32 ml in trial 2 ($P < 0.001$). The predose (trough) FEV1 also improved in trials 1 and 2 with tiotropium, as compared with placebo: a difference of 88 ± 31 ml ($P = 0.01$) and 111 ± 30 ml ($P < 0.001$), respectively. The addition of tiotropium increased the time to the first severe exacerbation (282 days vs. 226 days), with an overall reduction of 21% in the risk of a severe exacerbation (hazard ratio, 0.79; $P = 0.03$). No deaths occurred; adverse events were similar in the two groups.

Conclusions.—In patients with poorly controlled asthma despite the use of inhaled glucocorticoids and LABAs, the addition of tiotropium significantly increased the time to the first severe exacerbation and provided modest sustained bronchodilation. (Funded by Boehringer Ingelheim and Pfizer; ClinicalTrials.gov numbers, NCT00772538 and NCT00776984.) (Table 2).

▶ Here is another setback in classifying drugs for single use. Tiotropium, US Food and Drug Administration—approved for some years, is well known and used frequently for the treatment of chronic obstructive pulmonary disease. Tiotropium (5 micrograms) or placebo was delivered via a soft-mist inhaler daily for 48 weeks to severe uncontrolled asthmatics on inhaled corticosteroids and long-acting beta agonists. Table 2 details the mean difference between tiotropium and placebo in the change from baseline to Weeks 24 and 48 in 2 different trials. Statistically significant improvement was seen and maintained to 48 weeks in peak expiratory flow rate and forced expiratory volume in 1 second. Fig 2 in the original article demonstrates the total number of severe exacerbations per patient year to be significantly lower in the tiotropium group 0.53 versus the placebo group 0.66 ($P = .046$). The addition of tiotropium increased the time to first severe exacerbation (282 days vs 226 days), with an overall reduction of 21% in the risk of severe exacerbation (hazard ratio, 0.79; $P = .03$). Yes, we have something new in the chronic therapy armamentarium for chronic, uncontrolled asthma: tiotropium!

S. K. Willsie, DO, MA

24-h duration of the novel LABA vilanterol trifenatate in asthma patients treated with inhaled corticosteroids

Lötvall J, Bateman ED, Bleecker ER, et al (Univ of Gothenburg, Sweden; Univ of Cape Town, South Africa; Wake Forest Univ Health Sciences, Winston-Salem, NC; et al)
Eur Respir J 40:570-579, 2012

Current guidelines recommend adding a long-acting inhaled β_2-agonist (LABA) to inhaled corticosteroids (ICS) in patients with uncontrolled asthma. This study evaluated the novel, once-daily LABA vilanterol

TABLE 4.—Summary of Adverse Event (AE) Data (Intent-to-Treat population)

	Placebo	3 µg VI	6.25 µg VI	12.5 µg VI	25 µg VI	50 µg VI
Total subjects n	102	101	101	100	101	102
Any on-treatment AE	37 (36)	37 (37)	34 (34)	25 (25)	23 (23)	31 (30)
Any post-treatment AE[#]	6 (6)	4 (4)	5 (5)	0	5 (5)	2 (2)
Any drug-related AE	7 (7)	8 (8)	8 (8)	5 (5)	4 (4)	7 (7)
Any AE leading to permanent discontinuation of drug or withdrawal[¶]	1 (<1)	1 (<1)	2 (2)	1 (1)	1 (<1)	0
SAEs	0	0	0	0	0	0
Most frequent on-treatment AEs (≥3% in any treatment group)						
Headache	8 (8)	12 (12)	7 (7)	9 (9)	7 (7)	8 (8)
Upper respiratory tract infection	2 (2)	2 (2)	1 (<1)	3 (3)	2 (2)	2 (2)
Nasopharyngitis	4 (4)	2 (2)	2 (2)	0	0	2 (2)
Dizziness	2 (2)	1 (<1)	1 (<1)	1 (1)	0	3 (3)
Back pain	0	3 (3)	0	1 (1)	1 (<1)	0
Muscle spasms	0	0	2 (2)	0	0	3 (3)
Dyspnoea	3 (3)	0	0	0	0	0

Data are presented as n (%). VI: vilanterol trifenatate; SAE: serious adverse event.
[#]: During the week following the 28-day dosing period.
[¶]: Two patients were withdrawn due to AEs; four patients were withdrawn primarily due to protocol-defined stopping criteria, with AEs as a sub-reason.

trifenatate (VI) in asthma patients who remained symptomatic despite existing ICS therapy.

The study involved a randomised, double-blind, placebo-controlled trial of VI (3, 6.25, 12.5, 25 and 50 µg), administered once daily in the evening by dry powder inhaler for 28 days, in asthma patients aged ≥12 yrs symptomatic on current ICS therapy. The primary end-point was trough (24 h post-dose) forced expiratory volume in 1 s (FEV_1); secondary end-points were weighted mean FEV_1, peak expiratory flow (PEF), symptom-/rescue-free 24-h periods, and safety.

A significant relationship was observed between VI dose and improvements in trough FEV_1 ($p = 0.037$). Statistically significant increases in mean trough FEV_1, relative to placebo, were documented for VI 12.5—50 µg (121—162 mL; $p \leq 0.016$). Dose-related effects of VI were observed on weighted mean (0-24 h) FEV_1, morning/evening PEF, and symptom-/rescue-free 24-h periods. All doses of VI were well tolerated with low incidences of recognised LABA-related adverse events (tremor 0—2%; palpitations 0—2%; glucose effects 0-1%; potassium effects 0—<1%).

Once-daily VI 12.5—50 µg resulted in prolonged bronchodilation of at least 24 h with good tolerability in asthma patients receiving ICS. Based on the overall efficacy and adverse event profile from this study, the optimum dose of VI appears to be 25 µg (Table 4).

▶ Vilanterol (V), a long-acting beta agonist (LABA) with attested 24-hour duration, was administered (3, 6.25, 12.5, 25, and 50 micrograms) via dry powder inhaler in the evening only for 28 days to 614 asthmatics who remained uncontrolled despite baseline inhaled corticosteroids (ICS) therapy. Fig 2 in the original article demonstrates the adjusted mean change in trough forced expiratory volume in 1 second (FEV_1) vs placebo at Day 28 (intent-to-treat [ITT]). Fig 3 in the original article demonstrates by colored line the changes from baseline serial FEV_1-adjusted treatment difference from placebo from repeated measures model. Dosing of V was well-tolerated and not dose-related as demonstrated by Table 4 (adverse events in the ITT group). No serious adverse effects were reported for any group. The first significant increase in FEV_1 was observed at the first time point measured following the first dose (15 minutes after inhalation) and the maximum effect was noted at 3 to 4 hours after dose on Day 1, and within 1 to 2 hours after dose on Day 28. These are promising results for this 24-hour LABA, yet further studies are needed with ICS therapy versus standard of care.

S. K. Willsie, DO, MA

A Systematic Review of Long-Acting β2-Agonists Versus Higher Doses of Inhaled Corticosteroids in Asthma
Castro-Rodriguez JA, Rodrigo GJ (Pontificia Universidad Católica de Chile, Santiago, Chile; Hosp Central de Las Fuerzas Armadas, Montevideo, Uruguay)
Pediatrics 130:e650-e657, 2012

Objective.—To compare the efficacy of inhaled corticosteroids (ICS) plus long-acting β2 agonist (LABA) versus higher doses of ICS in children/adolescents with uncontrolled persistent asthma.

Methods.—Randomized, prospective, controlled trials published January 1996 to January 2012 with a minimum of 4 weeks of LABA+ICS versus higher doses of ICS were retrieved through Medline, Embase, Central, and manufacturer's databases. The primary outcome was asthma exacerbations requiring systemic corticosteroids; secondary outcomes were the pulmonary function test (PEF), withdrawals during the treatment period, days without symptoms, use of rescue medication, and adverse events.

Results.—Nine studies ($n = 1641$ patients) met criteria for inclusion (7 compared LABA+ICS versus double ICS doses and 2 LABA+ICS versus higher than double ICS doses). There was no statistically significant difference in the number of patients with asthma exacerbations requiring systemic corticosteroids between children receiving LABA+ICS and those receiving higher doses of ICS (odds ratio = 0.76; 95% confidence interval: 0.48–1.22, $P = .25$, $I^2 = 16\%$). In the subgroup analysis, patients receiving LABA+ICS showed a decreased risk of asthma exacerbations compared with higher than twice ICS doses (odds ratio = 0.48; 95% confidence interval: 0.28–0.82, $P = .007$, $I^2 = 0$). Children treated with LABA+ICS had significantly higher PEF, less use of rescue medication, and higher short-term growth than those on higher ICS doses. There were no other significant differences in adverse events.

Conclusions.—There were no statistically significant group differences between ICS+LABA and double doses of ICS in reducing the incidence of asthma exacerbations but it did decrease the risk comparing to higher than double doses of ICS.

▶ Very interesting meta-analysis reviewing studies of pediatric asthmatics treated with inhaled corticosteroids (ICS) plus long-acting beta agonist (LABA) compared with ICS alone (subdivided by ICS doubled or ICS greater than doubled dose). A subgroup analysis revealed a reduction in asthma exacerbations favoring the ICS plus LABA group. There were several surprises from this study: LABA plus ICS had significantly higher peak expiratory flow (PEF); used less rescue medicine; had higher short-term growth compared with the ICS—all more than a doubled dose of ICS. In addition, the ICS and LABA group had improved PEF compared with the higher dose ICS group. It is not known if this will enter into the continued dialogue about ICS alone or ICS plus LABA in a meaningful way, but this investigation has certainly added important information not well known in the literature.

S. K. Willsie, DO, MA

Asthma controller delay and recurrence risk after an emergency department visit or hospitalization
Stanford RH, Buikema AR, Riedel AA, et al (US Health Outcomes, Research Triangle Park, NC; OptumInsight, Eden Prairie, MN; et al)
Respir Med 106:1631-1638, 2012

Background.—Patients who have asthma-related emergency department (ED) visits or hospitalizations are at risk for recurrent exacerbation events. Our objectives were to assess whether receiving a controller medication at discharge affects risk of recurrence and whether delaying controller initiation alters this risk.

Methods.—Asthma patients with an ED visit or inpatient (IP) stay who received a controller dispensing within 6 months were identified from healthcare claims. Cox proportional hazards of the time to first recurrence of an asthma-related ED or IP visit in the 6-month period following the initial event were constructed, with time following discharge without controller medication as the primary predictor.

Results.—A total of 6139 patients met inclusion criteria, 78% with an ED visit and 22% with an IP visit; 15% had a recurrence within 6 months. The adjusted hazard ratio (HR) associated with not having controller medication at discharge was 1.79 (95% confidence interval [CI], 1.42–2.25). The controller-by-time interaction was significant ($P < 0.001$), with hazard rising as time-to-controller initiation increased. Delaying initiation by 1 day approximately tripled the risk (HR 2.95; 95% CI 1.48–5.88). Sensitivity analyses, including accounting for controller fills prior to the index event, did not substantially alter these results.

Conclusions.—This observational study shows that the risk of a recurrent asthma-related ED visit or IP stay increased as the time to initiate a

TABLE 2.—Medications During Follow-up

	Total (N = 6139)	0 Days (n = 1538)	Number of Days to Controller Initiation Following Index Event Discharge					
			1–30 Days (n = 2645)	31–60 Days (n = 673)	61–90 Days (n = 415)	91–120 Days (n = 344)	121–150 Days (n = 285)	151–180 Days (n = 239)
Index (first) controller medication[a]								
ICS[b]	4916 (80)	1322 (86)	2093 (79)	512 (76)	322 (78)	255 (74)	216 (76)	196 (82)
Leukotriene modifier	1801 (29)	413 (27)	778 (29)	212 (32)	132 (32)	110 (32)	90 (32)	66 (28)
Any follow-up controller medication[c]								
ICS[b]	5271 (86)	1408 (92)	2273 (86)	553 (82)	346 (83)	269 (78)	222 (78)	200 (84)
ICS monotherapy	3025 (49)	862 (56)	1337 (51)	282 (42)	186 (45)	140 (41)	114 (40)	104 (44)
Fluticasone/salmeterol	2550 (42)	655 (43)	1088 (41)	295 (44)	168 (40)	136 (40)	111 (39)	97 (41)
Budesonide/formoterol	11 (0.2)	2 (0.1)	8 (0.3)	1 (0.2)	0 (0)	0 (0)	0 (0)	0 (0)
Leukotriene modifiers	2338 (38)	588 (38)	1030 (39)	266 (40)	153 (37)	130 (38)	103 (36)	68 (28)
LABA monotherapy	26 (0.4)	8 (0.5)	12 (0.5)	3 (0.5)	3 (0.7)	0 (0)	0 (0)	0 (0)
Mast cell stabilizers	16 (0.3)	3 (0.2)	11 (0.4)	1 (0.2)	0 (0)	0 (0)	1 (0.4)	0 (0)
Methylxanthines	11 (0.2)	3 (0.2)	2 (0.1)	3 (0.5)	1 (0.2)	2 (0.6)	0 (0)	0 (0)
Omalizumab	6 (0.1)	1 (0.1)	3 (0.1)	2 (0.3)	0 (0)	0 (0)	0 (0)	0 (0)
Quick-relief medication								
SABA	5037 (82)	1270 (83)	2133 (81)	561 (83)	351 (85)	283 (82)	245 (86)	194 (81)
OCS	3641 (59)	685 (45)	1719 (65)	428 (64)	275 (66)	221 (64)	179 (63)	134 (56)

ICS, inhaled corticosteroid; LABA, long-acting beta-agonist; OCS, oral corticosteroid; SABA, short-acting beta-agonist.
[a]By definition, the first controller medication could be an inhaled corticosteroid or leukotriene modifier. Patients could have claims for both types of medication on the same date.
[b]Includes monotherapy and LABA combinations.
[c]Includes the first controller and any subsequent controller medications.

controller increased. Our findings support the importance of early controller initiation following an asthma-related ED or IP visit in reducing risk of recurrence (Table 2).

▶ Asthmatics requiring inpatient admissions (IP) or emergency department visits (ED) for asthma are at increased risk for recurrent exacerbations.[1,2] Accordingly, current practice guidelines recommend that discharge planning include preventive measures to address future exacerbations.[3,4] Use of controller medications after an acute exacerbation of asthma has been found to effectively reduce the risk of recurrent exacerbation.[5-7] Table 2 depicts the type of controller or no controller prescription after hospital admission or ED visit to the study cohort. The overall results of this study show that delay in use of controller medication by even 1 day increased the hazard ratio (HR) and nearly tripled the risk for exacerbation (HR 2.95; 95% confidence interval: 1.48–5.88). The significant controller-by-time interaction was $P < .001$, indicting the hazard for exacerbation increases with delay in controller initiation therapy. Perhaps most alarming, despite this investigation and others in the last decade, the majority of ED physicians still do not provide controller medication at the time of discharge.[8,9] ED physicians and hospitalists should be a primary target for education on the need to dispense controller medication at the time of discharge, rather than leaving this to the primary care provider.

S. K. Willsie, DO, MA

References

1. Miller MK, Lee JH, Miller DP, Wenzel SE. Recent asthma exacerbations: a key predictor of future exacerbations. *Respir Med.* 2007;101:481-489.
2. Adams RJ, Smith BJ, Ruffin RE. Factors associated with hospital admissions and repeat emergency department visits for adults with asthma. *Thorax.* 2000;55: 566-573.
3. National Asthma Education and Prevention Program. *Expert Panel Report 3: Guidelines for the Diagnosis and Management of Asthma.* National Heart Lung and Blood Institute; 2007. http://www.nhlbi.nih.gov/guidelines/asthma/asthgdln/pdf. Accessed July 26, 2012.
4. Global Initiative for Asthma (GINA). *Gina Report, Global Strategy for Asthma Management and Prevention.* Global Initiative for Asthma (GINA); 2011. http://www.ginasthma.org. Accessed July 26, 2012.
5. Silverman RA, Nowak RM, Korenblat PE, et al. Zafirlukast treatment for acute asthma: evaluation in a randomized, double-blind, multicenter trial. *Chest.* 2004;126:1480-1489.
6. Sin DD, Man SF. Low-dose inhaled corticosteroid therapy and risk of emergency department visits for asthma. *Arch Intern Med.* 2002;162:1591-1595.
7. Smith MJ, Rascati KL, McWilliams BC. Inhaled anti-inflammatory pharmacotherapy and subsequent hospitalizations and emergency department visits among patients with asthma in the Texas Medicaid program. *Ann Allergy Asthma Immunol.* 2004;92:40-46.
8. Scarfone RJ, Zorc JJ, Angsuco CJ. Emergency physicians' prescribing of asthma controller medications. *Pediatrics.* 2006;117:821e7.
9. Cydulka RK, Tamayo-Sarver JH, Wolf C, Herrick E, Gress S. Inadequate follow-up controller medications among patients with asthma who visit the emergency department. *Ann Emerg Med.* 2005;46:316e22.

A Cost-Effectiveness Analysis of Inhaled Corticosteroid Delivery for Children with Asthma in the Emergency Department

Andrews AL, Teufel RJ II, Basco WT Jr, et al (Med Univ of South Carolina, Charleston)
J Pediatr 161:903-907.e1, 2012

Objective.—To determine the clinical effectiveness and cost-effectiveness of 3 inhaled corticosteroid (ICS) delivery options for children with asthma treated in and discharged from the emergency department (ED).

Study Design.—We conducted cost-effectiveness analysis using a decision tree to compare 3 ED-based ICS delivery options: usual care (recommending outpatient follow-up), prescribe (uniformly prescribing ICS), and dispense (uniformly dispensing ICS). Accounting for expected follow-up rates, prescription filling, and medication compliance, we compared projected rates of ED relapse visits and hospitalizations within 1 month of ED visit across all 3 arms. Direct and indirect costs were compared.

Results.—The model predicts that the rate of return to ED per 100 patients within 1 month of the ED visit was 10.6 visits for the usual care arm, 9.4 visits for the prescription arm, and 8.4 visits for the medication-dispensing arm. Rates of hospitalization per 100 patients were 2.4, 2.2, and 1.9, respectively. Direct costs per 100 patients for each arm were $23 400, $20 800, and $19 100, respectively. Including indirect costs related to missed parental work, total costs per 100 patients were $27 100, $22 000, and $20 100, respectively. Total cost savings per 100 patients comparing the usual care arm with the medication dispensing arm was $7000.

Conclusions.—This decision analysis model suggests that uniform prescribing or dispensing of ICS at the time of ED visit for asthma may lead to a decreased number of ED visits and hospital admissions within 1 month of the sentinel ED visit and provides a substantial cost-savings (Fig 1).

▶ Emergency department (ED) treatment for asthma has been found to be lacking as anti-inflammatory therapy, particularly in the form of inhaled corticosteroids (ICS). This treatment is usually not offered at all, or the patient is told to follow up with his or her primary care provider (PCP) for further ICS treatment. The flaws in current logic are that many patients simply use the ED as their primary care provider or don't follow up with a PCP because they start to feel better and don't see the need for a follow-up appointment, which they equate with time and money spent. This investigation designed a model (Fig 1) to compare the cost effectiveness of usual ED care (no ICS given), ICS prescription provided/recommended, and ICS actually dispensed to the patient on discharge from the ED. This model resulted in a savings of $7000 per 100 subjects dispensed an ICS inhaler before discharge; this savings is due to reduced ED visits and hospitalizations. Being able to follow a recipe doesn't require a medical degree, and physician extenders as practitioners will likely become more prevalent in EDs. In

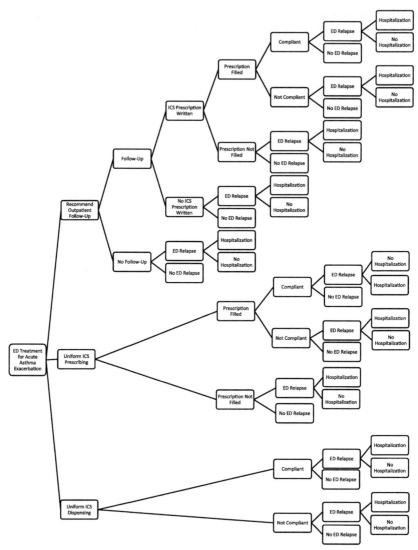

FIGURE 1.—Decision tree for ICS delivery in the ED. (Reprinted from Journal Pediatrics. Andrews AL, Teufel II RJ, Basco WT Jr, et al. A cost-effectiveness analysis of inhaled corticosteroid delivery for children with asthma in the emergency department. *J Pediatr.* 2012;161:903-907.e1, Copyright 2012, with permission from Elsevier.)

view of the looming Affordable Care Act, such cost savings modeling will likely soon become reality in an ED near you.

S. K. Willsie, DO, MA

Efficacy and safety of fluticasone/formoterol combination therapy in patients with moderate-to-severe asthma

Corren J, Mansfield LE, Pertseva T, et al (Allergy Med Clinic, Los Angeles, CA; Western Sky Med Res, El Paso, TX; Dniepropetrovsk State Med Academy, Ukraine; et al)
Respir Med 107:180-195, 2013

Background.—The inhaled corticosteroid, fluticasone propionate, and the long-acting β_2-adrenergic agonist, formoterol fumarate, are both highly effective treatments for bronchial asthma. This study (NCT00393952/ EudraCT number: 2006-005989-39) compared the efficacy and safety of fluticasone/formoterol combination therapy (*flutiform*®; 250/10 µg) administered twice daily (b.i.d.) via a single aerosol inhaler, with the individual components (fluticasone 250 µg b.i.d.; formoterol 10 µg b.i.d.), in adult and adolescent patients with moderate-to-severe asthma.

Methods.—This was a 12-week, double-blind, randomised, parallel-group, multicentre, placebocontrolled phase 3 study. The co-primary efficacy endpoints were: i) the mean change in the forced expiratory volume in the first second (FEV_1) from morning pre-dose at baseline to pre-dose at week 12 (fluticasone/formoterol 250/10 µg vs. formoterol), ii) the mean change in FEV_1 from morning pre-dose at baseline to 2 h post-dose at week 12 (fluticasone/formoterol 250/10 µg vs. fluticasone), and iii) the number of patients who discontinued prematurely due to lack of treatment efficacy (fluticasone/formoterol 250/10 µg vs. placebo). The secondary endpoints included measures of lung function, disease control, and asthma

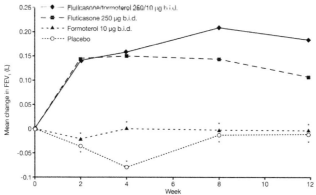

*p ≤0.05 versus fluticasone/formoterol 250/10 µg b.i.d. treatment group.
Baseline means were 2.085 L, 2.134 L, 2.143 L, and 2.066 L for the fluticasone/formoterol 250/10 µg b.i.d., fluticasone, formoterol, and placebo treatment groups, respectively, for all patients in the full analysis set.
b.i.d. = twice daily

FIGURE 3.—Mean change in FEV_1 (L) from pre-dose at baseline to pre-dose at weeks 2, 4, 8, and 12: the contribution from the fluticasone component of fluticasone component of fluticasone/formoterol 250/ 10 µg b.i.d. combination therapy, full analysis set using last observation carried forward imputation. (Reprinted from Respiratory Medicine. Corren J, Mansfield LE, Pertseva T, et al. Efficacy and safety of fluticasone/formoterol combination therapy in patients with moderate-to-severe asthma. *Respir Med.* 2013;107:180-195, Copyright 2012, with permission from Elsevier.)

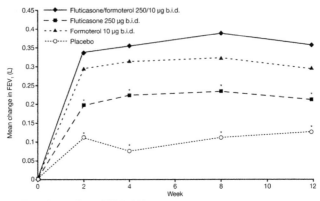

FIGURE 4.—Mean change in FEV₁ (L) from pre-dose at baseline to 2 h post-dose at weeks 2, 4, 8, and 12: the contribution from the formoterol component of fluticasone component of fluticasone/formoterol 250/10 µg b.i.d. combination therapy, full analysis set using last observation carried forward imputation. (Reprinted from Respiratory Medicine. Corren J, Mansfield LE, Pertseva T, et al. Efficacy and safety of fluticasone/formoterol combination therapy in patients with moderate-to-severe asthma. *Respir Med.* 2013;107:180-195, Copyright 2012, with permission from Elsevier.)

symptoms. Safety was assessed based on adverse events, vital signs, and clinical laboratory evaluations.

Results.—Overall, 395 (70.9%) patients completed the study. Fluticasone/formoterol 250/10 µg b.i.d. was superior to the individual components and placebo for all three co-primary endpoints and demonstrated numerically greater improvements for multiple secondary efficacy analyses. Fluticasone/formoterol combination therapy had a good safety profile over the 12 weeks.

Conclusion.—Fluticasone/formoterol combination therapy will provide clinicians with an efficacious alternative treatment option for patients with moderate-to-severe asthma (Figs 3 and 4, Table 4).

▶ This is an efficacy study comparing fluticasone propionate plus formoterol to fluticasone alone and formoterol alone. Fig 3 depicts predose at baseline and at Weeks 2, 4, 6, 8, 10, and 12; Fig 4 delineates predose to 2 hours postdose at Weeks 2, 4, 6, 8, 10, and 12. Table 4 compares efficacy over weeks of treatment, clearly favoring the combination product. The combination product, fluticasone plus formoterol, was shown to be safe and provide superior efficacy to its individual products. For asthmatics in which a combination product is needed with an inhaled corticosteroid (ICS) and a long-acting beta agonist (LABA), consideration should be given to this product. In the meantime, head-to-head studies with standard ICS and LABAs products should be undertaken.

S. K. Willsie, DO, MA

TABLE 4.—Overview of Secondary Efficacy Variables. Disease Control: Asthma Control Days, Rescue Medication-Free Days, Symptom-Free Days, and Awakening-Free Nights: Mean Change From Baseline to Week 12, Full Analysis Set

Characteristic	Treatment Group			
	Fluticasone/ Formoterol 250/10 µg b.i.d. N = 108	Placebo b.i.d. N = 105	Fluticasone 250 µg b.i.d. N = 109	Formoterol 10 µg b.i.d. N = 110
Asthma control days (%)	n = 103	n = 101	n = 102	n = 106
Baseline[a] mean (SD)	12.9 (20.48)	11.2 (19.09)	9.8 (18.72)	10.9 (22.02)
Week 12 mean (SD)	53.8 (42.69)	27.3 (35.25)	45.2 (41.47)	39.7 (39.18)
Change to week 12				
Mean (SD)	40.9 (40.98)	16.1 (37.08)	35.4 (38.90)	28.7 (43.20)
Difference from fluticasone/formoterol 250/10 µg b.i.d.[b]				
p-value		0.001[c]	0.027[c]	0.032[c]
Rescue medication free days (%)	n = 103	n = 104	n = 106	n = 109
Baseline[a] mean (SD)	19.8 (25.15)	17.6 (22.61)	15.2 (21.40)	21.9 (27.06)
Week 12 mean (SD)	60.4 (39.70)	34.9 (35.65)	50.6 (40.63)	47.2 (39.94)
Change to week 12				
Mean (SD)	40.6 (42.11)	17.3 (37.27)	35.5 (36.80)	25.3 (43.01)
Difference from fluticasone/formoterol 250/10 µg b.i.d.[b]				
p-value		0.009[c]	0.042[c]	0.013[c]
Symptom-free days (%)	n = 103	n = 104	n = 105	n = 108
Baseline[a] mean (SD)	24.3 (25.82)	24.3 (27.59)	20.3 (25.91)	24.5 (31.34)
Week 12 mean (SD)	61.1 (41.40)	38.6 (38.76)	53.9 (40.81)	51.8 (40.83)
Change to week 12				
Mean (SD)	36.8 (36.66)	14.3 (39.98)	33.6 (37.14)	27.4 (41.71)
Difference from fluticasone/formoterol 250/10 µg b.i.d.[b]				
p-value		0.007[c]	0.342	0.140
Awakening-free nights (%)	n = 103	n = 104	n = 104	n = 109
Baseline[a] mean (SD)	62.4 (35.36)	60.7 (31.59)	59.6 (35.34)	61.9 (34.77)
Week 12 mean (SD)	82.5 (30.27)	70.4 (34.15)	82.0 (29.94)	80.9 (28.20)
Change to week 12				
Mean (SD)	20.1 (40.74)	9.7 (38.95)	22.4 (38.91)	19.0 (37.69)
Difference from fluticasone/formoterol 250/10 µg b.i.d.[b]				
p-value		0.209	0.810	0.240

N = number of patients in treatment group, n = number of patients with data available, SD = standard deviation.
[a]Baseline was the 7-day average calculated on the last 7 days prior to the first dose of study drug.
[b]Analysis method was Cochran Mantel-Haenszel using van Elteren's method for combining Wilcoxon rank sum test results from independent strata, with baseline FEV_1 % predicted category and site as the strata for the analysis.
[c]$p \leq 0.050$ versus fluticasone/formoterol 250/10 µg b.i.d. but not statistically significant per sequential gatekeeping approach.

Status asthmaticus in the medical intensive care unit: A 30-year experience
Peters JI, Stupka JE, Singh H, et al (Univ of Texas Health Science Ctr San Antonio; et al)
Respir Med 106:344-348, 2012

Objectives.—To investigate the characteristics, trends in management (permissive hypercapnia; mechanical ventilation (MV); neuromuscular

TABLE 1.—Demographics and Characteristics of Subjects With SA ($n = 227$)

Variable	Data
Age[a]— yrs	37.3 ± 14.87 (range 16—77)
Sex — no. (%)	
Male	80 (35%)
Female	147 (65%)
Ethnicity — no. (%)	
Hispanic	118 (52%)
African American	51 (22%)
Caucasian	48 (21%)
Others	10 (4%)
Childhood asthma onset[b]	86 (38%)
Recurrent episodes	
Subjects— no. (%)	34 (15%)
Episodes — no. (%)[c]	53 (19%)
Oral corticosteroids use — no. (%)	
Steroid dependent	62 (27%)
Recent steroid taper[d]	41 (18%)

[a]Data are presented as mean ± SD or no. (%).
[b]Asthma onset before 17 yrs of age.
[c]Total 53 recurrent episodes in 34 subjects: 20 (2 episodes); 10 (3 episodes); 3 (4episodes); and 1 (5 episodes).
[d]Oral corticosteroid tapering within 4 weeks from SA.

TABLE 2.—Differences in Characteristics Between Intubated and Non-Intubated Patients

Characteristics	Non-Intubated	Intubated	p-Value
Age — yrs	36.0 ± 13.9	38.2 ± 13.5	$p = 0.37$
Ethnicity — no. (%)			
Hispanic	50	68 (58%)	
African American	12	39 (76%)	
Caucasian	15	33 (69%)	
Duration of symptoms — days	4.13 ± 3.92	3.04 ± 2.9	$p = 0.06$
Peak pCO_2 — (Torr)	40.55 ± 12.6	60.54 ± 18.1	$p \leq 0.001$
Lowest pH	7.36 ± 0.11	7.21 ± 0.15	$p = 0.01$
Hospitalization duration — days	5.3 ± 3.4	6.8 ± 4.21	$p = 0.07$

blockade) and their impact on complications and outcomes in Status Asthmaticus (SA).

Methods.—We performed a retrospective observational study of subjects admitted with SA to a single multidisciplinary MICU over a 30-year period. All laboratory, radiologic, respiratory care, physician notes and orders were extracted from an electronic medical record (EMR) maintained during the entire duration of the study.

Results.—Two hundred and twenty-seven subjects were admitted with 280 episodes of SA. While subjects reflected our regional population (52% Hispanic), African Americans were over-represented (22%) and Caucasians under-represented (21%). Thirty-eight percent reported childhood asthma, 27% were steroid dependent (10% in the last 10 years), and 18% had a recent steroid taper. One hundred and thirty-nine (61.2%) required intubation. The duration of hospitalization was similar between

TABLE 3.—Complications of Status Asthmaticus

Variable	First 20 yrs (1980–1999), n = 248	Number (%) Last 10 yrs (2000–2009), n = 32	Overall 30 yrs (1980–2009), n = 280
Death[a]	1 (0.4%)	0	1 (0.4%)
Anoxic encephalopathy	1 (0.4%)	0	1 (0.4%)
Pneumothorax	7 (2.8%)	0	7 (2.5%)
Myocardial infarction	4 (1.6%)	2 (6.3%)	6 (2.1%)
Hypotension	12 (4.8%)	3 (9.4%)	15 (5.4%)
Pneumonia	5 (2.0%)	3 (9.4%)	8 (2.9%)
Hypokalemia	89 (35%)	9 (28%)	98 (35%)
Hypophosphatemia	45 (18%)	3 (9.4%)	48 (17%)
Hyperglycemia[b]	114 (46%)	6 (18%)	120 (43%)

[a]From myocardial infarction with secondary massive GI after anticoagulation
[b]Glucose over 130 mg/dl.

mechanically ventilated and non-ventilated subjects (5.8 ± 4.41 vs. 6.8 ± 7.22 days; $p = 0.07$). The overall complication rate remained low irrespective of the use of permissive hypercapnia or mode of mechanical ventilation (overall mortality 0.4%; pneumothorax 2.5%; pneumonia 2.9%). The frequency of SA declined significantly in the last 10 years of the study (12.4 vs. 3.2 cases/year).

Conclusions.—Despite the frequent use of mechanical ventilation, mortality/complication rates remained extremely low. MV did not significantly increase the duration of hospitalization. At our institution, the frequency of SA significantly decreased despite an increase in emergency room visits for asthma (Tables 1-3).

▶ This is a retrospective review of 30 years of status asthmaticus cases treated in the medical intensive care unit at the University of Texas Health Science Center in San Antonio, Texas. Interesting aspects of this investigation are: The years included allowed comparison of outcomes between 10 and 12 mL/kg tidal volume versus low tidal volume ventilation; diversity of population; and use of neuromuscular blockade during the past 10 years of data collection. Tables 1 and 2 depict the demographics and differences in characteristics between nonintubated and intubated patients. Table 3 lists the complications for the first 20 years of data collection (1980-1999) and the past 10 years (2000-2010). Interestingly, there was a marked reduction in the numbers of cases of status asthmaticus during the past 10 years (12.4 per year compared with 3.2 cases per year) of the study with overrepresentation of African Americans and underrepresentation of Caucasians. A number of questions remain unanswered, including why in an area that is primarily Hispanic the numbers of Hispanics with status asthmaticus were lower than might be predicted.

S. K. Willsie, DO, MA

Association Between Evidence-Based Standardized Protocols in Emergency Departments With Childhood Asthma Outcomes: A Canadian Population-Based Study

Li P, To T, Parkin PC, et al (McGill Univ Health Centre, Montreal, Quebec, Canada; Univ of Toronto, Ontario, Canada)
Arch Pediatr Adolesc Med 166:834-840, 2012

Objective.—To determine whether children treated in emergency departments (EDs) with evidence-based standardized protocols (EBSPs) containing evidence-based content and format had lower risk of hospital admission or ED return visit and greater follow-up than children treated in EDs with no standardized protocols in Ontario, Canada.

Design.—Retrospective population-based cohort study of children with asthma. We used multivariable logistic regression to estimate risk of outcomes.

Setting.—All EDs in Ontario (N = 146) treating childhood asthma from April 2006 to March 2009.

Participants.—Thirty-one thousand one hundred thirty-eight children (aged 2 to 17 years) with asthma.

TABLE 1.—Evidence-Based Content in Standardized Protocols to Improve Hospitalizations, ED Return Visits, and Follow-Up

Evidence-Based Content According to Each Outcome

Hospital admission
  Required content
    1. Indication for steroids[6-8,12,a]
    2. Repeated β-agonist treatment for severe asthma[6-8,35,a]
    3. Inhaled anticholinergics with a selective β-agonist for severe asthma[6-8,a]
  Desired content
    1. Timely indication for steroids (within the first hour)[6-8,12,a]
    2. Continuous β-agonist treatment (1 nebulization every 15 min or >4 treatments/h) for severe asthma[6-8,35,a]
    3. >1 Dose of inhaled anticholinergics with a selective β -agonist for severe asthma[6-8,a]
ED return visits
  Required content
    Short course of steroids at discharge from ED[6-8,13,a]
  Desired content
    1. Short course of steroids at discharge from ED[6-8,13,a]
    2. Reminder for follow-up visit[6-8,b]
    3. Discharge instructions (including some or all of the following: written action plan, instructions for medications prescribed, instructions for increasing medications or seeking medical care if asthma worsened, and review of inhaler technique when possible)[6-8,b]
Outpatient follow-up
  Required content
    1. Reminder for follow-up visit with primary care physician, pediatrician, asthma education center, or outpatient clinic[6-8,b]

Abbreviation: ED, emergency department.
Editor's Note: Please refer to original journal article for full references.
[a]Evidence A: supported by randomized controlled trials.
[b]Evidence B (US National Asthma Education and Prevention Program) and D (Global Initiative for Asthma): supported by randomized controlled trials with limited body of data and panel consensus, respectively.

TABLE 2.—ED Outcomes for Children With Asthma by Type of SP Use in the ED

Type of SP	Hospital Admission	No. (%) ED Return Visits	Outpatient Follow-Up
EBSPs			
Eds[a]	16 (11.0)	10 (6.8)	15 (10.3)
Patients[b]	12 999 (28.0)	5033 (12.1)	6864 (16.2)
Other SPs			
Eds[a]	27 (18.5)	33 (22.6)	28 (19.2)
Patients[b]	5830 (12.5)	11 699 (28.1)	10 052 (23.8)
No SP			
Eds[a]	103 (70.5)	103 (70.5)	103 (70.5)
Patients[b]	27 681 (59.5)	24 907 (59 8)	25 383 (60.0)

Abbreviations: EBSP, evidence-based standardized protocol; ED, emergency department; SP, standardized protocol.
[a]N = 146 EDs.
[b]N = 46 510 for hospital admissions; N = 42 297 for ED return visits; and N = 42 299 for outpatient follow-up

Main Exposure.—Type of standardized protocol (EBSPs, other standardized protocols, or none).

Main Outcome Measures.—Hospital admission, high-acuity 7-day return visit to the ED, and 7-day outpatient follow-up visit.

Results.—The final cohort made 46 510 ED visits in 146 EDs. From the index ED visit, 4211 (9.1%) were admitted to the hospital. Of those discharged, 1778 (4.2%) and 7350 (17.4%) had ED return visits and outpatient follow-up visits, respectively. The EBSPs were not associated with hospitalizations, return visits, or follow-up (adjusted odds ratio, 1.17 [95% CI, 0.91-1.49]; adjusted odds ratio, 1.10 [95% CI, 0.86-1.41]; and adjusted odds ratio, 1.08 [95% CI, 0.87-1.35], respectively).

Conclusions.—The EBSPs were not associated with improvements in rates of hospital admissions, return visits to the ED, or follow-up. Our findings suggest the need to address gaps linking improved processes of asthma care with outcomes (Tables 1 and 2).

▶ Use of evidence-based standardized protocols (EBSPs) is frequently touted as improving outcomes, such as improved asthma care and reduced exacerbations. This large Canadian study evaluated the differences in emergency department (ED) visit outcomes among those EDs who applied EBSPs, local standardized protocols and routine care, meaning care provided by local practitioners not according to any particular protocol. Table 1 details EBSPs according to presentation (ED visit; hospitalization; 7-day follow-up visit). Table 2 provides ED outcomes for children with asthma by type of standard protocol use in the ED. Gaps remain in between optimal results and currently utilized therapy, as evidenced by this study. Further study should include the impact of bridge factors, including follow-up calls or reminders for provider visits, compliance, and action plans.

S. K. Willsie, DO, MA

Cystic Fibrosis

Personalized Medicine in Cystic Fibrosis: Dawning of a New Era

Clancy JP, Jain M (Cincinnati Children's Hosp Med Ctr and Univ of Cincinnati, OH; Northwestern Univ, Chicago, IL)
Am J Respir Crit Care Med 186:593-597, 2012

Life expectancy in cystic fibrosis (CF) has improved substantially over the last 75 years, with a median predicted survival now approaching 40 years. This improvement has resulted largely from therapies treating end-organ manifestations. In an effort to develop drugs that would target the underlying defects in the CF transmembrane conductance regulator (CFTR), the Cystic Fibrosis Foundation embarkedon a bold initiative in which it established collaborations with biopharmaceutical companies to support early-stage efforts to discover new medicines for CF. This has led to the development and clinical trial testing of several novel drugs targeting specific CFTR mutations. One drug, ivacaftor, was recently approved by the US Food and Drug Administration for the approximately 4% of patients with CF who have the G551D gating mutation. Drugs targeting F508 del CFTR and premature termination codons, which would be applicable to 90% of patients with CF, are undergoing clinical trials. The impact of such drugson CFTR biomarkers, such as sweat chloride and nasal potential difference, suggests that they may reset the clinical trajectory of CF, but their effect on long-term outcomes will remain unknown formany years. Nevertheless, development of CFTR-targeted drugs represents an important milestone in CF, perhaps revolutionizing the care of these patients in a fundamental way.

▶ If you read only a single article about cystic fibrosis (CF) this year, let this be the one. The authors artfully describe the historical advances over the past 75 years and highlight the unique partnership between industry and academia that led to the launch of the first step in "personalized therapy" or genetically directed therapy for CF patients. Fig 1 in the original article delineates the steps that have occurred since the 1950s; who can believe that it was in the late 1950s that the CF test was first invented, and that antibiotics to combat *Pseudomonas aeruginosa* came on the scene in the 1960s? Most important are the advances made leading up to the first cystic fibrosis transmembrane conductance regulator (CFTR) potentiator (Ivacaftor) to gain US Food and Drug Administration's approval. Currently, this drug is restricted for CF patients with the G551D mutation, present in approximately 4% of CF patients. Ivacaftor was extensively studied and led to rapid, dramatic, and sustained improvements in forced expiratory volume in 1 second (FEV_1) and biomarkers of CFTR function. Similar findings were seen in the phase III trial of patients aged 6 to 11 years, including absolute FEV_1 percent predicted improvement of greater than 12% and weight gain of 1.9 kg. This is particularly striking in younger patients with CF, confirming the suspicion of "silent" disease in seemingly normal patients with CF and providing support to the notion that early disease is reversible (and potentially preventable). Whether or not CFTR modulators will yield long-term results or a "cure" for CF remains to be seen, but I hope I piqued your interest enough to dig into this important article of 2012!

S. K. Willsie, DO, MA

Ivacaftor in Subjects With Cystic Fibrosis Who Are Homozygous for the *F508del-CFTR* Mutation
Flume PA, for the VX 08-770-104 Study Group (Med Univ of South Carolina, Charleston; et al)
Chest 142:718-724, 2012

Background.—Ivacaftor (VX-770) is a cystic fibrosis transmembrane conductance regulator (CFTR) potentiator that was approved in the United States for the treatment of cystic fibrosis (CF) in patients ≥ 6 years of age who have a G551D mutation; however, the most prevalent disease-causing *CFTR* mutation, F508del, causes a different functional defect. The objectives of this study were to evaluate the safety of ivacaftor in a larger population and for a longer time period than tested previously and to assess the efficacy of ivacaftor in subjects with CF who are homozygous for *F508del-CFTR*.

Methods.—This was a phase 2 study with a 16-week randomized (4:1), double-blind, placebo-controlled period (part A) and an open-label extension (part B) for subjects who met prespecified criteria.

TABLE 1.—Baseline Characteristics of Study Participants

Characteristic	Placebo (n = 28)	Ivacaftor (n = 112)
Female, No. (%)	12 (43)	54 (48)
Age, y		
Mean (SD)	25.0 (8.4)	22.8 (10.3)
Median	24.0	19.5
Range	12-39	12-52
Height, cm		
Median	170.7	164.0
Range	145.6-184.0	139.0-189.6
Weight, kg		
Median	64.9	55.9
Range	44.2-100.3	35.1-99.8
BMI, kg/m^2		
Median	21.5	20.4
Range	17.9-40.8	15.7-31.6
Sweat chloride, mmol/L		
Mean (SD)	102.4 (7.9)	101.4 (10.3)
Median	101.5	101.0
Range	91.0-122.0	79.5-135.5
FEV$_1$ % predicted		
Mean (SD)	74.8 (24.1)	79.7 (22.7)
Median	67.0	79.0
Range	43-127	40-129

None of the characteristics differed significantly between the groups (*P*>.05 for all comparisons).

TABLE 2.—Most Common Adverse Events Reported During the Study by Treatment Group

Adverse Event	Placebo (n = 28)	Ivacaftor (n = 112)
Subjects with any adverse event	25 (89.3)	98 (87.5)
Cough	4 (14.3)	34 (30.4)
Pulmonary exacerbation[a]	11 (39.3)	25 (22.3)
Nasal congestion	2 (7.1)	13 (11.6)
Headache	2 (7.1)	11 (9.8)
Upper respiratory tract infection	2 (7.1)	11 (9.8)
Nausea	1 (3.6)	10 (8.9)
Oropharyngeal pain	3 (10.7)	10 (8.9)
Fatigue	3 (10.7)	9 (8.0)
Productive cough	1 (3.6)	9 (8.0)
Pyrexia	2 (7.1)	9 (8.0)
Rash	0	9 (8.0)
Sinusitis	1 (3.6)	8 (7.1)
Upper abdominal pain	1 (3.6)	7 (6.3)
Increase in C-reactive protein	1 (3.6)	6 (5.4)
Contact dermatitis	0	6 (5.4)
Diarrhea	2 (7.1)	6 (5.4)

Data are presented as No. (%). Minimum frequency of 5% of subjects in the ivacaftor group.
[a]Coded as cystic fibrosis lung.

TABLE 3.—Other Clinically Relevant Measures

Measure	Placebo (n = 28)	Ivacaftor (n = 112)
Absolute change in FEV_1 % predicted	−0.2	1.5
Absolute change in CFQ-R respiratory domain score	−1.4	−0.1
Absolute change in weight, kg	0.96	0.84
Absolute change in BMI, kg/m^2	0.25	0.21
Absolute change in weight-for-age z score	0.0007	0.43
Absolute change in BMI-for-age z score	−0.002	0.73
Pulmonary exacerbation,[a] No. (%)	10 (32)	25 (21)
Antibiotic treatment of sinopulmonary signs or symptoms,[b] No. (%)	16 (56)	48 (43)

P values for all measures were not significant. CFQ-R = Cystic Fibrosis Questionnaire-Revised.
[a]Treatment with new or changed antibiotic therapy for ≥4 sinopulmonary signs/symptoms.
[b]Events requiring new or changed antibiotic therapy for ≥1 sinopulmonary sign/symptom.

Results.—Part A: The safety profile of ivacaftor was comparable to that of the placebo. The overall adverse event frequency was similar in the ivacaftor (87.5%) and placebo (89.3%) groups through 16 weeks. The difference in the change of FEV_1 % predicted from baseline through week 16 (primary end point) between the ivacaftor and placebo groups was 1.7% ($P = .15$). Sweat chloride, a biomarker of CFTR activity, showed a small reduction in the ivacaftor vs placebo groups of −2.9 mmol/L ($P = .04$) from baseline through week 16. Part B: No new safety signals were identified. The changes in FEV_1 or sweat chloride in part A were not sustained with ivacaftor treatment from week 16 to week 40.

Conclusions.—These results expand the safety information for ivacaftor and support its continued evaluation. Lack of a clinical effect suggests that a CFTR potentiator alone is not an effective therapeutic approach for patients who have CF and are homozygous for *F508del-CFTR*.

Trial Registry.—ClinicalTrials.gov; No.: NCT00953706; URL: www.clinicaltrials.gov (Tables 1-3).

▶ Ivacaftor is a cystic fibrosis transmembrane conductance regulator (CFTR) potentiator approved for patients ≥ 6 years of age who have a G551D mutation. The most frequent disease causing cystic fibrosis (CF) mutation, F509del, causes a different functional cellular effect. This study aimed to administer ivacaftor in higher doses to evaluate efficacy in homozygotes for F508del-CFTR and to obtain additional safety data. Table 1 depicts baseline characteristics of all subjects, none of which were statistically different. Fig 2 in the original article depicts the reduction over time through 16 weeks of the sweat chloride versus placebo (*P* = .0240). Table 3 shows changes over time in the placebo and ivacaftor groups with regard to pulmonary function, CF questionnaire, weight, exacerbations, and need for antibiotic treatment for sinopulmonary signs or symptoms. This table shows no clinically significant change in the ivacaftor group versus placebo group for any marker. The most common adverse events were mild or moderate. Several serious adverse events occurred in both the ivacaftor and placebo groups. Clearly, based on these data, ivacaftor alone offers little to patients with the most common mutation causing CF. Further studies are in order with other agents to determine best therapies for the F508del-CFTR subpopulation.

S. K. Willsie, DO, MA

Role of Cystic Fibrosis Transmembrane Conductance Regulator in Patients With Chronic Sinopulmonary Disease

Gonska T, Choi P, Stephenson A, et al (Univ of Toronto, Ontario, Canada; St Michael's Hosp and Univ of Toronto, Ontario, Canada; et al)
Chest 142:996-1004, 2012

Background.—Previous studies report a high frequency of mutations in the cystic fibrosis (CF) transmembrane conductance regulator gene (*CFTR*) in patients with idiopathic bronchiectasis. However, most studies have based their findings on preselected patient groups or have performed limited testing for CF transmembrane conductance regulator (CFTR) dysfunction. The objective of our study was to evaluate the prevalence of *CFTR* gene mutations and/or CFTR-related ion channel abnormalities among subjects with idiopathic chronic sinopulmonary disease and the prevalence of CF or a CFTR-related disorder in this population.

Methods.—We evaluated 72 prospectively enrolled patients from 1995 to 2005 at the Hospital for Sick Children and St. Michael's Hospital with idiopathic chronic sinopulmonary disease for evidence of CFTR-mediated abnormalities. We performed *CFTR* genotyping and assessed CFTR function using sweat testing and nasal potential difference testing. The results

TABLE 2.—CFTR Genotypes Identified in Subjects With Idiopathic Sinopulmonary Disease

CF Causing/CF Causing	CF Causing/CFTR Mutation	CFTR Mutation/ CFTR Mutation	CF Causing/ Unknown	CFTR Mutation/ Unknown
F508del/A455E 3x	F508del /D1152H 2x	D579G/D579G 2x	F508del /−6x	R764X/ −
	F508del/S1251N	R75X/V456A		758delC/ −
	F508del/L967S	1716G>A/5T		1716G>A/ −
	F508del/5T	R75Q/5T		R117H (7T)/ − 3x
	F508del/3212T>C			5T/ − 3x
	G542X/D1152H			
	1717-1G>A/Q1291H			

Patients are grouped according to the identified CFTR alterations on allele 1/allele 2. "CF causing" refers to CFTR mutations that are known to cause CF disease, whereas " CFTR mutation" refers to any molecular alteration in CFTR regardless of consequences. These may cause CF, a CFTR-related disorder, or have benign consequences. In some patients, no CFTR mutation was found for the second allele, "unknown" or (−).

CF = cystic fibrosis; CFTR = cystic fibrosis transmembrane conductance regulator; CFTR = cystic fibrosis transmembrane conductance regulator gene.

were compared with data from healthy control subjects, CF heterozygotes, and patients with CF.

Results.—The CFTR functional tests in idiopathic sinopulmonary patients showed a continuous spectrum, ranging from normal to values typically seen in individuals with CF. Forty-eight patients (66%) demonstrated *CFTR* mutations and/or abnormalities of CFTR function. Twenty-two (31%) fulfilled criteria for a diagnosis of CF and 26 (36%) for a CFTR-related disorder with a strong female preponderance. Functional tests, more than genotyping, were instrumental in establishing a CF diagnosis. Clinical features failed to distinguish subjects with CF from those with CFTR-related or idiopathic disease.

Conclusions.—The high prevalence of CF and CFTR dysfunction among patients with idiopathic chronic sinopulmonary disease underscores the need for extensive diagnostic evaluation for CF (Table 2).

▶ This is an extremely important investigation that is a must-read for all pediatricians, allergists, and chest clinicians. A group of 72 individuals with chronic sinopulmonary disease were evaluated for the presence of cystic fibrosis transmembrane conductance regulator (CFTR) or CFTR-mediated ion channel dysfunction. Table 2 provides a listing of CFTR genotypes identified in this group of patients with chronic sinopulmonary disease (49 mutant CFTR alleles were discovered). Table 2 demonstrates the High Resolution Computed Tomography scores of patients with idiopathic bronchiectasis, CFTR-related disease, and cystic fibrosis (CF). Thirty-three subjects carried at least 1 mutant CFTR allele and 39 had no mutant alleles. CF was diagnosed in 22 subjects solely on the basis of the sweat test or nasal potential difference measurement or both. Six individuals diagnosed with CF had no CFTR mutations. Either 26% or 36% of the group met diagnostic criteria for CFTR-related disorder. In summary, this investigation points out the need for a comprehensive and CF center—driven diagnostic approach to patients with idiopathic sinopulmonary disease to ensure that appropriate treatments are applied as early as possible to patients who actually have CF or CFTR-related disease. Failure to do so may not only lead to a missed diagnosis, particularly because the sinopulmonary disease was the main presentation in these patients, but also a missed opportunity to intervene before the disease has progressed significantly. Until we have CF testing at birth, this is the best possible way to ensure correct diagnosis of CF and CFTR-related disease, a condition not well understood by many.

S. K. Willsie, DO, MA

Understanding the natural progression in %FEV₁ decline in patients with cystic fibrosis: a longitudinal study

Taylor-Robinson D, Whitehead M, Diderichsen F, et al (Univ of Liverpool, UK; Univ of Copenhagen, Denmark; et al)

Thorax 67:860-866, 2012

Background.—Forced expiratory volume in 1 s as a percentage of predicted ($\%FEV_1$) is a key outcome in cystic fibrosis (CF) and other lung diseases. As people with CF survive for longer periods, new methods are required to understand the way $\%FEV_1$ changes over time. An up to date approach for longitudinal modelling of $\%FEV_1$ is presented and applied to a unique CF dataset to demonstrate its utility at the clinical and population level.

Methods and Findings.—The Danish CF register contains 70 448 $\%FEV_1$ measures on 479 patients seen monthly between 1969 and 2010. The variability in the data is partitioned into three components (between patient, within patient and measurement error) using the empirical variogram. Then a linear mixed effects model is developed to explore factors influencing $\%FEV_1$ in this population. Lung function measures are correlated for over 15 years. A baseline $\%FEV_1$ value explains 63% of the variability in $\%FEV_1$ at 1 year, 40% at 3 years, and about 30% at 5 years. The model output smooths out the short-term variability in $\%FEV_1$ (SD 6.3%), aiding clinical interpretation of changes in $\%FEV_1$. At the population level significant effects of birth cohort, pancreatic status and *Pseudomonas aeruginosa* infection status on $\%FEV_1$ are shown over time.

Conclusions.—This approach provides a more realistic estimate of the $\%FEV_1$ trajectory of people with chronic lung disease by acknowledging the imprecision in individual measurements and the correlation structure of repeated measurements on the same individual over time. This method has applications for clinicians in assessing prognosis and the need for treatment intensification, and for use in clinical trials (Table 1).

▶ Unique data mining from the Danish Cystic Fibrosis (CF) registry, which contains 70 448 forced expiration volumes in 1 second (FEV₁s) performed on 479 patients between 1960, and 2010, allows correlation of lung function for a minimal of 15 years. Table 1 depicts the CF population's data collection, beginning in 1948, adding another decade of data through 1998. This dataset allows continuous and longitudinal logging of the variability of lung function,

TABLE 1.—Baseline Characteristics of the Danish Cystic Fibrosis (CF) Population

			Birth Cohort				Total
	≥1948	≥1958	≥1968	≥1978	≥1988	≥1998	
N (%)	7 (1.5)	42 (8.8)	110 (23)	105 (21.9)	141 (29.4)	74 (15.4)	479 (100)
Women	1 (14.3)	19 (45.2)	48 (43.6)	52 (49.5)	74 (52.5)	42 (56.8)	236 (49.3)
No. Delta F508 = 0	0 (0)	0 (0)	1 (0.9)	4 (3.8)	5 (3.5)	5 (6.8)	15 (3.1)
No. Delta F508 = 1	2 (28.6)	14 (33.3)	26 (23.6)	24 (22.9)	42 (29.8)	19 (25.7)	127 (26.5)
No. Delta F508 = 2	5 (71.4)	28 (66.7)	83 (75.5)	77 (73.3)	94 (66.7)	50 (67.6)	337 (70.4)
Developed chronic *Pseudomonas*	6 (85.7)	31 (73.8)	84 (76.4)	55 (52.4)	20 (14.2)	5 (6.8)	201 (42)
Missing infection information	0 (0)	5 (11.9)	2 (1.8)	2 (1.9)	1 (0.7)	0 (0)	10 (2.1)
Pancreatic insufficient	7 (100)	42 (100)	105 (95.5)	99 (94.3)	133 (94.3)	73 (98.6)	459 (95.8)
Copenhagen	4 (57.1)	38 (90.5)	83 (75.5)	72 (68.6)	79 (56)	50 (67.6)	329 (68.7)
Alive	4 (57.1)	27 (64.3)	79 (71.8)	77 (73.3)	132 (93.6)	74 (100)	393 (82)
Developed CFRD	3 (42.9)	21 (50)	41 (37.3)	31 (29.5)	22 (15.6)	1 (1.4)	119 (24.8)

CFRD, cystic fibrosis related diabetes.

providing the possibility to project or generate a potential data curve, based on trajectory. This information can assist the care provider during times of reduced lung function to have a more realistic prognosis of the patient's pulmonary function based on past lung function. This is a much more reliable picture than prognosticating on a single FEV_1; this type of database information allows prediction of future lung function based on past peaks and valleys in addition to worsening and improvements in lung function, which are not infrequent in CF patients.

S. K. Willsie, DO, MA

2 Chronic Obstructive Pulmonary Disease

Introduction

Over the past few years, significant progress has been made in the ability to predict prognosis in COPD. This year's chapter begins with a few additional studies that add tweaks to our ability to predict mortality. A diverse set of factors—spirometric measures in early disease, emphysema scores on computerized tomography, inflammatory biomarkers, and a patient's level of physical activity—are addressed in four separate studies. A fifth study in this group extends this theme; it is a literature review of the frequency and adequacy of end-of-life conversations with COPD patients.

Acute exacerbation management continues to be an active area of research. One of the tools widely used in community-acquired pneumonia, but not available for COPD, are predictive algorithms or tools to help understand severity of exacerbation and prognosis. The first article in this section describes a tool for this purpose, which is currently in validation trials and looks very promising. Other studies address the use of blood eosinophilia in exacerbations to direct steroid treatment in a randomized trial, and the efficacy of antibiotic treatment in mild and moderate exacerbations of COPD. This is a perennial study topic, and the current study, a blinded, randomized controlled trial comes in on the side of using antibiotics. But read critically, the study—even with what appears to be a robust approach— has some major methodological issues. A possibly related topic is a description of the microbiome of the respiratory tract. A really "hot" research area in multiple organ systems, the microbiome, describes a population of multiple microbes identified by modern RNA fragment technology from various organs that suggests a heterogenous population of microbes rather than sterility. The impact of these recent findings remains unclear.

An article is included on the use of bronchodilator treatment in chronic management. One is a systematic review of a new once-a-day beta-agonist, indacaterol, used in comparison to several different long-acting bronchodilators in different studies.

Since COPD has been recognized as a systemic illness with chronic inflammatory markers and high rates of comorbid disease, new studies appear each year addressing the impact of these co-morbidities on morbidity and mortality. Studies included in this edition include the impact of COPD on myocardial infarction management and outcome, venous thromboembolism in COPD patients, and a systematic review of the impact of COPD on cognitive function.

The final three reports in COPD this year address the impact of occupational exposure in the development of COPD from a large Swiss Cohort. A second investigation reports on some new genetic susceptibility findings from the large genetic study group performing genome wide association studies. The ultimate impact of these findings is not yet known. The final article I included is one in which the investigators tried to use a bronchodilator-responsive phenotype of COPD to see if the phenotype was stable and could predict outcomes. They found the bronchodilator-responsiveness was not stable. The approach of using genotypes and phenotypes to predict outcomes and target therapy will undoubtedly be very valuable, but it will also undoubtedly have many false starts along the way. More to come!

Janet R. Mauer, MD, MBA

Spirometric Predictors of Lung Function Decline and Mortality in Early Chronic Obstructive Pulmonary Disease

Drummond MB, Hansel NN, Connett JE, et al (Johns Hopkins Univ, Baltimore, MD; Univ of Minnesota, Minneapolis; et al)
Am J Respir Crit Care Med 185:1301-1306, 2012

Rationale.—The course of lung function decline for smokers with early airflow obstruction remains undefined. It is also unclear which early spirometric characteristics identify individuals at risk for rapid decline and increased mortality.

Objectives.—To determine the association between spirometric measures and 5-year decline in FEV_1 and 12-year mortality.

Methods.—We analyzed longitudinal data from the Lung Health Study, a clinical trial of intensive smoking cessation intervention with or without bronchodilator therapy in 5,887 smokers with mild to moderate airflow obstruction. Participants were stratified into bins of baseline FEV_1 to FVC ratio, using bins of 5%, and separately into bins of Z-score (difference between actual and predicted FEV_1/FVC, normalized to SD of predicted FEV_1/FVC). Associations between spirometric measures and FEV_1 decline and mortality were determined after adjusting for baseline characteristics and time-varying smoking status.

Measurements and Main Results.—The cohort was approximately two-thirds male, predominantly of white race (96%), and with mean age of 49 ± 7 years. In general, individuals with lower lung function by any metric had more rapid adjusted FEV_1 decline. A threshold for differential decline was present at FEV_1/FVC less than 0.65 ($P < 0.001$) and Z-score less than −2 (2.3 percentile) ($P < 0.001$). At year 12, 575 (7.2%) of the cohort had died. Lower thresholds of each spirometric metric were associated with increasing adjusted hazard of death.

Conclusions.—Smokers at risk or with mild to moderate chronic obstructive pulmonary disease have accelerated lung function decline. Individuals with lower baseline FEV_1/FVC have more rapid decline and worse mortality.

▶ Declining forced expiration in 1 second (FEV_1) levels in patients with chronic obstructive lung disease (COPD) has for a long time been a primary marker of declining lung function; FEV_1 was felt to relentlessly decline at a rate several times that of decline in persons without COPD until death. More recently, it has been demonstrated that FEV_1 does not reliably relentlessly decline and may, in fact, stabilize or even improve for a time.[1,2] Thus it's no longer considered a reliable predictor of mortality and now combination indices, which include FFV_1, but also other parameters, such as BODE (body mass index, FEV_1, dyspnea, exercise capacity), are much more accurate and predictive of mortality. Most of the indices predictive of mortality concentrate on patients with severe and very severe disease. Combination indices have not been validated in patients with early disease, and it is even unclear which spirometric (or if spirometric) values are useful. To determine if there were useful spirometric indices to follow in patients with mild and moderate disease, the authors used data from the multicenter Lung Health Study, a study in which the spirometry was very closely quality controlled. In this study, all participants were smokers at entry. Smoking cessation was encouraged. Not surprisingly, continuous smokers had a more accelerated decline in function, but also those patients with mild or moderate disease who had lower FEV_1/forced vital capacity ratios or lower FEV_1% predicted had more rapid declines and a higher risk of death. These findings support a variable course of disease progression in mild and moderate disease patients as has been reported in more severe disease. However, it has not previously been documented in this group of patients. We still don't understand well patients with moderate or mild disease and need to better determine how to stratify and manage these patients beyond smoking cessation.

J. R. Maurer, MD

References

1. Vestbo J, Edwards LD, Scanlon PD, et al. Changes in forced expiratory volume in 1 second over time in COPD. *N Engl J Med.* 2011;365:1184-1192.
2. Casanova C, de Torres JP, Aguirre-Jaíme A, et al. The progression of chronic obstructive pulmonary disease is heterogeneous: the experience of the BODE cohort. *Am J Respir Crit Care Med.* 2011;184:1015-1021.

Emphysema Scores Predict Death From COPD and Lung Cancer
Zulueta JJ, Wisnivesky JP, Henschke CI, et al (Univ of Navarra, Pamplona, Spain; Mount Sinai School of Medicine, NY; et al)
Chest 141:1216-1223, 2012

Objective.—Our objective was to assess the usefulness of emphysema scores in predicting death from COPD and lung cancer.

Methods.—Emphysema was assessed with low-dose CT scans performed on 9,047 men and women for whom age and smoking history were documented. Each scan was scored according to the presence of emphysema as follows: none, mild, moderate, or marked. Follow-up time was calculated from time of CT scan to time of death or December 31, 2007, whichever came first. Cox regression analysis was used to calculate the hazard ratio (HR) of emphysema as a predictor of death.

Results.—Median age was 65 years, 4,433 (49%) were men, and 4,133 (46%) were currently smoking or had quit within 5 years. Emphysema was identified in 2,637 (29%) and was a significant predictor of death from COPD (HR, 9.3; 95% CI, 4.3-20.2; $P < .0001$) and from lung cancer (HR, 1.7; 95% CI, 1.1-2.5; $P = .013$), even when adjusted for age and smoking history.

Conclusions.—Visual assessment of emphysema on CT scan is a significant predictor of death from COPD and lung cancer.

▶ The most valuable current prognostic indicators for mortality in chronic obstructive pulmonary disease (COPD) such as the BODE (body mass index, airway obstruction, dyspnea, and exercise capacity) or ODA (airway obstruction, dyspnea, and age) use clinical and symptom parameters, but not imaging parameters. Some studies have shown a correlation between advanced disease or lung cancer and their computed tomography (CT) finding of emphysema. However, these studies were small and focused on specific populations.[1,2] The authors of this study sought to use the general population of asymptomatic smokers and ex-smokers presenting for low-dose CT lung cancer screening to determine if CT findings of emphysema in a diverse group of at-risk patients could predict mortality. There were 9047 patients in the study, and the median pack year history was 43. During the study, 147 patients died from either COPD or lung cancer, and the mortalities of each disease increased with increased amounts of emphysema detected on CT. Most of the deaths occurred in patients with some degree of emphysema on CT. In these asymptomatic patients, prevalence of emphysema on CT was 30% for men and 28% for women and was present more often in current smokers. This study supports previous more targeted studies that correlate emphysema and risk of death. It has implications for those interested in cancer screening programs in that the finding of emphysema may suggest the need for more frequent screening. Certainly this finding on an at-risk patient's CT should be followed up with a conversation about that person's increased risk of mortality, particularly if he or she is still smoking.

J. R. Maurer, MD

References

1. Ueda K, Jinbo M, Li TS, Yagi T, Suga K, Hamano K. Computed tomography-diagnosed emphysema, not airway obstruction, is associated with the prognostic outcome of early-stage lung cancer. *Clin Cancer Res.* 2006;12:6730-6736.
2. Haruna A, Muro S, Nakano Y, et al. CT scan findings of emphysema predict mortality in COPD. *Chest.* 2010;138:635-640.

Inflammatory Biomarkers Improve Clinical Prediction of Mortality in Chronic Obstructive Pulmonary Disease

Celli BR, for the ECLIPSE Investigators (Brigham and Women's Hosp, Boston, MA; et al)

Am J Respir Crit Care Med 185:1065-1072, 2012

Rationale.—Accurate prediction of mortality helps select patients for interventions aimed at improving outcome.

Objectives.—Because chronic obstructive pulmonary disease is characterized by low-grade systemic inflammation, we hypothesized that addition of inflammatory biomarkers to established predictive factors will improve accuracy.

Methods.—A total of 1,843 patients enrolled in the Evaluation of COPD Longitudinally to Identify Predictive Surrogate Endpoints study were followed for 3 years. Kaplan-Meier curves, log-rank analysis, and Cox proportional hazards analyses determined the predictive value for mortality of clinical variables, while C statistics assessed the added discriminative power offered by addition of biomarkers.

Measurements and Main Results.—At recruitment we measured anthropometrics, spirometry, 6-minute walk distance, dyspnea, BODE index, history of hospitalization, comorbidities, and computed tomography scan emphysema. White blood cell and neutrophil counts, serum or plasma levels of fibrinogen, chemokine ligand 18, surfactant protein D, C-reactive protein, Clara cell secretory protein-16, IL-6 and -8, and tumor necrosis factor-α were determined at recruitment and subsequent visits. A total of 168 of the 1,843 patients (9.1%) died. Nonsurvivors were older and had more severe air flow limitation, increased dyspnea, higher BODE score, more emphysema, and higher rates of comorbidities and history of hospitalizations. The best predictive model for mortality using clinical variables included age, BODE, and hospitalization history (C statistic of 0.686; $P < 0.001$). One single biomarker (IL-6) significantly improved the C statistic to 0.708, but this was further improved to 0.726 ($P = 0.003$) by the addition of all biomarkers.

Conclusions.—The addition of a panel of selected biomarkers improves the ability of established clinical variables to predict mortality in chronic obstructive pulmonary disease.

Clinical trial registered with www.clinicaltrials.gov (NCT00292552).

▶ In recent years, longitudinal studies in large groups of chronic obstructive pulmonary disease (COPD) patients have resulted in the identification of fairly accurate predictors of mortality. The best of these predictors seems to be those that combine multiple parameters. These include, for example, the BODE (body mass index, airway obstruction or forced expiratory volume in 1 second [FEV$_1$], dyspnea, and exercise capacity), ADO (age, dyspnea, and FEV$_1$), and DOSE (dyspnea, FEV$_1$, smoking status, and frequency of exacerbations).[1] A very recent study also singles out level of physical activity as an independent significant predictor of mortality.[2] Interestingly, none of these predictive indices includes any biomarkers even though a number of inflammatory biomarkers have been identified in patients with COPD so that it is now recognized as a systemic inflammatory illness. Some of the biomarkers that have been identified in these patients include interleukin (IL)-6, IL-8, C-reactive protein (CRP), tumor necrosis factor alpha, Clara Cell secretory protein 16, CCL-18/PARC, and surfactant protein D. Before this report, these inflammatory markers had not been studied as a group or in large enough populations to be able to determine if they add any value to the clinical predictive indices. The authors theorized that the addition of a panel of some combination of these biomarkers would improve the accuracy of the clinical variable indices that are currently the primary predictive tools. They were fortunate to be able to access the database of the large ECLIPSE (Evaluation of COPD Longitudinally to Identify Predictive Surrogate Endpoints) study in which there was available biomarker data on 1843 patients, 168 of whom died during the 3-year follow-up. Although the data show that adding the results of the "panel" of biomarkers increases predictive power to the clinical indices, most of the improvement in predictive power comes from a single marker, IL-6. Also, some biomarkers identified as present in COPD patients were not tested here (eg, metalloproteinases and growth factors), so their utility is not known. Biomarkers, singly or in various combinations, are promising in increasing the accuracy of clinical models and should be further evaluated.

J. R. Maurer, MD

References

1. Jones RC, Donaldson GC, Chavannes NH, et al. Derivation and validation of a composite index of severity in chronic obstructive pulmonary disease: the DOSE Index. *Am J Respir Crit Care Med.* 2009;180:1189-1195.
2. Waschki B, Kirsten A, Holz O, et al. Physical activity is the strongest predictor of all-cause mortality in patients with COPD: a prospective cohort study. *Chest.* 2011;140:331-342.

Physical Activity Is the Strongest Predictor of All-Cause Mortality in Patients With COPD: A Prospective Cohort Study

Waschki B, Kirsten A, Holz O, et al (Pulmonary Res Inst at Hosp Grosshansdorf, Germany; Hosp Grosshansdorf Ctr for Pneumology and Thoracic Surgery, Germany; et al)

Chest 140:331-342, 2011

Background.—Systemic effects of COPD are incompletely reflected by established prognostic assessments. We determined the prognostic value of objectively measured physical activity in comparison with established predictors of mortality and evaluated the prognostic value of noninvasive assessments of cardiovascular status, biomarkers of systemic inflammation, and adipokines.

Methods.—In a prospective cohort study of 170 outpatients with stable COPD (mean FEV_1, 56% predicted), we assessed lung function by spirometry and body plethysmography; physical activity level (PAL) by a multisensory armband; exercise capacity by 6-min walk distance test; cardiovascular status by echocardiography, vascular Doppler sonography (ankle-brachial index [ABI]), and N-terminal pro-B-type natriuretic peptide level; nutritional and muscular status by BMI and fat-free mass index; biomarkers by levels of high-sensitivity C-reactive protein, IL-6, fibrinogen, adiponectin, and leptin; and health status, dyspnea, and depressive symptoms by questionnaire. Established prognostic indices were calculated. The median follow-up was 48 months (range, 10-53 months).

Results.—All-cause mortality was 15.4%. After adjustments, each 0.14 increase in PAL was associated with a lower risk of death (hazard ratio [HR], 0.46; 95% CI, 0.33-0.64; $P < .001$). Compared with established predictors, PAL showed the best discriminative properties for 4-year survival (C statistic, 0.81) and was associated with the highest relative risk of death per standardized decrease. Novel predictors of mortality were adiponectin level (HR, 1.34; 95% CI, 1.06-1.71; $P = .017$), leptin level (HR, 0.81; 95% CI, 0.65-0.99; $P = .042$), right ventricular function (Tei-index) (HR, 1.26; 95% CI, 1.04-1.54; $P = .020$), and ABI < 1.00 (HR, 3.87; 95% CI, 1.44-10.40; $P = .007$). A stepwise Cox regression revealed that the best model of independent predictors was PAL, adiponectin level, and ABI. The composite of these factors further improved the discriminative properties (C statistic, 0.85).

Conclusions.—We found that objectively measured physical activity is the strongest predictor of all-cause mortality in patients with COPD. In addition, adiponectin level and vascular status provide independent prognostic information in our cohort.

▶ Daily physical activity has clearly been associated with mortality in several common diseases such as cardiovascular disease and diabetes.[1,2] Exercise capacity is a component of the commonly used and validated mortality predictor—body mass index, airflow obstruction, dyspnea, and exercise capacity (BODE)—in chronic obstructive pulmonary disease as well. In patients with chronic obstructive pulmonary disease (COPD), reduced physical activity is related to the degree of airway limitation as well as extrapulmonary effects such as cardiac disease and impaired muscle function. Pulmonary rehabilitation is recognized as an important component of management of COPD patients with the presumption that improved physical functioning will improve quality of life, but has not been shown to definitively reduce mortality. However, direct associations between level of physical activity and mortality in this disease are poorly documented.[3] The purpose of this study was to determine if objectively measured physical activity could be correlated with all-cause mortality as it has been in other diseases. In addition, the authors sought to compare physical activity with several other predictors of mortality such as BODE and also further evaluate the predictive value of biomarkers and adipokines. It is important to distinguish measures of exercise capacity (such as the 6-minute walk test) from the actual amount of daily physical activity that patients were completing, which was the measurement in this study. Patients were followed for a mean of 48 months. Level of daily physical activity, as a single entity, was more predictive of all-cause mortality than other well-accepted predictors such as muscle wasting, age and malnutrition, or biomarkers or adipokines (Fig 1 in the original article). This is consistent with observations in other disease states. It emphasizes the importance of pulmonary rehabilitation programs and argues for aggressive continuing home regimens—a simple, but rarely stressed component of comprehensive COPD care.

J. R. Maurer, MD

References

1. Katzmarzyk PT, Church TS, Craig CL, Bouchard C. Sitting time and mortality from all causes, cardiovascular disease, and cancer. *Med Sci Sports Exerc*. 2009; 41:998-1005.
2. Rask K, O'Malley E, Druss B. Impact of socioeconomic, behavioral and clinical risk factors on mortality. *J Public Health (Oxf)*. 2009;31:231-238.
3. Garcia-Aymerich J, Lange P, Benet M, Schnohr P, Antó JM. Regular physical activity reduces hospital admission and mortality in chronic obstructive pulmonary disease: a population based cohort study. *Thorax*. 2006;61:772-778.

Discussing an uncertain future: end-of-life care conversations in chronic obstructive pulmonary disease. A systematic literature review and narrative synthesis
Momen N, Hadfield P, Kuhn I, et al (Univ of Cambridge, UK; North Street Med Practice, Peterborough, UK)
Thorax 67:777-780, 2012

Background.—Guidelines recommend open discussions between patients and healthcare professionals as the end-of-life (EOL) approaches. Much of the knowledge about the EOL is based on the needs of patients with cancer and the applicability of this to other diseases is often queried. A literature review was undertaken concerning EOL care (EOLC) conversations in chronic obstructive pulmonary disease (COPD).

Design.—A systematic literature review and narrative synthesis obtained papers reporting on EOLC conversations between patients with COPD and their healthcare professionals with respect to the prevalence of conversations; each party's preferences for timing and content; and the facilitators and blockers. Inclusion criteria were articles published in peer-reviewed journals, written in English, reporting studies of adult patients with COPD and/or their healthcare professionals concerning discussions of care at the EOL.

Results.—30 papers were identified. Most patients reported that they have not had EOLC discussions with healthcare professionals. While many patients would like these conversations, a potentially large minority would not; the proportions varied among studies. Healthcare professionals find these discussions difficult and many prefer patients to initiate them.

Conclusions.—Patients' preferences for EOLC conversations vary greatly. Healthcare professionals need to respect the wishes of those not wanting to discuss EOLC and provide multiple opportunities for those who do wish to have these discussions. Recommendations on how to approach the conversation are made.

▶ It was gratifying to see a number of studies in 2012 focus on the end-of-life of patients with chronic obstructive pulmonary disease (COPD).[1,2] Notably, almost all of the research in this area has been published since 2000. It was also somewhat dismaying, particularly in this review of 30 studies, to be reminded that most physicians and other health care providers do not have appropriate end-of-life conversations with their COPD patients. In fact, the authors describe these conversations as "rare." For unclear reasons, health providers continue to consider cancer the primary illness that requires discussions around end-of-life even as the life span increases and more and more people develop and die of other chronic illnesses. Other barriers are less obscure. The authors identify difficulty in prognosticating remaining life span in COPD, poor understanding of COPD among the public, and providers not identifying end-of-life discussions as their responsibility. There are increasing data, however, that more patients want to discuss these issues, and that the end-of-life discussions result in perceived overall quality of and satisfaction with care.[2] There are other important benefits to recognition by both the caregivers and the patient that the end of life is near. These discussions and documentations allow for the implementation of appropriate palliative measures at an appropriate time and ensure that unwanted invasive approaches to prolonging life are not used in patients who do not desire them. End-of-life protocols should be part of the management strategy of every physician caring for patients with chronic, progressive disease.

J. R. Maurer, MD

References

1. Janssen DJ, Curtis JR, Au DH, et al. Patient-clinician communication about end-of-life care for Dutch and US patients with COPD. *Eur Respir J*. 2011;38:268-276.
2. Leung JM, Udris EM, Uman J, Au DH. The effect of end-of-life discussions on perceived quality of care and health status among patients with COPD. *Chest*. 2012;142:128-133.

Usefulness of the Chronic Obstructive Pulmonary Disease Assessment Test to Evaluate Severity of COPD Exacerbations
Mackay AJ, Donaldson GC, Patel AR, et al (Univ College London Med School, UK; et al)
Am J Respir Crit Care Med 185:1218-1224, 2012

Rationale.—The Chronic Obstructive Pulmonary Disease (COPD) Assessment Test (CAT) is an eight-item questionnaire designed to assess and quantify the impact of COPD symptoms on health status. COPD exacerbations impair quality of life and are characterized by worsening respiratory symptoms from the stable state. We hypothesized that CAT scores at exacerbation relate to exacerbation severity as measured by exacerbation duration, lung function impairment, and systemic inflammation.

Objectives.—To evaluate the usefulness of the CAT to assess exacerbation severity.

Methods.—One hundred sixty-one patients enrolled in the London COPD cohort completed the CAT at baseline (stable state), exacerbation, and during recovery between April 2010 and June 2011.

Measurements and Main Results.—Frequent exacerbators had significantly higher baseline CAT scores than infrequent exacerbators (19.5 ± 6.6 vs. 16.8 ± 8.0, $P = 0.025$). In 152 exacerbations, CAT scores rose from an average baseline value of 19.4 ± 6.8 to 24.1 ± 7.3 ($P < 0.001$) at exacerbation. Change in CAT score from baseline to exacerbation onset was significantly but weakly related to change in C-reactive protein (rho = 0.26, $P = 0.008$) but not to change in fibrinogen (rho = 0.09, $P = 0.351$) from baseline to exacerbation. At exacerbation, rises in CAT score were significantly associated with falls in FEV_1 (rho = −0.20, $P = 0.032$). Median recovery time as judged by symptom diary cards was significantly related to the time taken for the CAT score to return to baseline (rho = 0.42, $P = 0.012$).

Conclusions.—The CAT provides a reliable score of exacerbation severity. Baseline CAT scores are elevated in frequent exacerbators. CAT scores increase at exacerbation and reflect severity as determined by lung function and exacerbation duration.

▶ The chronic obstructive pulmonary disease (COPD) Assessment Test (CAT) was developed to understand the health status of patients in a routine clinical practice setting. Other quality-of-life instruments, such as the Saint George Respiratory Questionnaire (SGRQ) and Chronic Respiratory Questionnaire (CRQ), are used primarily in clinical trials and have not been incorporated into clinical practice because they are long and hard to use. The CAT is an eight 8-question instrument that is easily understood by the patients and easy to complete (Fig 1 in the original article) and can be easily filled out at each office visit.[1] Scores can be trended over time or reviewed on a visit by visit basis. Initial validation of this instrument showed good correlation with SGRQ and with response to pulmonary rehabilitation.[1,2] It is currently being tested and validated in other clinical COPD settings. In the current study, the investigators attempted to use it in an acute setting by evaluating exacerbation severity. The CAT scores were able to help characterize exacerbations. The authors suggest CAT may be useful not only in routine management of patients, but also in clinical studies to help "objectively assess the ability of novel interventions to reduce exacerbation severity." Jones et al[3]—one of the original CAT developers—studied the use of CAT during exacerbations and its ability to assess health status and came to similar conclusions as the Mackay et al investigators. The CAT looks like a valuable tool that can be easily used in routine management of stable and acutely ill COPD patients to help guide therapy and help clinicians better understand impact of their disease management on their patients.

J. R. Maurer, MD

References

1. Jones PW, Harding G, Berry P, Wiklund I, Chen WH, Kline Leidy N. Development and first validation of the COPD Assessment Test. *Eur Respir J.* 2009;34:648-654.
2. Dodd JW, Hogg L, Nolan J, et al. The COPD assessment test (CAT): response to pulmonary rehabilitation. A multicentre, prospective study. *Thorax.* 2011;66: 425-429.
3. Jones PW, Harding G, Wiklund I, et al. Tests of the responsiveness of the COPD assessment test following acute exacerbation and pulmonary rehabilitation. *Chest.* 2012;142:134-140.

Blood Eosinophils to Direct Corticosteroid Treatment of Exacerbations of Chronic Obstructive Pulmonary Disease: A Randomized Placebo-Controlled Trial

Bafadhel M, McKenna S, Terry S, et al (Univ of Leicester, UK; et al)
Am J Respir Crit Care Med 186:48-55, 2012

Rationale.—Exacerbations of chronic obstructive pulmonary disease (COPD) and responses to treatment are heterogeneous.

Objectives.—Investigate the usefulness of blood eosinophils to direct corticosteroid therapy during exacerbations.

Methods.—Subjects with COPD exacerbations were entered into a randomized biomarker-directed double-blind corticosteroid versus standard therapy study. Subjects in the standard arm received prednisolone for 2 weeks, whereas in the biomarker-directed arm, prednisolone or matching placebo was given according to the blood eosinophil count biomarker. Both study groups received antibiotics. Blood eosinophils were measured in the biomarker directed and standard therapy arms to define biomarker-positive and -negative exacerbations (blood eosinophil count > and $\leq 2\%$, respectively). The primary outcome was to determine noninferiority in health status using the chronic respiratory questionnaire (CRQ) and in the proportion of exacerbations associated with a treatment failure between subjects allocated to the biomarker-directed and standard therapy arms.

Measurements and Main Results.—There were 86 and 80 exacerbations in the biomarker-directed and standard treatment groups, respectively. In the biomarker-directed group, 49% of the exacerbations were not treated with prednisolone. CRQ improvement after treatment in the standard and biomarker-directed therapy groups was similar (0.8 vs. 1.1; mean difference, 0.3; 95% confidence interval, 0.0−0.6; $P = 0.05$). There was a greater improvement in CRQ in biomarker-negative exacerbations given placebo compared with those given prednisolone (mean difference, 0.45; 95% confidence interval, 0.01−0.90; $P = 0.04$). In biomarker-negative exacerbations, treatment failures occurred in 15% given prednisolone and 2% of those given placebo ($P = 0.04$).

Conclusions.—The peripheral blood eosinophil count is a promising biomarker to direct corticosteroid therapy during COPD exacerbations, but larger studies are required.

▶ Guidelines for the management of acute exacerbations of chronic obstructive pulmonary disease (COPD) support the use of systemic corticosteroids along with other types of bronchodilation and, in some cases, antibiotics. Only certain types of inflammatory cells, however, are responsive to corticosteroid treatment. Among the most responsive are eosinophils, a primary inflammatory cell in many asthmatics and recently recognized as a primary cause of inflammation in some exacerbations of COPD.[1,2] Because corticosteroids have many side effects, it would be useful to identify those patients most likely to respond to them and target those patients with corticosteroid therapy; alternatively, it may be wise not to use these drugs in patients who are not likely to respond. Bafadhel et al undertook a well-designed study to determine if withholding prednisone in patients with less than 2% peripheral eosinophilia resulted in excessive treatment failures. It did not. The authors conclude that it is safe to use non—steroid-containing regimens in patients without eosinophilia. Interestingly, there were as many treatment failures in the patients with elevated levels of eosinophilia who were treated with prednisone. Thus, the study does not provide definitive evidence supporting a positive impact of steroid treatment in eosinophilia-positive patients. Further, larger prospective studies are needed to better define the usefulness of peripheral eosinophilia as a marker for targeted therapy of exacerbations. One weakness of the study is that most of the exacerbations were mild to moderate and did not require hospitalization. It may be that studying a more diverse group including severe exacerbations will help better define the role of eosinophilia as a marker for steroid use.

J. R. Maurer, MD

References

1. Saha S, Brightling CE. Eosinophilic airway inflammation in COPD. *Int J Chron Obstruct Pulmon Dis.* 2006;1:39-47.
2. Siva R, Green RH, Brightling CE, et al. Eosinophilic airway inflammation and exacerbations of COPD: a randomised controlled trial. *Eur Respir J.* 2007;29: 906-913.

Efficacy of Antibiotic Therapy for Acute Exacerbations of Mild to Moderate Chronic Obstructive Pulmonary Disease
Llor C, Moragas A, Hernández S, et al (Univ Rovira i Virgili, Spain; Primary Care Ctr Jaume I, Tarragona, Spain; et al)
Am J Respir Crit Care Med 186:716-723, 2012

Rationale.—Antimicrobial therapy remains a controversial issue in non-severe exacerbations of chronic obstructive pulmonary disease (COPD).

Objectives.—To evaluate the efficacy of antibiotic therapy in moderate exacerbations of mild-to-moderate COPD.

Methods.—This study involved a multicenter, parallel, double-blind, placebo-controlled, randomized clinical trial. Patients aged 40 years or older, smokers, or ex-smokers of 10 pack-years or more with spirometrically confirmed mild-to-moderate COPD ($FEV_1 > 50\%$ predicted and FEV_1/FVC ratio < 0.7) and diagnosed with an exacerbation were enrolled in the study. The patients were randomized to receive amoxicillin/clavulanate 500/125 mg three times a day or placebo three times a day for 8 days.

Measurements and Main Results.—The primary outcome measure was clinical cure at end of therapy visit (EOT) at Days 9 to 11. A total of 310 subjects fulfilled all the criteria for efficacy analysis. A total of 117 patients with amoxicillin/clavulanate (74.1%) and 91 with placebo (59.9%) were considered cured at EOT (difference, 14.2%; 95% confidence interval, 3.7−24.3). The median time to the next exacerbation was significantly longer in patients receiving antibiotic compared with placebo (233 d [interquartile range, 110−365] compared with 160 d [interquartile range, 66−365]; $P < 0.05$). The best C-reactive protein serum cut-off for predicting clinical failure with placebo was 40 mg/L, with an area under the curve of 0.732 (95% confidence interval, 0.614−0.851).

Conclusions.—Treatment of ambulatory exacerbations of mild-to-moderate COPD with amoxicillin/clavulanate is more effective and significantly prolongs the time to the next exacerbation compared with placebo.

▶ Just when it seems there can't possibly be another article addressing when/if to use antibiotics in acute exacerbations of chronic obstructive pulmonary disease (COPD), we have this multicenter prospective, parallel, randomized, double-blinded, placebo-controlled study suggesting that those patients to whom almost no one gives antibiotics any longer for their exacerbations—mild to moderate COPD with exacerbations treatable as an outpatient—may actually do better with antibiotics! Current management approaches are based on the lack of support (lack of good studies, actually) for use of antibiotics in patients with mild and moderate disease.[1-4] The authors state the purpose of their study is to rectify this lack of studies—and they come to the opposite conclusion that antibiotics are beneficial in these patients. But, on close inspection, it is not clear that the authors have created a case for antibiotic use in exacerbations in the studied population. A major concern is some of the study's faults, one of which is the study's inability to recruit the full cohort of patients originally hoped. To meet the authors' power calculations, they required 667 patients, more than double the actual recruited sample. Another is that symptoms were not objectively assessed at the end of therapy. Yet another is that the definition of exacerbation was based on only 1 of the typical criteria rather than 2 or 3.[5] This study should not be interpreted as a green light to treat everyone with a mild COPD exacerbation with antibiotics. Rather, it should raise questions of whether there is a subset of patients in this population that might benefit from antibiotics. The next study should be to try to sort this out: Are there biomarkers that can guide treatment? Are there specific patient characteristics that can guide treatment? Are there specific exacerbation characteristics that can guide treatment?

J. R. Maurer, MD

References

1. Puhan MA, Vollenweider D, Steurer J, Bossuyt P, Ter Riet G. Where is the supporting evidence for treating mild to moderate chronic obstructive pulmonary disease exacerbations with antibiotics? A systematic review. *BMC Med*. 2008;6:28.
2. Ram FS, Rodriguez-Roisin R, Granados-Navarte A, Garcia-Aymerich J, Barnes NC. Antibiotis for exacerbations of chronic obstructive pulmonary disease. *Cochrane Database Syst Rev*. 2006;(2):CD004403.
3. Puhan MA, Vollenweider D, Latshang T, Steurer J, Steurer-Stey C. Exacerbations of chronic obstructive pulmonary disease: when are antibiotics indicated? A systematic review. *Respir Res*. 2007;8:30.
4. Saint S, Bent S, Vittinghoff E, Grady D. Antibiotics in chronic obstructive pulmonary disease exacerbations. A meta-analysis. *JAMA*. 1995;273:957-960.
5. Anthonisen NR, Manfreda J, Warren CP, Hershfielf ES, Harding GKM, Nelson NA. Antibiotic therapy in exacerbations of chronic obstructive pulmonary disease. *Ann Intern Med*. 1987;106:196-204.

Significance of the microbiome in obstructive lung disease

Han MK, Huang YJ, Lipuma JJ, et al (Univ of Michigan Health System, Ann Arbor; Univ of California San Francisco; et al)
Thorax 67:456-463, 2012

The composition of the lung microbiome contributes to both health and disease, including obstructive lung disease. Because it has been estimated that over 70% of the bacterial species on body surfaces cannot be cultured by currently available techniques, traditional culture techniques are no longer the gold standard for microbial investigation. Advanced techniques that identify bacterial sequences, including the 16S ribosomal RNA gene, have provided new insights into the depth and breadth of microbiota present both in the diseased and normal lung. In asthma, the composition of the microbiome of the lung and gut during early childhood development may play a key role in the development of asthma, while specific airway microbiota are associated with chronic asthma in adults. Early bacterial stimulation appears to reduce asthma susceptibility by helping the immune system develop lifelong tolerance to innocuous antigens. By contrast, perturbations in the microbiome from antibiotic use may increase the risk for asthma development. In chronic obstructive pulmonary disease, bacterial colonisation has been associated with a chronic bronchitic phenotype, increased risk of exacerbations, and accelerated loss of lung function. In cystic fibrosis, studies utilising culture-independent methods have identified associations between decreased bacterial community diversity and reduced lung function; colonisation with *Pseudomonas aeruginosa* has been associated with the presence of certain CFTR mutations. Genomic analysis of the lung microbiome is a young field, but has the potential to define the relationship between lung microbiome composition and disease course. Whether we can manipulate bacterial communities to improve clinical outcomes remains to be seen.

▶ Despite the long-held belief that the lower respiratory tract is sterile, the burgeoning technology that has allowed the in-depth analysis of small pieces of genetic material has completely changed that perception. Measurement of small snippets of bacteria genetic material, typically ribosomal RNA, obtained by sampling both lung and airways, has identified a previously unknown population of many microbes that live within the respiratory tract. This is termed the *microbiome*, and it is thought that as many as 70% of the species identified have not been cultured and cannot be cultured by currently available techniques.[1] So much remains unknown about them. The discovery of the lung microbiome has led to many questions: What is the role of the microbiome in health and disease? How does it differ from person to person? How does it differ in people without and with lung disease? Is it different in different diseases? Han et al review the general approaches to identifying these elusive microorganisms and some of the data that are known about the microbiome of different diseases. Other research published in the last year included an analysis of the lung tissue microbiome (as opposed to airway) in obstructive lung disease[2] and an analysis of the microbiome[3] at different levels of the bronchial tree in obstructive disease. The pulmonary microbiome is an emerging area of research and holds great promise as a useful tool in helping understand disease progression and possibly disease heterogeneity. It may lead to the development of exciting new treatment approaches to pulmonary disease. Look for many more exciting discoveries in the next few years.

J. R. Maurer, MD

References

1. Hayashi H, Sakamoto M, Benno Y. Phylogenetic analysis of the human gut microbiota using 16S rDNA clone libraries and strictly anaerobic culture-based methods. *Microbiol Immunol.* 2002;46:535-548.
2. Sze MA, Dimitriu PA, Hayashi S, et al. The lung tissue microbiome in chronic obstructive pulmonary disease. *Am J Respir Crit Care Med.* 2012;185:1073-1080.
3. Cabrera-Rubio R, Garcia-Núñez M, Setó L, et al. Microbiome diversity in the bronchial tracts of patients with chronic obstructive pulmonary disease. *J Clin Microbiol.* 2012;50:3562-3568.

Comparison of Indacaterol With Tiotropium or Twice-Daily Long-Acting β-Agonists for Stable COPD: A Systematic Review

Rodrigo GJ, Neffen H (Hospital Central de las Fuerzas Armadas, Montevideo, Uruguay; Hospital de Niños "O. Allassia," Santa Fe, Argentina)
Chest 142:1104-1110, 2012

Background.—Bronchodilators are central to the symptomatic management of patients with COPD. Previous data have shown that inhaled indacaterol improved numerous clinical outcomes over placebo.

Methods.—This systematic review explored the efficacy and safety of indacaterol in comparison with tiotropium or bid long-acting β₂-agonists

(TD-LABAs) for treatment of moderate to severe COPD. Randomized controlled trials were identified after a search of different databases of published and unpublished trials.

Results.—Five trials (5,920 participants) were included. Compared with tiotropium, indacaterol showed statistically and clinically significant reductions in the use of rescue medication and dyspnea (43% greater likelihood of achieving a minimal clinically important difference [MCID] in the transitional dyspnea index [TDI]; number needed to treat for benefit [NNTB] = 10). Additionally, the MCID in health status was more likely to be achieved with indacaterol than with tiotropium (OR = 1.43; 95% CI, 1.22−1.68; $P = .00001$; NNTB = 10). Trough FEV_1 was significantly higher at the end of treatment with indacaterol than with TD-LABAs (80 mL, $P = .00001$). Similarly, indacaterol significantly improved dyspnea (61% greater likelihood of achieving an MCID in TDI, $P = .008$) and health status (21% greater likelihood of achieving an MCID in St George's Respiratory Questionnaire, $P = .04$) than TD-LABA. Indacaterol showed similar levels of safety and tolerability to both comparators.

Conclusions.—Available evidence suggests that indacaterol may prove useful as an alternative to tiotropium or TD-LABA due to its effects on health status, dyspnea, and pulmonary function.

▶ Long-acting bronchodilators are one of the mainstays of treatment for patients with moderate and severe obstructive lung disease. Many studies have linked bronchodilator therapy with improved dyspnea and health status and, in some cases, fewer exacerbations.[1] Long-acting bronchodilators include the twice-daily anticholinergic tiotropium as well as several long-acting beta-agonists: twice-daily dosed formoterol and salmeterol and once-daily dosed indacaterol. Indacaterol is in use in a number of countries and was approved by the US Food and Drug Administration on July 1, 2011. The potential benefit to a once-daily dosed drug—if it has equivalent positive impact on parameters such as forced expiratory volume in 1 second (FEV_1), health status, use of rescue inhalers, etc.—is adherence. Compared with placebo, indacaterol has been shown to improve FEV_1, achieve symptom control, improve health status, and reduce exacerbations.[2,3] It has an acceptable safety profile. This meta-analysis looked at studies comparing indacaterol, not with placebo, but with other long-acting beta agonists or tiotropium. Five well-designed studies were identified. Two trials compared indacaterol with tiotropium and 3 with twice-daily dosing long-acting beta agonists. In all cases, indacaterol performed at similar levels of benefit. This makes it an attractive alternative for patients who have difficulties adhering to medication regimens.

J. R. Maurer, MD

References

1. Vogelmeier C, Hederer B, Glaab T, et al; POET-COPD Investigators. Tiotropium versus salmeterol for the prevention of exacerbations of COPD. *N Engl J Med.* 2011;364:1093-1103.
2. Chapman KR, Rennard SI, Dogra A, Owen R, Lassen C, Kramer B; INDORSE Study Investigators. Long-term safety and efficacy of indacaterol, a long-acting

β₂ agonist, in subjects with COPD: a randomized, placebo-controlled study. *Chest.* 2011;140:68-75.

3. Feldman G, Siler T, Prasad N, et al; INLIGHT 1 study group. Efficacy and safety of indacaterol 150 microg once-daily in COPD: a double-blind, randomised, 12-week study. *BMC Pulm Med.* 2010;10:11.

Cognitive dysfunction in patients with chronic obstructive pulmonary disease — A systematic review

Schou L, Østergaard B, Rasmussen LS, et al (Frederiksberg Univ Hosp, Copenhagen F, Denmark; Univ of Southern Denmark, Odense C; Univ Hosp of Copenhagen, Østerbro, Denmark; et al)
Respir Med 106:1071-1081, 2012

Background.—Substantial healthcare resources are spent on chronic obstructive pulmonary disease (COPD). In addition, the involvement of patients in monitoring and treatment of their condition has been suggested. However, it is important to maintain a view of self-care that takes differences in cognitive ability into account.

The aim of this study was to determine the occurrence and severity of cognitive dysfunction in COPD patients, and to assess the association between severity of COPD and the level of cognitive function.

Methods.—We conducted a systematic review, and a search in the following databases: Medline, PsychINFO, Cochrane Library, EMBASE, CINAHL, and SweMed up to July 2010. The articles were included if participants were patients with COPD, relevant outcome was cognitive function investigated by a neuropsychological test battery, and the severity of COPD had been assessed.

Results.—Fifteen studies were included, involving 655 COPD patients and 394 controls. Cognitive function was impaired in COPD patients as compared to healthy controls, but the level of functioning was better than in patients with Alzheimer's disease. There was a significant association between severity of COPD, as measured by lung function and blood gases, and cognitive dysfunction, but only in patients with severe COPD.

Conclusions.—Cognitive impairment can be detected in severe COPD patients, but the clinical relevance of the cognitive dysfunction is not yet known. Future studies should concentrate on the consequences of cognitive dysfunction for daily living in these patients, and solutions involving a high degree of self-care might require special support.

▶ In an environment of increasing emphasis on patient-centered care and patient self-management, it is important to understand if/when the patient is both willing to and capable of accepting more responsibility for self-care. This is particularly relevant in older patients who have increasing levels of cognitive dysfunction. In the general population, the prevalence of mild cognitive impairment is 10% in those age 70 to 79 and 25% in those age 80 to 89.[1] This information is very relevant in managing chronic obstructive pulmonary disease (COPD) patients because they are generally older patients and have additional factors/comorbidities that might increase their chances of having mild or greater cognitive impairment. These include generalized vascular disease and potential episodes of hypoxemia. Reduced cognitive functioning has been associated with poor compliance with treatment regimens.[2,3] Schou et al, in this systematic review of published studies documenting the occurrence and severity of cognitive dysfunction and the association with the severity of COPD, were only able to find 15 usable published studies. There were a total of 655 COPD patients and 394 controls in the final studies selected. The data the authors were able to glean are fairly sparse. COPD patients functioned significantly better than Alzheimer patients, but not at the level of the general population. There was a correlation with cognitive dysfunction and severity of COPD only in severe and very severe disease. All of these findings should be considered preliminary because the studies were heterogeneous, fairly small, and not all included the severity of COPD and the evaluation studies used very variable. Much larger studies encompassing the spectrum of information necessary to make reasonable conclusions about cognitive function are greatly needed. In the meantime, we continue to care for patients and to offload increasing responsibility for their care to them and their families. It is prudent to do at least a minimal preassessment of the family and patient's ability to handle that responsibility.

J. R. Maurer, MD

References

1. Roberts RO, Geda YE, Knopman DS, et al. The Mayo Clinic Study of Aging: design and sampling, participation, baseline measures and sample characteristics. *Neuroepidemiology.* 2008;30:58-69.
2. Allen SC, Jain M, Ragab S, Malik N. Acquisition and short-term retention of inhaler techniques require intact executive function in elderly subjects. *Age Ageing.* 2003;32:299-302.
3. Incalzi RA, Gemma A, Marra C, Capparella O, Fuso L, Carbonin P. Verbal memory impairment in COPD: its mechanisms and clinical relevance. *Chest.* 1997;112: 1506-1513.

Venous Thromboembolism in Patients with Chronic Obstructive Pulmonary Disease

Piazza G, Goldhaber SZ, Kroll A, et al (Harvard Med School, Boston, MA; Univ of Massachusetts Med School, Worcester; et al)
Am J Med 125:1010-1018, 2012

Objective.—Our aim was to compare the clinical characteristics, prophylaxis, treatment, and outcomes of venous thromboembolism in patients with and without previously diagnosed chronic obstructive pulmonary disease.

Methods.—We analyzed the population-based Worcester Venous Thromboembolism Study of 2488 consecutive patients with validated venous thromboembolism to compare clinical characteristics, prophylaxis, treatment, and outcomes in patients with and without chronic obstructive pulmonary disease.

Results.—Of 2488 patients with venous thromboembolism, 484 (19.5%) had a history of clinical chronic obstructive pulmonary disease and 2004 (80.5%) did not. Patients with chronic obstructive pulmonary disease were older (mean age 68 vs 63 years) and had a higher frequency of heart failure (35.5% vs 12.9%) and immobility (53.5% vs 43.3%) than patients without chronic obstructive pulmonary disease (all $P < .0001$). Patients with chronic obstructive pulmonary disease were more likely to die in hospital (6.8% vs 4%, $P = .01$) and within 30 days of venous thromboembolism diagnosis (12.6% vs 6.5%, $P < .0001$). Patients with chronic obstructive pulmonary disease demonstrated increased mortality despite a higher frequency of venous thromboembolism prophylaxis. Immobility doubled the risk of in-hospital death (adjusted odds ratio, 2.21; 95% confidence interval, 1.35-3.62) and death within 30 days of venous thromboembolism diagnosis (adjusted odds ratio, 2.04; 95% confidence interval, 1.43 2.91).

Conclusion.—Patients with chronic obstructive pulmonary disease have an increased risk of dying during hospitalization and within 30 days of venous thromboembolism diagnosis. Immobility in patients with chronic obstructive pulmonary disease is an ominous risk factor for adverse outcomes.

▶ Chronic obstructive pulmonary disease (COPD) is now widely recognized as a systemic disease in which inflammatory biomarkers typically are present. In addition, researchers have found elevated levels of tissue factor procoagulant activity and increased levels of fibrinogen and factor XIII in patients with COPD.[1] The prevalence of pulmonary embolism (PE) is higher than that in the general population and in autopsy studies of patients admitted for acute exacerbations, PE has been reported at 30%.[2] Pulmonary embolic disease is often missed in patients with COPD because it is hard to distinguish many of the symptoms of an acute exacerbation from those of PE. In hospitalized patients, particularly, it may portend a poor prognosis and prolonged hospitalization.[3] However, overall outcomes and impact on COPD patients who develop PE are not well delineated. The authors of this study took advantage of a large database of independently confirmed venous thromboembolism from a population-based study in central Massachusetts, The Worcester Venous Thromboembolism study. They were able to compare various characteristics of COPD patients with PE and non-COPD patients with PE. The impact of PE in the COPD population, particularly the immobile COPD population, is sobering. Bertoletti et al,[4] in a separate study using a large multinational European registry of confirmed thromboembolic disease (RIETE [Registro Informatizado de la Enfermedad TromboEmbolica]) confirmed Piazza et al's findings of a higher mortality in COPD patients. These investigators also found that COPD patients more often present with PE rather than deep venous thrombosis. Confirmation of not only the high rate of thromboembolic disease, but also the high risks and poor outcomes in patients with COPD, should remind us to always consider this potentially preventable disease in the differential diagnosis, not only in hospitalized patients but also in patients presenting with increased symptoms in the outpatient setting.

J. R. Maurer, MD

References

1. Vaidyula VR, Criner GJ, Grabianowski C, Rao AK. Circulating tissue factor pro-coagulant activity is elevated in stable moderate to severe chronic obstructive pulmonary disease. *Thromb Res.* 2009;124:259-261.
2. Ambrosetti M, Ageno W, Spanevello A, Salerno M, Pedretti RF. Prevalence and prevention of venous thromboembolism in patients with acute exacerbations of COPD. *Thromb Res.* 2003;112:203-207.
3. Gunen H, Gulbas G, In E, Yetkin O, Hacievliyagil SS. Venous thromboemboli and exacerbations of COPD. *Eur Respir J.* 2010;35:1243-1248.
4. Bertoletti L, Quenet S, Mismetti P, et al; Monreal M & the RIETE Investigators. Clinical presentation and outcome of venous thromboembolism in COPD. *Eur Respir J.* 2012;39:862-868.

The Impact of COPD on Management and Outcomes of Patients Hospitalized With Acute Myocardial Infarction: A 10-Year Retrospective Observational Study

Stefan MS, Bannuru RR, Lessard D, et al (Baystate Med Ctr, Springfield, MA; Tufts Univ School of Medicine, Boston, MA; Univ of Massachusetts Med School, Worcester, MA)
Chest 141:1441-1448, 2012

Background.—There are limited data describing contemporary trends in the management and outcomes of patients with COPD who develop acute myocardial infarction (AMI).

Methods.—The study population consisted of patients hospitalized with AMI at all greater Worcester, Massachusetts, medical centers between 1997 and 2007.

Results.—Of the 6,290 patients hospitalized with AMI, 17% had a history of COPD. Patients with COPD were less likely to be treated with β-blockers or lipid-lowering therapy or to have undergone interventional procedures during their index hospitalization than patients without COPD. Patients with COPD were at higher risk for dying during hospitalization (13.5% vs 10.1%) and at 30 days after discharge (18.7% vs 13.2%), and their outcomes did not improve during the decade-long period under study. After multivariable adjustment, the adverse effects of COPD remained on both in-hospital (OR, 1.25; 95% CI, 0.99-1.50) and 30-day all-cause mortality (OR, 1.31; 95% CI, 1.10-1.58). The use of evidence-based therapies for all patients with AMI increased between 1997 and 2007, with a particularly marked increase for patients with COPD.

Conclusions.—Our results suggest that the gap in medical care between patients with and without COPD hospitalized with AMI narrowed substantially between 1997 and 2007. Patients with COPD, however, remain less aggressively treated and are at increased risk for hospital adverse outcomes than patients without COPD in the setting of AMI. Careful consideration is necessary to ensure that these high-risk complex patients are not denied the benefits of effective cardiac therapies.

▶ Cardiovascular disease is a common comorbidity of chronic obstructive lung disease (COPD) because smoking is a major risk factor for both. Thus, many patients with COPD will have cardiac events, which has been shown to be the leading cause of death in these patients.[1] Interestingly, it has also been reported that despite the frequency of acute cardiac events in COPD patients, they often do not receive optimal treatment for their cardiac disease.[2] There are several reasons that might explain this. First, it may be difficult to differentiate between cardiac problems such as worsening congestive heart failure and acute exacerbations of COPD because of confusing chest x-ray changes and similar symptoms. However, the use of natriuretic peptide measurements has been very helpful over the past few years in helping to distinguish heart failure and should lead physicians to the correct diagnosis.[3] Second, physicians have often been reluctant to use beta blockers—a major therapeutic approach in patients with cardiac disease including myocardial infarction—because of fear of worsening their respiratory status. Recent studies also have debunked this and suggested strongly that beta blockers have a positive effect on survival of COPD patients with acute cardiac events, and they should be used.[4] Finally, optimal treatment may be withheld because of the degree of comorbidity conferred on the patient by the concomitant COPD. This can only be justified in the most severely impaired COPD patients with limited life expectancy. It is encouraging to see that the gap in care of acute cardiac events identified in the early phase of Stefan et al's study is improving. However, it is also concerning that the death rate of those with COPD remains higher whereas the level of care is still not at the level received be non-COPD patients.

J. R. Maurer, MD

References

1. Anthonisen NR, Connett JE, Enright PL, Manfreda J; Lung Health Study Research Group. Hospitalizations and mortality in the Lung Health Study. *Am J Respir Crit Care Med.* 2002;166:333-339.
2. Albouaini K, Andron M, Alahmar A, Egred M. Beta-blockers use in patients with chronic obstructive pulmonary disease and concomitant cardiovascular conditions. *Int J Chron Obstruct Pulmon Dis.* 2007;2:535-540.
3. Le Jemtel TH, Padeletti M, Jelic S. Diagnostic and therapeutic challenges in patients with coexistent chronic obstructive pulmonary disease and chronic heart failure. *J Am Coll Cardiol.* 2007;49:171-180.
4. Salpeter S, Ormiston T, Salpeter E. Cardioselective beta-blockers for chronic obstructive pulmonary disease. *Cochrane Database Syst Rev.* 2005;(4):CD003566.

Bronchodilator responsiveness as a phenotypic characteristic of established chronic obstructive pulmonary disease

Albert P, Agusti A, Edwards L, et al (Univ Hosp Aintree, Liverpool, UK; Hosp Clínic, Barcelona, Spain; GlaxoSmithKline Res and Development, Research Triangle Park, NC; et al)
Thorax 67:701-708, 2012

Background.—Bronchodilator responsiveness is a potential phenotypic characteristic of chronic obstructive pulmonary disease (COPD). We studied whether change in lung function after a bronchodilator is abnormal in COPD, whether stable responder subgroups can be identified, and whether these subgroups experience different clinical outcomes.

Methods.—1831 patients with COPD, 285 smoking (SC) and 228 non-smoking (NSC) controls from the Evaluation of COPD Longitudinally to Identify Predictive Surrogate Endpoints (ECLIPSE) cohort. Spirometric reversibility to 400 µg inhaled salbutamol was assessed on four occasions over 1 year.

Results.—Forced expiratory volume in 1 s (FEV_1) increase after salbutamol was similar in SC (mean 0.14 litres (SD 0.15)) and COPD (0.12 litres (0.15)) and was significantly greater than NSC (0.08 litres (0.14)). Reversibility status varied with repeated testing in parallel with the day-to-day variation in pre-bronchodilator FEV_1, which was similar in control subjects and patients with COPD. Absolute FEV_1 change decreased by Global initiative for chronic Obstructive Lung Disease (GOLD) stage in patients with COPD (GOLD II, mean 0.16 litres (SD 0.17); III, 0.10 litres (0.13); IV, 0.05 litres (0.08) as did chances of being classified as reversible. CT-defined emphysema was weakly related to the absolute change in FEV_1 post salbutamol. Consistently reversible patients (n = 227) did not differ in mortality, hospitalisation or exacerbation experience from irreversible patients when allowing for differences in baseline FEV_1.

Limitations.—Reversibility only assessed with salbutamol and defined by FEV_1 criteria. The COPD population was older than the control populations.

Conclusions.—Post-salbutamol FEV_1 change is similar in patients with COPD and smoking controls but is influenced by baseline lung function and the presence of emphysema. Bronchodilator reversibility status varies temporally and does not distinguish clinically relevant outcomes, making it an unreliable phenotype.

▶ Genome-wide analysis in large populations of chronic obstructive pulmonary disease (COPD) patients has identified a number of potential genetic markers that confer increased risk of developing the disease. This emphasizes the genetic heterogeneity of chronic airway disease. In this context, multiple phenotypes—described as "a single or combination of disease attributes that describe differences among individuals with COPD as they relate to clinically meaningful outcomes"[1]—of COPD have been described and are now being studied. One such phenotype is that of frequent exacerbators. This research has been aided by the creation of networks of pulmonary physicians from multiple countries willing to participate in large prospective trials, which is the only way to accumulate enough data for this type of study. One COPD phenotype are those COPD patients who have a component of reversibility of their airway disease defined by at least a 12% and a 200 mL in FEV_1 following bronchodilator challenge. Studying specific phenotypes has several purposes. These include determining overall prognosis relative to the population of COPD as a whole; determining whether specific targeted therapy results in improved responses or outcomes; and determining whether specific genetic markers relate to specific phenotypes. The authors here did not look at specific genetic markers but were interested in determining whether the bronchodilator phenotype is a stable phenotype that could be used to predict outcomes. They used a database from a large clinical trial and were able to show that reversibility is not a stable characteristic over the population studied and was not useful in predicting outcomes over a 3-year period of follow up. From a practical standpoint, the authors note that "reversibility status on one occasion is an unreliable basis on which to make clinical decisions (in the COPD population), no additional clinically useful data—beyond that provided by pre-test FEV_1—are obtained when testing on multiple occasions." Reversibility in COPD, at least without a more genetically or otherwise specifically selected subpopulation, appears not to be a phenotype that can help predict outcome or target therapy.

J. R. Maurer, MD

Reference

1. Han MK, Agusti A, Calverley PM, et al. Chronic obstructive pulmonary disease phenotypes: the future of COPD. *Am J Respir Crit Care Med.* 2010;182:598-604.

Occupational Exposure to Dusts, Gases, and Fumes and Incidence of Chronic Obstructive Pulmonary Disease in the Swiss Cohort Study on Air Pollution and Lung and Heart Diseases in Adults

Mehta AJ, the SAPALDIA Team (Swiss Tropical and Public Health Inst, Basel, Switzerland; et al)
Am J Respir Crit Care Med 185:1292-1300, 2012

Rationale.—There is limited evidence from population-based studies demonstrating incidence of spirometric-defined chronic obstructive pulmonary disease (COPD) in association with occupational exposures.

Objectives.—We evaluated the association between occupational exposures and incidence of COPD in the Swiss Cohort Study on Air Pollution and Lung and Heart Diseases in Adults (SAPALDIA).

Measurements and Main Results.—Prebronchodilator ratio of forced expiratory volume in 1 second over forced vital capacity (FEV_1/FVC) was measured in 4,267 nonasthmatic SAPALDIA participants ages 18–62 at baseline in 1991 and at follow-up in 2001–2003. COPD was defined by the Global Initiative for Chronic Obstructive Lung Disease (GOLD) criterion ($FEV_1/FVC < 0.70$) and Quanjer reference equation ($FEV_1/FVC <$ lower limit of normal [LLN]), and categorized by severity ($\geq$ 80% and < 80% predicted FEV_1 for stage I and stage II+, respectively). Using a job-exposure matrix, self-reported occupations at baseline were assigned exposures to biological dusts, mineral dusts, gases/fumes, and vapors, gases, dusts, or fumes (VGDF) (high, low, or unexposed as reference). Adjusted incident rate ratios (IRRs) of stage I and stage II+ COPD were estimated in mixed Poisson regression models. Statistically significant (P < 0.05) IRRs of stage II+ GOLD and LLN-COPD, indicating risks between two- and fivefold, were observed for all occupational exposures at high levels. Occupational exposure-associated risk of stage II+ COPD was observed mainly in males and ages $\geq$ 40 years and remained elevated when restricted to nonsmokers.

Conclusions.—In a Swiss working adult population, occupational exposures to biological dusts, mineral dusts, gases/fumes, and VGDF were associated with incidence of COPD of at least moderate severity.

▶ Many experts believe that a significant amount of chronic obstructive lung disease in a population is attributable to occupational exposure. This would, in part, explain the finding in several population spirometry screening studies of a significant group of people (10+%) who have no smoking history or other known cause of airway disease. Several cross-sectional and case-controlled studies have associated obstructive disease and occupational exposure,[1-3] but prospective evaluation of a causal relationship using objective parameters has been sparse. The difference between those studies and the current one is that this is prospective, population-based methodology in which baseline data were collected from a large, random sample of the population, and they were then followed over at least a 10-year period. Detailed surveys were used to record occupational histories and smoking histories. Correlation of the measured spirometry over at least a 10-year period (both ever-smokers and nonsmokers) and their occupational exposures allowed the authors to attribute an appreciable amount of the chronic obstructive pulmonary disease in the population to occupational exposures. It is important to note limitations of the study: asthmatics were not specifically excluded from the study using bronchodilator testing (though patients reporting a diagnosis of asthma were excluded); some variations from the recorded exposure may exist because of participants changing jobs and a potential short time in the "current" job, the job used to record level of exposure. At any rate, despite limitations, this study is one of the best relating occupational exposure to development of lung disease. It helps better understand the excess burden of chronic lung disease in many populations and, hopefully, can be used to influence public policy around cleaner work environments.

J. R. Maurer, MD

References

1. Blanc PD, Iribarren C, Trupin L, et al. Occupational exposures and the risk of COPD: dusty trades revisited. *Thorax.* 2009;64:6-12.
2. Matheson MC, Benke G, Raven J, et al. Biological dust exposure in the workplace is a risk factor for chronic obstructive pulmonary disease. *Thorax.* 2005;60: 645-651.

3. Weinmann S, Vollmer WM, Breen V, et al. COPD and occupational exposures: a case-control study. *J Occup Environ Med.* 2008;50:561-569.

Genome-Wide Association Studies Identify *CHRNA5/3* and *HTR4* in the Development of Airflow Obstruction

Wilk JB, Shrine NRG, Loehr LR, et al (Brigham and Women's Hosp and Harvard Med School, Boston, MA; Univ of Leicester, UK; Univ of North Carolina at Chapel Hill; et al)

Am J Respir Crit Care Med 186:622-632, 2012

Rationale.—Genome-wide association studies (GWAS) have identified loci influencing lung function, but fewer genes influencing chronic obstructive pulmonary disease (COPD) are known.

Objectives.—Perform meta-analyses of GWAS for airflow obstruction, a key pathophysiologic characteristic of COPD assessed by spirometry, in population-based cohorts examining all participants, ever smokers, never smokers, asthma-free participants, and more severe cases.

Methods.—Fifteen cohorts were studied for discovery (3,368 affected; 29,507 unaffected), and a population-based family study and a meta-analysis of case-control studies were used for replication and regional follow-up (3,837 cases; 4,479 control subjects). Airflow obstruction was defined as FEV_1 and its ratio to FVC (FEV_1/FVC) both less than their respective lower limits of normal as determined by published reference equations.

Measurements and Main Results.—The discovery meta-analyses identified one region on chromosome 15q25.1 meeting genome-wide significance in ever smokers that includes *AGPHD1, IREB2*, and *CHRNA5/CHRNA3* genes. The region was also modestly associated among never smokers. Gene expression studies confirmed the presence of *CHRNA5/3* in lung, airway smooth muscle, and bronchial epithelial cells. A single-nucleotide polymorphism in *HTR4*, a gene previously related to FEV_1/FVC, achieved genome-wide statistical significance in combined meta-analysis. Top single-nucleotide polymorphisms in *ADAM19, RARB, PPAP2B*, and *ADAMTS19* were nominally replicated in the COPD meta-analysis.

Conclusions.—These results suggest an important role for the *CHRNA5/3* region as a genetic risk factor for airflow obstruction that may be independent of smoking and implicate the *HTR4* gene in the etiology of airflow obstruction.

▶ I would be remiss in not including in this yearly update some of the ongoing research that is better defining the genetic susceptibility to lung disease, particularly chronic obstructive pulmonary disease (COPD). This study extends our knowledge in this area. Several genomewide association studies in the past few years have looked for genetic markers that correlate with lung function abnormalities, particularly forced expiratory velocity in 1 second (FEV_1) and forced vital capacity (FVC). At least 16 genetic loci have been associated to date with FEV_1 or FEV_1/FVC values.[1] Two specific loci, *HHIP* and *FAM13A*, have been found in genomewide association studies at statistically significant levels to influence risk of developing COPD.[2,3] The current study sought to further evaluate a region on chromosome 15 in which single nucleotide polymorphism (SNPs) have been shown to be associated with COPD. This area includes the cholinergic nicotinic receptor genes (CHRNA5-CHRNA3-CHRNB4).[5] The authors were able to confirm this association as well as implicate the HTR4 gene in the pathogenesis of airflow obstruction. Another area of genetic research in airway disease, beyond genetic risk of pathogenesis, is defining genetic markers that may increase or reduce susceptibility to certain pharmacological agents. It has been demonstrated, for example, that a SNP resulting in an amino acid change at position 16 of the b2 adrenergic receptor gene (ADRB2) is associated with airway diseases.[4] Studies investigating the impact on response to bronchodilators when polymorphisms exist because of a SNP in the ADRB2 receptor have been small and inconsistent, however. Bleeker et al combined data from 2 large studies with the goal of specifically evaluating the impact of a Gly16Arg polymorphism on the efficacy and tolerability of budesonide/formoterol treatment in patients with moderate to severe COPD.[5] Patients with this polymorphism were compared with responses of those with Gly/Gly and Arg/Arg genotypes. The Gly16Arg polymorphism did not seem to influence response or rate of exacerbation for either combination or monotherapy with either drug. These types of data will hopefully help tailor specific therapeutic approaches in these patients.

J. R. Maurer, MD

References

1. Soler Artigas M, Loth DW, Wain LV, et al. Genome-wide association and large-scale follow up identifies 16 new loci influencing lung function. *Nat Genet.* 2011,43.1082 1090.
2. Cho MH, Boutaoui N, Klanderman BJ, et al. Variants in FAM13A are associated with chronic obstructive pulmonary disease. *Nat Genet.* 2010;42:200-202.
3. Van Durme YM, Eijgelsheim M, Joos GF, et al. Hedgehog-interacting protein is a COPD susceptibility gene: the Rotterdam Study. *Eur Respir J.* 2010;36:89-95.
4. Matheson MC, Ellis JA, Raven J, Johns DP, Walters EH, Abramson MJ. Beta2-adrenergic receptor polymorphisms are associated with asthma and COPD in adults. *J Hum Genet.* 2006;51:943-951.
5. Bleecker ER, Meyers DA, Bailey WC, et al. ADRB2 polymorphisms and budesonide/formoterol responses in COPD. *Chest.* 2012;142:320-328.

3 Lung Cancer

Introduction

Lung cancer claimed an estimated 160 000 lives in the United States in 2012 and is the leading cause of cancer death around the world.[1] Mortality rates continue to decline in American men and may finally be declining finally in women, but lung cancer still causes more deaths per year in this country than the total number caused by breast, colorectal, and prostate cancers combined. The number of lung cancer deaths in women (72 590) continues to creep toward the number of deaths in men (87 750). Recent data demonstrating that mortality rates may be plateauing or even increasing in young and middle aged women across the nation and particularly in southern and midwestern states raise the grim possibility that the favorable trends seen over the past decade may reverse if these groups continue to smoke as they age.[2] Given widespread public health educational interventions already in place, legislation supporting efforts to limit tobacco exposure should remain at the forefront of health policy initiatives.

At present, about 21% of adult Americans (approximately 46 million individuals) continue to smoke cigarettes.[3] We have known about the causal link of smoking to lung cancer for over 60 years, but clearly the addictive capacity of cigarettes in many cases is more powerful than the knowledge of their health consequences. The few reliable tools we have to aid smoking cessation should therefore be used liberally. The three first-line classes of tobacco cessation pharmacotherapy approved by the Food and Drug Administration (FDA) include nicotine replacement therapy, buproprion, and varenicline. A recent systematic review and meta-analysis addressed concern about the potential cardiovascular side effects of varenicline and concluded that no increase in serious adverse cardiovascular events is associated with its use.[4] Readers should recognize that a study reporting that smokers using nicotine replacement were more likely to relapse to smoking[5] was firmly rebutted by the Association for the Treatment of Tobacco Use and Dependence, and that this therapy is still a cornerstone of cessation for nicotine-dependent smokers. We should be aware that patients who have turned to electronic cigarettes may be exposing themselves to adverse outcomes that are as yet poorly defined, since these devices are not yet regulated by the FDA.[6] Counseling our patients is still a powerful intervention; many of us may underestimate what 3 minutes of our time addressing smoking cessation might achieve.[7]

Lung cancer screening was a topic of intense interest this year. In 2011, both the National Lung Screening Trial (NLST) and the Prostate, Lung, Colorectal, and Ovarian (PLCO) Trial published their results, demonstrating that screening for lung cancer with low-dose computed tomography (LDCT) scanning does result in a reduction in lung cancer mortality, as opposed to screening with plain chest radiography, which was no better than no screening.[8,9] To achieve the 20% relative reduction in lung cancer mortality seen in the NLST, the entry criteria of the study would need to be met (ages 55-74, with $\geq$ 30 pack-years of smoking history, either currently smoking or having quit within the previous 15 years). However, as discussed in a thoughtful commentary by Bach and Gould, wide variation in mortality benefit is seen even within the NLST population, highlighting the importance of physician evaluation and counseling before a screening study is ever ordered.[10] Screening in a population meeting the NLST criteria is endorsed by all the major national medical societies invested in lung cancer care, but at least two of these organizations have broadened their screening recommendations to include other population groups.[11,12] The lack of an evidence base to support the latter recommendations is problematic, but the recognition that there are tens of millions of people in this country who are at risk for lung cancer and for whom screening is not recommended is also a significant problem. This makes the current efforts to develop reliable risk predictive models an important priority, both for people who fit the NLST criteria and those who do not but have other recognized and significant risk factors, and for whom it is unlikely that large clinical trials on the NLST scale can ever realistically be done.[13-16] Further, the NLST highlighted the potential harms associated with screening, including the high rate of false positive findings, the likelihood of further imaging studies and procedures triggered by those abnormalities, and the potential for associated complications and higher radiation exposure. All of these contribute to the recommendation that lung cancer screening should ideally be performed in the context of a multidisciplinary program that can adequately address the indications, the benefits, and also the potential harms of screening, to ensure that patients receive appropriate education, counseling, and evaluation.[11,17]

From a diagnostic standpoint, a number of interesting studies were published this year on exhaled breath analysis. Exhaled breath contains a variety of substances, including volatile organic compounds, proteins, DNA, and RNA, which can be collected and analyzed in several ways. The concept of using breath "biosignatures" is appealing in that exhaled breath is a noninvasive and easily accessible sample of the whole lung. While the human nose is incapable of adequately analyzing such samples, trained dogs appear to be able to do so, and the electronic "nose" or other chemical sensing arrays may provide reliable automated means of accomplishing this.[18,19] Breath analysis is being looked at as a tool potentially applicable to lung cancer risk prediction, nodule assessment, and cancer prognostication.

Finally, treatment options for lung cancer continue to expand. As we rapidly understand more about the molecular and genetic characteristics of individual lung cancers, the identification of potential future targets for therapies, both personalized and broad, has accelerated. *ROS1* is an example of a new potential target; rearrangements of this gene appear to be associated with a subset of adenocarcinomas and are distinct from mutations in *EGFR* or *ALK* rearrangements[20] In contrast, work on harnessing the immune system's innate anti-tumor capabilities has identified the programmed death-1 (PD-1) pathway as potentially broadly mechanistically important in lung cancer. Inhibition of this pathway in Phase I trials appears to be of benefit in a subpopulation of patients with non-small cell lung cancer, particularly those with tumors that express the ligand PD-L1.[21,22] Improving our understanding of the cellular and molecular changes associated with individual tumors as well as histologic lung cancer subsets will continue to enhance the development of more focused and effective therapies.

Lynn T. Tanoue, MD

References

1. Siegel R, Naishadham D, Jemal A. Cancer statistics, 2012. *CA Cancer J Clin.* 2012;62:10-29.
2. Jemal A, Ma J, Rosenberg PS, Siegel R, Anderson WF. Increasing lung cancer death rates among young women in southern and midwestern States. *J Clin Oncol.* 2012;30:2739-2744.
3. Dube S, McClave A, James C, Caralblllo R, Kaufmann R, Pechacek T. Vital signs: current cigarette smoking among adults aged > 18 years - United States, 2009. *MMWR Morb Mortal Wkly Rep.* 2010;59:1-6.
4. Prochaska JJ, Hilton JF. Risk of cardiovascular serious adverse events associated with varenicline use for tobacco cessation: systematic review and meta-analysis. *BMJ.* 2012;344:e2856.
5. Alpert HR, Connolly GN, Biener L. A prospective cohort study challenging the effectiveness of population-based medical intervention for smoking cessation. *Tob Control.* 2013;22:32-37.
6. Vardavas CI, Anagnostopoulos N, Kougias M, Evangelopoulou V, Connolly GN, Behrakis PK. Short-term pulmonary effects of using an electronic cigarette: impact on respiratory flow resistance, impedance, and exhaled nitric oxide. *Chest.* 2012;141:1400-1406.
7. Fiore MC, Jaén CR. A clinical blueprint to accelerate the elimination of tobacco use. *JAMA.* 2008;299:2083-2085.
8. Aberle DR, Adams AM, Berg CD, et al. Reduced lung-cancer mortality with low-dose computed tomographic screening. *N Engl J Med.* 2011;365:395-409.
9. Oken MM, Hocking WG, Kvale PA, et al. Screening by chest radiograph and lung cancer mortality: the Prostate, Lung, Colorectal, and Ovarian (PLCO) randomized trial. *JAMA.* 2011;306:1865-1873.
10. Bach PB, Gould MK. When the average applies to no one: personalized decision making about potential benefits of lung cancer screening. *Ann Intern Med.* 2012; 157:571-573.
11. Bach PB, Mirkin JN, Oliver TK, et al. Benefits and harms of CT screening for lung cancer: a systematic review. *JAMA.* 2012;307:2418-2429.
12. Wood DE, Eapen GA, Ettinger DS, et al. Lung cancer screening. *J Natl Compr Canc Netw.* 2012;10:240-265.
13. Tammemagi CM, Pinsky PF, Caporaso NE, et al. Lung cancer risk prediction: Prostate, Lung, Colorectal and Ovarian Cancer Screening Trial models and validation. *J Natl Cancer Inst.* 2011;103:1058-1068.
14. Raji OY, Duffy SW, Agbaje OF, et al. Predictive accuracy of the Liverpool Lung Project risk model for stratifying patients for computed tomography screening for

lung cancer: a case-control and cohort validation study. *Ann Intern Med.* 2012; 157:242-250.
15. Spitz MR, Etzel CJ, Dong Q, et al. An expanded risk prediction model for lung cancer. *Cancer Prev Res (Phila).* 2008;1:250-254.
16. Bach PB, Kattan MW, Thornquist MD, et al. Variations in lung cancer risk among smokers. *J Natl Cancer Inst.* 2003;95:470-478.
17. Arenberg D, Kazerooni EA. Setting up a lung cancer screening program. *J Natl Compr Canc Netw.* 2012;10:277-285.
18. Ehmann R, Boedeker E, Friedrich U, et al. Canine scent detection in the diagnosis of lung cancer: revisiting a puzzling phenomenon. *Eur Respir J.* 2012;39: 669-676.
19. Mazzone PJ, Wang XF, Xu Y, et al. Exhaled breath analysis with a colorimetric sensor array for the identification and characterization of lung cancer. *J Thorac Oncol.* 2012;7:137-142.
20. Bergethon K, Shaw AT, Ou SH, et al. ROS1 rearrangements define a unique molecular class of lung cancers. *J Clin Oncol.* 2012;30:863-870.
21. Topalian SL, Hodi FS, Brahmer JR, et al. Safety, activity, and immune correlates of anti-PD-1 antibody in cancer. *N Engl J Med.* 2012;366:2443-2454.
22. Brahmer JR, Tykodi SS, Chow LQ, et al. Safety and activity of anti-PD-L1 antibody in patients with advanced cancer. *N Engl J Med.* 2012;366:2455-2465.

Epidemiology of Lung Cancer

Cancer Statistics, 2012

Siegel R, Naishadham D, Jemal A (American Cancer Society, Atlanta, GA)
CA Cancer J Clin 62:10-29, 2012

Each year, the American Cancer Society estimates the numbers of new cancer cases and deaths expected in the United States in the current year and compiles the most recent data on cancer incidence, mortality, and survival based on incidence data from the National Cancer Institute, the Centers for Disease Control and Prevention, and the North American Association of Central Cancer Registries and mortality data from the National Center for Health Statistics. A total of 1,638,910 new cancer cases and 577,190 deaths from cancer are projected to occur in the United States in 2012. During the most recent 5 years for which there are data (2004-2008), overall cancer incidence rates declined slightly in men (by 0.6% per year) and were stable in women, while cancer death rates decreased by 1.8% per year in men and by 1.6% per year in women. Over the past 10 years of available data (1999-2008), cancer death rates have declined by more than 1% per year in men and women of every racial/ethnic group with the exception of American Indians/Alaska Natives, among whom rates have remained stable. The most rapid declines in death rates occurred among African American and Hispanic men (2.4% and 2.3% per year, respectively). Death rates continue to decline for all 4 major cancer sites (lung, colorectum, breast, and prostate), with lung cancer accounting for almost 40% of the total decline in men and breast cancer accounting for 34% of the total decline in women. The reduction in overall cancer death rates since 1990 in men and 1991 in women translates to the avoidance of about 1,024,400 deaths from cancer. Further progress can be accelerated by applying existing cancer control knowledge

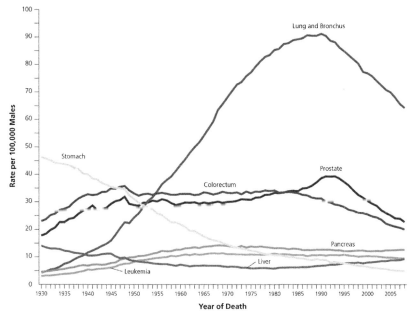

FIGURE 4.—Trends in death rates among males for selected cancers, United States, 1930 to 2008. Rates are age adjusted to the 2000 US standard population. Due to changes in International Classification of Diseases (ICD) coding, numerator information has changed over time. Rates for cancers of the lung and bronchus, colorectum, and liver are affected by these changes. (Reprinted from Siegel R, Naishadham D, Jemal A. Cancer statistics, 2012. *CA Cancer J Clin.* 2012;62:10-29, with permission from CA: A Cancer Journal for Clinicians and John Wiley and Sons, www.interscience.wiley.com.)

across all segments of the population, with an emphasis on those groups in the lowest socioeconomic bracket (Figs 4-6).

▶ In the United States, 1 of every 4 deaths is cancer-related, with lung cancer being the leading cause of cancer death in both men and women. In 2012, lung cancer claimed an estimated 160 340 American lives (87 750 men and 72 590 women), more than the next 3 leading causes of cancer death combined (breast, colorectal, and prostate cancers). These 4 cancers account for nearly half of all cancer deaths in the United States. In men, both lung cancer incidence and death rates have been steadily declining since the early 1990s (Fig 4). In women, lung cancer incidence and death rates have been relatively stable over the past decade, though perhaps for the first time we are seeing a favorable bending of the mortality curve (Fig 5). The 2 figures point out that mortality for all 4 major causes of cancer death has been decreasing over that period; in fact, overall cancer death rates have decreased, as demonstrated in Fig 6. It is worth noting that the reductions in lung cancer death rates among both men and women are largely due to reduction in tobacco use.[1] In contrast, the decreases in death rates for

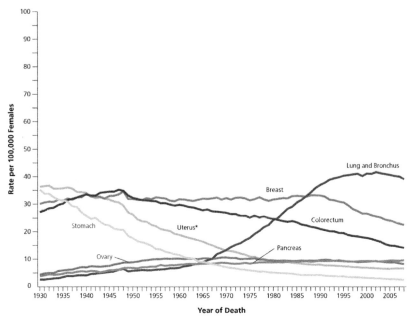

FIGURE 5.—Trends in death rates among females for selected cancers, United States, 1930 to 2008. Rates are age adjusted to the 2000 US standard population. Due to changes in International Classification of Diseases (ICD) coding, numerator information has changed over time. Rates for cancers of the uterus, ovary, lung and bronchus, and colorectum are affected by these changes. *Uterus includes uterine cervix and uterine corpus. (Reprinted from Siegel R, Naishadham D, Jemal A. Cancer statistics, 2012. *CA Cancer J Clin.* 2012;62:10-29, with permission from CA: A Cancer Journal for Clinicians and John Wiley and Sons, www.interscience.wiley.com.)

prostate, colorectal, and breast cancers are generally attributed to improvements in early detection and treatment.[2-4]

L. T. Tanoue, MD

References

1. Jemal A, Thun MJ, Ries LA, et al. Annual report to the nation on the status of cancer, 1975–2005, featuring trends in lung cancer, tobacco use, and tobacco control. *J Natl Cancer Inst.* 2008;100:1672-1694.
2. Berry DA, Cronin KA, Plevritis SK, et al. Effect of screening and adjuvant therapy on mortality from breast cancer. *N Engl J Med.* 2005;353:1784-1792.
3. Etzioni R, Tsodikov A, Mariotto A, et al. Quantifying the role of PSA screening in the US prostate cancer mortality decline. *Cancer Causes Control.* 2008;19:175-181.
4. Edwards BK, Ward E, Kohler BA, et al. Annual report to the nation on the status of cancer, 1975–2006, featuring colorectal cancer trends and impact of interventions (risk factors, screening, and treatment) to reduce future rates. *Cancer.* 2010;116:544-573.

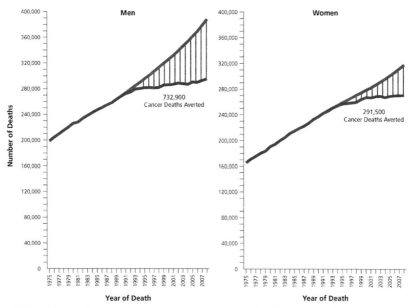

FIGURE 6.—Total number of cancer deaths averted from 1991 to 2008 in men and from 1992 to 2008 in women. The blue line represents the actual number of cancer deaths recorded in each year, and the red line represents the expected number of cancer deaths if cancer mortality rates had remained at their peak (1990 in men and 1991 in women). For interpretation of the references to color in this figure legend, the reader is referred to web version of this article. (Reprinted from Siegel R, Naishadham D, Jemal A. Cancer statistics, 2012. *CA Cancer J Clin*. 2012;62:10-29, with permission from CA: A Cancer Journal for Clinicians and John Wiley and Sons, www.interscience.wiley.com.)

Increasing Lung Cancer Death Rates Among Young Women in Southern and Midwestern States

Jemal A, Ma J, Rosenberg PS, et al (American Cancer Society, Atlanta, GA; Natl Cancer Inst, Rockville, MD)
J Clin Oncol 30:2739-2744, 2012

Purpose.—Previous studies reported that declines in age-specific lung cancer death rates among women in the United States abruptly slowed in women younger than age 50 years (ie, women born after the 1950s). However, in view of substantial geographic differences in antitobacco measures and sociodemographic factors that affect smoking prevalence, it is unknown whether this change in the trend was similar across all states.

Methods.—We examined female age-specific lung cancer death rates (1973 through 2007) by year of death and birth in each state by using age-period-cohort models. Cohort relative risks adjusted for age and period effects were used to compare the lung cancer death rate for a given birth cohort to a referent birth cohort (ie, the 1933 cohort herein).

Results.—Age-specific lung cancer death rates declined continuously in white women in California, but the rates declined less quickly or even increased in the remaining states among women younger than age 50 years and women born after the 1950s, especially in several southern and midwestern states. For example, in some southern states (eg, Alabama), lung cancer death rates among women born in the 1960s were approximately double those of women born in the 1930s.

Conclusion.—The unfavorable lung cancer trend in white women born after circa 1950 in southern and midwestern states underscores the need for additional interventions to promote smoking cessation in these high-risk populations, which could lead to more favorable future mortality trends for lung cancer and other smoking-related diseases.

▶ Over the past several years, a hopeful plateauing of mortality rates resulting from lung cancer has been observed in women.[1] However, this report by Jemal and colleagues documents a concerning decrease in the rate of decline and an even more alarming increase in mortality rates in young and middle-aged women in nearly all the states examined. Of the 23 states included in the study, only California demonstrated a consistent decline in age-specific lung cancer death rates. Fig 1 in the original article shows trends in lung cancer death rates by year of death and stratified by age cohort in white women in California, New York, and Alabama; the increase in death rates is most obvious in the 2 younger age cohorts in Alabama. The authors speculate that geographic differences in public policies against tobacco use and socioeconomic factors influencing smoking may be strong contributors to these differences, because cigarette use is felt to be a causative agent in 70% of lung cancers in women.[2] The state of California has been a pioneer in antitobacco initiatives such as higher cigarette excise taxes and smoking bans in public spaces and workplaces. In contrast, such public policies aimed at decreasing tobacco use and exposure are less supported in Southern states, where tobacco is a more important factor in local economy and perhaps intrinsically more accepted in local culture. These trends are worrisome. Although the number of deaths in younger age groups is not high enough yet to impact the overall lung cancer death rate, if these groups continue to smoke as they grow older, there is the unfortunate and grim likelihood that the overall mortality rate resulting from lung cancer in women will actually increase.

L. T. Tanoue, MD

References

1. Siegel R, Naishadham D, Jemal A. Cancer statistics, 2012. *CA Cancer J Clin.* 2012; 62:10-29.
2. Centers for Disease Control and Prevention (CDC). Smoking-attributable mortality, years of potential life lost, and productivity losses—United States, 2000-2004. *MMWR Morb Mortal Wkly Rep.* 2008;57:1226-1228.

Lung Cancer Incidence and Mortality Among HIV-Infected and HIV-Uninfected Injection Drug Users

Shiels MS, Cole SR, Mehta SH, et al (Johns Hopkins Bloomberg School of Public Health, Baltimore, MD; Univ of North Carolina at Chapel Hill)
J Acquir Immune Defic Syndr 55:510-515, 2010

Objectives.—To examine the impact of HIV on lung cancer incidence and survival.

Design.—Prospective study of 2495 HIV-infected and HIV-uninfected injection drug users in Baltimore, MD.

Methods.—Cancer data were obtained from the Maryland Cancer Registry. We estimated hazard ratios (HRs) and 95% confidence intervals (CIs) for lung cancer in 2 strata of packs of cigarettes smoked per day by HIV serostatus, and for mortality by HIV serostatus.

Results.—HIV-infected participants had twice the risk (HR = 2.3; 95% CI: 1.1 to 5.1) of lung cancer. There was no evidence of an interaction between HIV and packs of cigarettes smoked per day (*P* interaction = 0.18). Compared with participants who smoked <1.43 packs per day, among HIV-uninfected individuals lung cancer risk was 6 times greater (HR = 5.9; 95% CI: 2.1 to 17) and among HIV-infected individuals lung cancer risk was doubled (HR = 2.1; 95% CI: 0.63 to 6.8) in persons who smoked ≥1.43 per day. Additionally, HIV was associated with 4 times the risk of death (HR = 3.8; 95% CI: 0.92 to 15) in lung cancer cases.

Conclusions.—HIV was associated with increased risk of lung cancer, after adjusting for smoking. However, no evidence was observed for synergistic effects of HIV and smoking. Further, HIV was associated with poorer lung cancer survival after accounting for cancer stage.

▶ Lung cancer incidence rates in the HIV-infected population are estimated to be 2 to 3 times higher than in the general population.[1,2] To some extent, this may be related to the higher prevalence of cigarette smoking observed in HIV-infected individuals. This study examined the incidence and outcomes of lung cancer among 2495 subjects in a large prospective cohort of injection drug users in Baltimore, MD. Nearly all had a history of smoking. After adjustment for age, gender, and cigarette exposure, HIV infection was an independent risk factor for lung cancer. The hazard ratio for development of lung cancer was 2.3 (95% CI: 1.1-5.1). Moreover, HIV-infected lung cancer cases had a lower 1-year survival rate (18 vs 42%). No synergistic effect of HIV infection with cigarettes on lung cancer risk was felt to be present.

HIV infection is not on the typical list of modifiable lung cancer risk factors. In light of these and other similar reports, a discussion of HIV risk or testing should be considered in the evaluation of patients known to have or are being evaluated for the possibility of lung cancer. Additionally, as HIV-infected individuals are anticipated to live longer lives, lung cancer may be an increasingly important cause of their mortality.

L. T. Tanoue, MD

References

1. Engels EA, Biggar RJ, Hall HI, et al. Cancer risk in people infected with human immunodeficiency virus in the United States. *Int J Cancer.* 2008;123:187-194.
2. Long JL, Engels EA, Moore RD, Gebo KA. Incidence and outcomes of malignancy in the HAART era in an urban cohort of HIV-infected individuals. *AIDS.* 2008;22: 489-496.

Tobacco-Related Issues

Risk of cardiovascular serious adverse events associated with varenicline use for tobacco cessation: systematic review and meta-analysis

Prochaska JJ, Hilton JF (Univ of California, San Francisco)
BMJ 344:e2856, 2012

Objective.—To examine the risk of treatment emergent, cardiovascular serious adverse events associated with varenicline use for tobacco cessation.

Design.—Meta-analysis comparing study effects using four summary estimates.

Data Sources.—Medline, Cochrane Library, online clinical trials registries, and reference lists of identified articles.

Review Methods.—We included randomised controlled trials of current tobacco users of adult age comparing use of varenicline with an inactive control and reporting adverse events. We defined treatment emergent, cardiovascular serious adverse events as occurring during drug treatment or within 30 days of discontinuation, and included any ischaemic or arrhythmic adverse cardiovascular event (myocardial infarction, unstable angina, coronary revascularisation, coronary artery disease, arrhythmias, transient ischaemic attacks, stroke, sudden death or cardiovascular related death, or congestive heart failure).

Results.—We identified 22 trials; all were double blinded and placebo controlled; two included participants with active cardiovascular disease and 11 enrolled participants with a history of cardiovascular disease. Rates of treatment emergent, cardiovascular serious adverse events were 0.63% (34/5431) in the varenicline groups and 0.47% (18/3801) in the placebo groups. The summary estimate for the risk difference, 0.27% (95% confidence interval −0.10 to 0.63; $P = 0.15$), based on all 22 trials, was neither clinically nor statistically significant. For comparison, the relative risk (1.40, 0.82 to 2.39; $P = 0.22$), Mantel-Haenszel odds ratio (1.41, 0.82 to 2.42; $P = 0.22$), and Peto odds ratio (1.58, 0.90 to 2.76; $P = 0.11$), all based on 14 trials with at least one event, also indicated a non-significant difference between varenicline and placebo groups.

Conclusions.—This meta-analysis—which included all trials published to date, focused on events occurring during drug exposure, and analysed findings using four summary estimates—found no significant increase in cardiovascular serious adverse events associated with varenicline use. For rare outcomes, summary estimates based on absolute effects are recommended and estimates based on the Peto odds ratio should be avoided.

▶ Three first-line classes of tobacco cessation pharmacotherapy are approved by the US Food and Drug Administration: (1) nicotine replacement therapy; (2) bupropion; and (3) varenicline. Varenicline is a partial agonist to nicotine receptors and appears to attenuate the symptoms of nicotine withdrawal. In randomized trials, varenicline has proved effective compared with placebo in achieving sustained nicotine abstinence in a significant, albeit small, number of smokers.[1] However, a recent meta-analysis by Singh and colleagues[2] reported an excess of serious cardiovascular effects associated with varenicline use, a concerning finding in light of the fact that smokers are already at increased cardiovascular risk. This new systematic review and meta-analysis by Prochaska and Hilton included 22 trials evaluating varenicline, and in contrast concluded that no increase in serious cardiovascular events was associated with its use. They point out methodological issues in the prior meta-analysis by Singh et al, specifically the inclusion of adverse events well beyond the treatment period, exclusion of trials without cardiovascular adverse events, and use of a statistical approach that might induce bias when evaluating rare events. Based on their results, these authors conclude that the risk of serious cardiovascular events related to varenicline use is "statistically and clinically insignificant."

More smokers die from cardiovascular disease than any other cause, including lung cancer.[3,4] Based on the results of this meta-analysis, varenicline should remain a first-line pharmacologic approach to achieving smoking cessation.

L. T. Tanoue, MD

References

1. Rigotti NA, Pipe AL, Benowitz NL, Arteaga C, Garza D, Tonstad S. Efficacy and safety of varenicline for smoking cessation in patients with cardiovascular disease: a randomized trial. *Circulation.* 2010;121:221-229.
2. Singh S, Loke YK, Spangler JG, Furberg CD. Risk of serious adverse cardiovascular events associated with varenicline: a systematic review and meta-analysis. *CMAJ.* 2011;183:1359-1366.
3. Doll R, Peto R, Boreham J, Sutherland I. Mortality in relation to smoking: 50 years' observations on male British doctors. *BMJ.* 2004;328:1519.
4. Centers for Disease Control and Prevention (CDC). Smoking-attributable mortality, years of potential life lost, and productivity losses—United States, 2000-2004. *MMWR Morb Mortal Wkly Rep.* 2008;57:1226-1228.

Short-term Pulmonary Effects of Using an Electronic Cigarette: Impact on Respiratory Flow Resistance, Impedance, and Exhaled Nitric Oxide

Vardavas CI, Anagnostopoulos N, Kougias M, et al (Harvard School of Public Health, Boston, MA; Smoking and Lung Cancer Res Ctr, Athens, Greece)
Chest 141:1400-1406, 2012

Background.—Debate exists over the scientific evidence for claims that electronic cigarettes (e-cigarettes) have no health-related ramifications.

This study aimed to assess whether using an e-cigarette for 5 min has an impact on the pulmonary function tests and fraction of exhaled nitric oxide (FENO) of healthy adult smokers.

Methods.—Thirty healthy smokers (aged 19-56 years, 14 men) participated in this laboratory-based experimental vs control group study. Ab lib use of an e-cigarette for 5 min with the cartridge included (experimental group, n = 30) or removed from the device (control group, n = 10) was assessed.

Results.—Using an e-cigarette for 5 min led to an immediate decrease in FENO within the experimental group by 2.14 ppb (*P* = .005) but not in the control group (*P* = .859). Total respiratory impedance at 5 Hz in the experimental group was found to also increase by 0.033 kPa/(L/s) (*P* < .001), and flow respiratory resistance at 5 Hz, 10 Hz, and 20 Hz also statistically increased. Regression analyses controlling for baseline measurements indicated a statistically significant decrease in FENO and an increase in impedance by 0.04 kPa/(L/s) (*P* = .003), respiratory resistance at 5 Hz by 0.04 kPa/(L/s) (*P* = .003), at 10 Hz by 0.034 kPa/(L/s) (*P* = .008), at 20 Hz by 0.043 kPa/(L/s) (*P* = .007), and overall peripheral airway resistance (β, 0.042 kPa/[L/s]; *P* = .024), after using an e-cigarette.

Conclusions.—e-Cigarettes assessed in the context of this study were found to have immediate adverse physiologic effects after short-term use that are similar to some of the effects seen with tobacco smoking; however, the long-term health effects of e-cigarette use are unknown but potentially adverse and worthy of further investigation.

▶ Electronic cigarettes (e-cigarettes), also known as electronic nicotine delivery systems (ENDS), are not yet regulated by the US Food and Drug Administration. Unless marketed as "therapeutic," for example to accomplish smoking cessation, they are not considered drugs, and neither are they regulated as devices. There has thus far been little rigorous evaluation of their potential health consequences. This report evaluated the immediate physiologic airway effects in healthy cigarette smokers after 5 minutes of ad lib e-cigarette inhalation. Of note, although no changes were detected in spirometry (forced expiratory volume in 1 second [FEV₁], forced vital capacity [FVC], FEV₁/FVC ratio), flow resistance increased with even this brief exposure. Flow resistance changes precede changes in peak expiratory flow and FEV₁ in experimental models of airways obstruction.[1] Additionally, exhaled nitric oxide levels (FENO), which are felt to reflect oxidative stress in the airways, also immediately decreased.[2] This change in FENO parallels that seen after short-term inhalation of tobacco smoke.[3] The clear concern is that e-cigarette use over long periods might, as with usual cigarettes, result in sustained adverse physiologic consequences.

E-cigarettes vary in design as well as ingredients. The lack of regulation of ENDS makes it difficult if not impossible to identify substances that might induce airway irritation and/or inflammation. Moreover, the pulmonary effects of inhaling these substances may vary in individuals who have also been habitually exposed to tobacco smoke. If e-cigarettes are used over a limited period to accomplish sustained smoking cessation, the long-term health benefits may outweigh any short-term adverse effects. However, health consequences of long-term use of ENDS are unknown. This lack of scientific data in a product that may be associated with both addiction and disease will only be addressed by further research and tighter regulation of these products.[4]

L. T. Tanoue, MD

References

1. Kanda S, Fujimoto K, Komatsu Y, Yasuo M, Hanaoka M, Kubo K. Evaluation of respiratory impedance in asthma and COPD by an impulse oscillation system. *Intern Med.* 2010;49:23-30.
2. American Thoracic Society Workshop. ATS Workshop Proceedings: exhaled nitric oxide and nitric oxide oxidative metabolism in exhaled breath condensate: executive summary. *Am J Respir Crit Care Med.* 2006;173:811-813.
3. Karrasch S, Ernst K, Behr J, et al. Exhaled nitric oxide and influencing factors in a random population sample. *Respir Med.* 2011;105:713-718.
4. Avdalovic MV, Murin S. Electronic cigarettes: no such thing as a free lunch...Or puff. *Chest.* 2012;141:1371-1372.

An Unexpected Consequence of Electronic Cigarette Use
McCauley L, Markin C, Hosmer D (Legacy Good Samaritan Med Ctr, Portland, OR)
Chest 141:1110-1113, 2012

Background.—Lipoid pneumonia is rare and usually chronic. It occurs as an inflammatory reaction triggered by lipid substances in the lungs and marked by the uptake by alveolar macrophages and accumulation in the interstitium. Endogenous cases occur when fat is deposited in lung tissue in vivo and are related to proximal obstructive lesions, fat embolism, necrotic tissue, lipid storage disease, or hyperlipidemia. Exogenous cases are associated with the aspiration of mineral oil-n-based laxatives in children or occupational exposures in adults. Older patients with underlying debility, achalasia, reflux, and neuromuscular disorder of the pharynx and esophagus are affected more often than others. A case was found in a smoker of electronic cigarettes (e-cigarettes).

Case Report.—Woman, 47, came for care after 7 months of experiencing dyspnea, productive cough, and subjective fevers. She visited the emergency department several times for similar complaints and taken several antibiotic courses. She recently began using e-cigarettes, and the history of problems began about the same time. Her history included asthma, reported rheumatoid arthritis, fibromyalgia, schizoaffective disorder, and hypertension. She was also taking amlodipine, albuterol metered dose inhaler, lovastatin, lisinopril, multiple vitamins, cyclobenzaprine, citalopram, and multiple psychiatric medications. Vital signs revealed mild tachycardia and a pulse oximetric saturation of 94% on room air. Laboratory tests were largely normal, but CT imaging showed new multifocal bilateral opacities, with extensive bilateral upper- and lower-lobe patchy ground glass pulmonary opacities in a "crazy paving" pattern. Bronchoalveolar lavage (BAL) cytologic examination showed abundant lipid-laden macrophages. Based on these findings the patient was diagnosed with lipoid pneumonia and advised to avoid using e-cigarettes. Subsequently, her symptoms improved, her chest radiograph was normal, and her pulmonary function tests revealed only mild diffusion impairment.

Results.—Many patients with lipoid pneumonia have no symptoms, but cough, dyspnea, fever, weight loss, chest pain, pleurisy, hemoptysis, chills, and night sweats can also be present. Hypoxia or respiratory alkalosis is often the presenting complaint. Pulmonary function tests reveal restrictive ventilator defect and/or diffusion impairment, but often are normal. Chest radiographs usually show extensive bilateral alveolar consolidations and ground glass opacities in dependent lung areas, but unilateral involvement is also noted. Fibrosis can lead to volume loss, and solid lesions can occur, but adenopathy is rare. The diagnosis often depends on high-resolution computed tomography (CT), which reveals bilateral posterior and lower-lobe-predominant alveolar consolidation, ground-glass opacities, and a "crazy paving" pattern. CT scan angiography can confirm that the consolidated lung has considerably lower attenuation than enhancing vessels. Finding lipid-laden macrophages in the sputum or BAL fluid is a key diagnostic component. Vacuolated macrophages stain orange with Sudan stain or red with Oil-Red-O stain. An inflammatory picture reminiscent of foreign body reaction is common. Once the diagnosis is confirmed, the patient is advised to avoid recurrent oil exposures and stop aspiration. Only severe cases should be treated with systemic corticosteroids.

Conclusions.—The health analysis and empirical research on e-cigarettes is limited, but many of the compounds found in them are carcinogenic and harmful to humans. Vegetable glycerin may be added to these nicotine solutions to make the visual smoke when the solution is vaporized. The glycerin can be produced using heated palm or coconut oil, or animal fat and soap. Since exogenous lipoid pneumonia is associated with mineral oil or lipid-based substance aspiration, it should be considered a risk for patients using e-cigarettes.

▶ Electronic cigarettes (e-cigarettes) typically are composed of battery-operated heating elements that vaporize nicotine solutions contained in replaceable cartridges. They are marketed as alternatives to traditional cigarettes, and sometimes therapeutically as beneficial in aiding smoking cessation. Although little analysis is available on the contents of e-cigarettes other than nicotine, it is clear that the solutions in the cartridges contain carrier compounds including, for example, N-nitrosamines and polycyclic aromatic hydrocarbons, which are harmful and potentially carcinogenic. Relevant to this case report, vegetable glycerin or other oils are commonly included in the nicotine solutions to generate visible "smoke." This report describes a case in which a patient developed progressive lipoid pneumonia, presumably from exogenous lipid inhalation related to use of e-cigarettes over several months. Clearly, these devices are not without potential harm.

Regulation of e-cigarettes has been an area of controversy. Because most of these devices are not marketed as "therapeutic," they do not fall under the traditional purview of the US Food and Drug Administration (FDA). However, under the Tobacco Control Act, the FDA can and intends to exert authority over e-cigarettes as tobacco products.[1]

L. T. Tanoue, MD

Reference

1. Electronic Cigarettes (e-Cigarettes). U.S. Department of Health and Human Services, 2012. http://www.fda.gov/newsevents/publichealthfocus/ucm172906. hun. Accessed January 6, 2013.

A prospective cohort study challenging the effectiveness of population-based medical intervention for smoking cessation
Alpert HR, Connolly GN, Biener L (Harvard School of Public Health, Boston, MA; Univ of Massachusetts, Boston)
Tob Control 22:32-37, 2013

Objective.—To examine the population effectiveness of nicotine replacement therapies (NRTs), either with or without professional counselling, and provide evidence needed to better inform healthcare coverage decisions.

Methods.—A prospective cohort study was conducted in three waves on a probability sample of 787 Massachusetts adult smokers who had recently quit smoking. The baseline response rate was 46%; follow-up was completed with 56% of the designated cohort at wave 2 and 68% at wave 3. The relationship between relapse to smoking at follow-up interviews and assistance used, including NRT with or without professional help, was examined.

Results.—Almost one-third of recent quitters at each wave reported to have relapsed by the subsequent interview. Odds of relapse were unaffected by use of NRT for > 6 weeks either with ($p = 0.117$) or without ($p = 0.159$) professional counselling and were highest among prior heavily dependent persons who reported NRT use for any length of time without professional counselling (OR 2.68).

Conclusions.—This study finds that persons who have quit smoking relapsed at equivalent rates, whether or not they used NRT to help them in their quit attempts. Cessation medication policy should be made in the larger context of public health, and increasing individual treatment coverage should not be at the expense of population evidence-based programmes and policies.

▶ The purpose of identifying this study is primarily to highlight the response to its findings from the Association for the Treatment of Tobacco Use and Dependence

(ATTUD, www.attud.org), an organization representing nearly 450 tobacco treatment specialists worldwide. Alpert and colleagues reported that smokers who used over-the-counter nicotine replacement therapy (NRT) in the past year were less likely to have sustained smoking cessation the following year. This report was widely disseminated in the lay press as demonstrating that over-the-counter NRTs are ineffective. ATTUD responded to this report out of concern that people who might well achieve smoking cessation with NRT would be discouraged from trying. The response points out that more than 100 randomized studies have demonstrated that NRT increases short-term abstinence and improves initial quit rates. ATTUD acknowledges that after NRT is discontinued, the rate of relapse to smoking does not differ from smokers who quit without NRT, which is not inconsistent with the Alpert study.

Nicotine replacement is one of the first-line pharmacologic approaches to smoking cessation and is approved by the US Food and Drug Administration. NRT is readily accessible, does not require a prescription, is relatively inexpensive, and has been demonstrated to be effective in aiding initial quitting in smokers. We should continue to recommend NRT when appropriate as we counsel our patients to stop smoking.

L. T. Tanoue, MD

Lung Cancer Screening

Benefits and Harms of CT Screening for Lung Cancer: A Systematic Review

Bach PB, Mirkin JN, Oliver TK, et al (Memorial Sloan-Kettering Cancer Ctr, NY; SUNY Downstate Med Ctr, Brooklyn, NY; American Society of Clinical Oncology, Alexandria, VI; et al)
JAMA 307:2418-2429, 2012

Context.—Lung cancer is the leading cause of cancer death. Most patients are diagnosed with advanced disease, resulting in a very low 5-year survival. Screening may reduce the risk of death from lung cancer.

Objective.—To conduct a systematic review of the evidence regarding the benefits and harms of lung cancer screening using low-dose computed tomography (LDCT). A multisociety collaborative initiative (involving the American Cancer Society, American College of Chest Physicians, American Society of Clinical Oncology, and National Comprehensive Cancer Network) was undertaken to create the foundation for development of an evidence-based clinical guideline.

Data Sources.—MEDLINE (Ovid: January 1996 to April 2012), EMBASE (Ovid: January 1996 to April 2012), and the Cochrane Library (April 2012).

Study Selection.—Of 591 citations identified and reviewed, 8 randomized trials and 13 cohort studies of LDCT screening met criteria for inclusion. Primary outcomes were lung cancer mortality and all-cause mortality, and secondary outcomes included nodule detection, invasive procedures, follow-up tests, and smoking cessation.

Data Extraction.—Critical appraisal using predefined criteria was conducted on individual studies and the overall body of evidence. Differences in data extracted by reviewers were adjudicated by consensus.

Results.—Three randomized studies provided evidence on the effect of LDCT screening on lung cancer mortality, of which the National Lung Screening Trial was the most informative, demonstrating that among 53 454 participants enrolled, screening resulted in significantly fewer lung cancer deaths (356 vs 443 deaths; lung cancer–specific mortality, 274 vs 309 events per 100 000 person-years for LDCT and control groups, respectively; relative risk, 0.80; 95% CI, 0.73-0.93; absolute risk reduction, 0.33%; $P =.004$). The other 2 smaller studies showed no such benefit. In terms of potential harms of LDCT screening, across all trials and cohorts, approximately 20% of individuals in each round of screening had positive results requiring some degree of follow-up, while approximately 1% had lung cancer. There was marked heterogeneity in this finding and in the frequency of follow-up investigations, biopsies, and percentage of surgical procedures performed in patients with benign lesions. Major complications in those with benign conditions were rare.

Conclusion.—Low-dose computed tomography screening may benefit individuals at an increased risk for lung cancer, but uncertainty exists about the potential harms of screening and the generalizability of results (Tables 1 and 4).

▶ The National Lung Screening Trial (NLST) was the first randomized controlled trial (RCT) to demonstrate a mortality benefit with lung cancer screening with low-dose chest computed tomography (LDCT).[1] This important article by Bach and colleagues is a systematic review of the evidence regarding the benefits and harms of LDCT screening for lung cancer, and was a joint initiative of the American Cancer Society (ACS), the American College of Chest Physicians (ACCP), the American Society of Clinical Oncology (ASCO), and the National Comprehensive Cancer Network (NCCN), and is the basis for the clinical practice guidelines of the ACCP and ASCO. The NCCN and ACS have or will publish their own lung cancer screening guidelines.[2]

After an extensive search of the medical literature, this systematic review included 8 RCTs and 13 cohort studies. It provides a balanced and thorough discussion of the benefits and, perhaps more importantly, the potential harms of LDCT screening. Table 1 outlines the 8 RCTs included in the study. Smoking was a consistent requirement for eligibility (15 to > 30 pack-year smoking history), and the majority of participants were male. Only 3 RCTs provide data on the effect of screening on lung cancer mortality: the NLST (United States), the Danish Lung Cancer Screening Trial (Denmark), and the Detection and Screening of Early Lung Cancer by Novel Imaging Technology and Molecular Essays (Milan, Italy).[1,3,4] As can be seen in Table 4, only the NLST demonstrated the gold standard benefit of screening, specifically a reduction in lung cancer deaths, with 320 persons needing to be screened to prevent 1 lung cancer death.

The article discusses the evidence review of the potential harms of LDCT screening, which are several: (1) There is a very a high rate of detection

TABLE 1.—Randomized Controlled Trials Identified in the Search of the Literature

Source	No. Randomized (% Screened or Followed Up at Baseline)		Screening With LDCT[a]		Study Duration			Participant Characteristics		Smoking History Eligibility (Current or Former)	
	LDCT	Control	Collimation, mm	Nodule Size Warranting Workup, mm[b]	Years of Accrual	Planned Follow-up From Baseline, y	No. of Screens, Planned/Completed (at Last Report)[c]	Male, %	Age Range, y	Pack-years[d]	Years Since Quit
				LDCT vs Usual Care (No Screening)							
NELSON,[18] 2009	7907 (95)[e]	7915 (100)[e]	0.75	≥4.6, >9.8	2004-NR[e]	10	3/2	84	50-75	>15	≤10
DLCST,[19,20] 2012	2052 (100)	2052 (100)	0.75[f]	≥5, >15	2004-2006	10	5/5	55	50-70	≥20	<10[g]
ITALUNG,[21] 2009	1613 (87)	1593 (100)	1-1.25	≥5, ≥8[h]	NR	NR	4/1	65	55-69	≥20	<10
DANTE,[22] 2009	1276 (91)	1196 (85)	5	Any, ≥6	2001-2006	NR	5/5[i]	100	60-74	≥20	<10
Garg et al,[16] 2002	92 (100)[j]	98 (100)[j]	5	Any, >10	2001-NR[j]	NR	2/1	75	50-80	≥30	NR[k]

Study	LDCT vs Chest Radiograph										
NLST[23,24] 2011	26 722 (98)	26 732 (97)	≤2.5	≥4	2002-2004	>7	3/3	59	55-74	≥30	≤15
LSS[25,26] 2005	1660 (96)	1658 (93)	5	Any[l]	2000	2	2/2[m]	59	55-74	≥30	<10
Dépiscan[27] 2007	385 (86)[n]	380 (77)	1-1.5	>5, ≥10	2002-2004	NR	3/1	71	47-76	≥15	<15

Abbreviations: DLCST, Danish Lung Cancer Screening Trial; LDCT, low-dose computed tomography; LSS, Lung Screening Study; NELSON Dutch Belgian Randomised Lung Cancer Screening Trial; NLST, National Lung Screening Trial; NR, not reported.

Editor's Note: Please refer to original journal article for full references.

[a] All studies had a protocol in place except LSS. Studies by NELSON, DANTE, and Garg et al had a protocol reported; however, specific details on adherence or deviation from the protocol or actual procedures used were not reported. For NLST, "... trial radiologists developed guidelines for diagnostic follow-up, but no specific evaluation approach was mandated."[23]

[b] Indicates first the largest-size nodule warranting additional imaging and, second, the largest-size nodule warranting diagnostic testing.

[c] All studies had screening conducted annually except the study by NELSON, which had planned screening at years 1, 2, and 4.

[d] Defined as the number of cigarette packs (20 cigarettes per pack) smoked per day multiplied by the number of years smoked.

[e] Randomization is ongoing with a target accrual of 16000 participants.

[f] Collimation = 16 × 0.75 mm.

[g] Former smokers had to have quit after the age of 50 years and less than 10 years ago.

[h] Diagnostic workup was a referral to a positron emission tomography scan.

[i] The median follow-up was 33.7 months and only 161 participants (6.5% of those screened or followed up at baseline) had 5 or more years of follow-up. Baseline data are mainly reported.

[j] Target accrual of 400 participants in total was planned.

[k] Study does not specify a maximum time since quitting.

[l] The size of the noncalcified nodule to warrant further imaging was increased to ≥4 mm at year 1 to reflect evolving practice.

[m] In the original design, 1 screen was planned; however, it was later amended to 2 screens (baseline and 1 repeat).

[n] Six patients randomized to chest radiography crossed over to receive LDCT at baseline.

TABLE 4.—Mortality Due to All Causes, Lung Cancer, and All Causes Other Than Lung Cancer in Randomized Trials: Rates and Relative Risk

Source	Events, No. (%)		Rate of Events per 100 000 Person-years		Relative Risk (95% CI)	Rate Ratio	Absolute Difference, %	No. Needed to Screen to Prevent 1 Event
	LDCT	Control	LDCT	Control				
All-Cause Mortality								
DANTE,[22] 2009	46 (3.6)	45 (3.8)	NR	NR	0.97 (0.80-1.20)[a,b]	NR	0.2	635
NLST,[23] 2011	1877 (7.0)	2000 (7.5)	1303[b]	1395[b]	0.93 (0.86-0.99)	0.93[b]	0.5	219
DLCST,[19] 2012	61 (3.0)	42 (2.0)	NR	NR	1.19 (1.01-1.40)	NR	-1.0	NR
Lung Cancer–Specific Mortality								
DANTE,[22] 2009	20 (1.6)	20 (1.7)	NR	NR	0.97 (0.71-1.32)[a,b]	NR	0.1	954
NLST,[23] 2011	356 (1.3)	443 (1.7)	247	309	0.80 (0.73-0.93)	0.80[b]	0.3	320
DLCST,[19] 2012	15 (0.7)	11 (0.5)	NR	NR	1.15 (0.83-1.61)	NR	-0.2	NR
Mortality Not Due to Lung Cancer								
DANTE,[22] 2009	26 (2.0)	25 (2.1)	NR	NR	0.99 (0.75-1.30)[b]	NR	0.1[b]	1898[b]
NLST,[23] 2011	1521 (5.7)	1557 (5.8)	1056[b]	1086[b]	0.99 (0.95-1.02)[b]	0.97[b]	0.1[b]	755[b]
DLCST,[19] 2012	46 (2.2)	31 (1.5)	NR	NR	1.20 (1.00-1.44)[b]	NR	-0.7[b]	NR

Abbreviations: DLCST, Danish Lung Cancer Screening Trial; NLST, National Lung Screening Trial; LDCT, low-dose computed tomography; NR, not reported.
Editor's Note: Please refer to original journal article for full references.
[a]Based on count data.
[b]Calculated by authors.

of abnormalities, the vast majority of which are false-positive findings. The average nodule detection rate was 20% per round of screening. Those abnormal findings generate (2) further imaging studies, with (3) resultant higher radiation exposure, (4) the possibility of invasive diagnostic procedures with (5) the possibility of complications from those procedures, (6) the potential for higher costs of care, and (7) possible adverse effects on quality of life.

Based on this comprehensive systematic review, the ACCP and ASCO have made the following 2 recommendations relating to LDCT screening for lung cancer.

"1. For smokers and former smokers aged 55 to 74 years who have smoked for 30 pack-years or more and either continue to smoke or have quit within the past 15 years, we suggest that annual screening with low-dose computed tomography (LDCT) should be offered over both annual screening with chest radiograph or no screening, but only in settings that can deliver the comprehensive care provided to National Lung Screening Trial (NLST) participants. (Grade of Recommendation: 2B).

2. For individuals who have accumulated fewer than 30 pack-years of smoking or are either younger than 55 years or older than 74 years, or individuals who quit smoking more than 15 years ago, and for individuals with severe comorbidities that would preclude potentially curative treatment, limit life expectancy, or both, we suggest that [computed tomography] screening should not be performed. (Grade of recommendation: 2C)"

L. T. Tanoue, MD

References

1. Aberle DR, Adams AM, Berg CD, et al. Reduced lung-cancer mortality with low-dose computed tomographic screening. *N Engl J Med.* 2011;365:395-409.
2. Wood DE, Eapen GA, Ettinger DS, et al. Lung cancer screening. *J Natl Compr Canc Netw.* 2012;10:240-265.
3. Infante M, Cavuto S, Lutman FR, et al. A randomized study of lung cancer screening with spiral computed tomography: three-year results from the DANTE trial. *Am J Respir Crit Care Med.* 2009;180:445-453.
4. Saghir Z, Dirksen A, Ashraf H, et al. CT screening for lung cancer brings forward early disease. The randomised Danish Lung Cancer Screening Trial: status after five annual screening rounds with low-dose CT. *Thorax.* 2012;67:296-301.

When the Average Applies to No One: Personalized Decision Making About Potential Benefits of Lung Cancer Screening
Bach PB, Gould MK (Memorial Sloan-Kettering Cancer Ctr, NY; Kaiser Permanente Southern California, Pasadena, CA)
Ann Intern Med 157:571-573, 2012

Background.—In 2011 the results of the National Lung Screening Trial (NLST) were published. This trial found that for high-risk persons, three rounds of annual screening with low-radiation-dose computed tomography

TABLE.—Projected Likelihood Over 6 Years of Lung Cancer Death With or Without Screening per 1000 Persons Screened*

Participant	Risk Factors	Deaths From Lung Cancer (Without Screening) per 1000 Persons, n	Deaths From Lung Cancer (With Screening) per 1000 Persons, n	Lung Cancer Deaths Averted per 1000 Persons, n	Persons Needed to Be Screened Annually for 3 y to Prevent 1 Death From Lung Cancer Over 6 y, n
"Typical" participant in the NLST	62-year-old male current 1.5-PPD smoker for 35 y	19.5	15.6	3.9	256
Minimum eligible participant in the NLST	55-year-old female former 1-PPD smoker for 30 y who just quit	4.0	3.2	0.8	1236
High-risk participant eligible for the NLST	70-year-old current 2-PPD smoker for 55 y	60.9	48.7	12.2	82
Minimum eligible participant by NCCN guidelines	50-year-old male former 1-PPD smoker for 20 y who quit 10 y ago with an occupational asbestos exposure history	1.6	1.3	0.3	3180
Low-risk eligible participant for Sequoia Hospital lung screening program	40-year-old female former 1-PPD smoker for 10 y who quit 15 y ago	0.10	0.08	0.02	35 186

NCCN = National Comprehensive Cancer Network; NLST = National Lung Screening Trial; PPD = packs per day.
*Assuming the program includes 3 annual y of screening.

(CT) reduced the relative risk of death from lung cancer by 20% compared with screening using chest radiographs. Practice guidelines now recommend CT screening for patients at risk for lung cancer in a way that promotes informed patient consent. Practitioners must explain to patients the potential risks and benefits of screening and convey that information in a way that is meaningful to the patient. Patients appear to understand absolute benefits better than relative benefits. Trial results were expressed in terms of absolute benefit to help guide these discussions. In addition, models and limitations were described.

Communicating Benefits and Risks.—The NLST's relative risk reduction of 20% translates to a reduction in risk of lung cancer death from about 1.7% for chest radiographs to 1.4% for CT screening—a difference of 0.3 percentage points. The advantage is limited to patients who were age 55 to 74 years at study entry, had 30 pack-years of smoking history, and, for former smokers, had quit within 15 years. Patients can be told that for every 1000 patients screened using CT 3 deaths may be averted.

Models and Limitations.—Two models can demonstrate the benefits and risks for patients. A "typical" person eligible for the NLST would be a 62-year-old man with a 52-year-pack smoking history who currently smokes. Over 6 years, for every 1000 persons like this, 19.5 lung cancer deaths would occur if screening is not done and 15.6 lung cancer deaths would occur even with screening. Persons at high risk or low risk for lung cancer but who still qualify for the NLST would have substantially higher or lower benefits, respectively. The low-risk person would have a risk of lung cancer death one fifth that of the typical person; the high-risk person would have a risk 15 times that of the low-risk patient.

The models do not consider all important predictors of lung cancer risk; are based on uncertain inputs, with confidence limits between 7% and 27%; and were developed using participants at high risk for cancer, with other risk profiles extrapolated from these risk estimates. In addition, there is no consideration of the probability of harm from screening and whether this will increase or diminish along with a person's risk for lung cancer death.

Conclusions.—The main finding from the NLST is that the potential benefit of screening varies widely depending on the participant's baseline risk of dying from lung cancer without screening. The underlying chance that a person will benefit from CT screening should be carefully considered when educating patients about screening for lung cancer (Table).

▶ The National Lung Screening Trial (NLST) demonstrated a 20% reduction in the relative risk for lung cancer death in high-risk individuals (ages 55–74, with a smoking history of at least 15 years, currently smoking or having quit within the past 15 years) with 3 rounds of annual screening with low-dose computed tomography of the chest (LDCT).[1] The potential harms and benefits of screening with LDCT are extensively examined in the systematic review by Bach and colleagues discussed previously in this section, as well as many other articles.[2] In this opinion piece, Bach and Gould provide an insightful and practical look at how clinicians should talk to patients about the benefit of lung cancer screening in terms that may be more meaningful than the commonly cited decrease in relative risk. In practical terms, screening an NLST population would avert 3 lung cancer deaths for every 1000 participants; among those 1000 persons, there would still be 14 lung cancer deaths even with screening. Moreover, the translation of the NLST results into practical terms is more complicated than the quoted 20% statistic because the magnitude of benefit will vary depending on individual characteristics of a given patient.

The table demonstrates this point: A "typical" participant in the NLST was defined as a 62-year-old male current smoker with a 52 pack-year smoking history.[3] For an individual with these characteristics, 3.9 lung cancer deaths would be averted per 1000 persons screened, and 256 persons would need to undergo annual screening for 3 years to save 1 lung cancer death. In contrast, for individuals who are younger and have less of a smoking history, the number of lung cancer deaths averted per 1000 persons screened would be lower, and the number of persons needed to be screened to save 1 lung cancer death would be higher. Conversely, for individuals who are older and have a more extensive smoking history, the number of lung cancer deaths averted per 1000 persons screened would be higher, and the number of persons needed to be screened to save 1 lung cancer death would be less. The table points out that the lower the risk, the less the benefit, and at some point the benefit becomes so small as to be of questionable value.

The conclusion of the report is that the potential benefit of screening varies by several orders of magnitude among persons who fit the NLST criteria. Appropriate application of the NLST results requires that we be able to interpret the findings in the context of an individual patient and to counsel patients about benefits and potential harms of screening with that information in mind.

L. T. Tanoue, MD

References

1. Aberle DR, Adams AM, Berg CD, et al. Reduced lung-cancer mortality with low-dose computed tomographic screening. *N Engl J Med.* 2011;365:395-409.
2. Bach PB, Mirkin JN, Oliver TK, et al. Benefits and harms of CT screening for lung cancer: a systematic review. *JAMA.* 2011;307:2418-2429.
3. Gohagan JK, Marcus PM, Fagerstrom RM, et al. Final results of the Lung Screening Study, a randomized feasibility study of spiral CT versus chest X-ray screening for lung cancer. *Lung Cancer.* 2005;47:9-15.

Lung Cancer Screening

Wood DE, Eapen GA, Ettinger DS, et al (Univ of Washington/Seattle Cancer Care Alliance; The Univ of Texas MD Anderson Cancer Ctr, Houston; The Sidney Kimmel Comprehensive Cancer Ctr at Johns Hopkins, Baltimore, MD; et al)
J Natl Compr Canc Netw 10:240-265, 2012

Background.—Most patients have advanced-stage lung cancer when first diagnosed, contributing to the low 5-year survival rate of about 15.6%. Studies are under way to identify screening tools to detect early-stage

TABLE.—

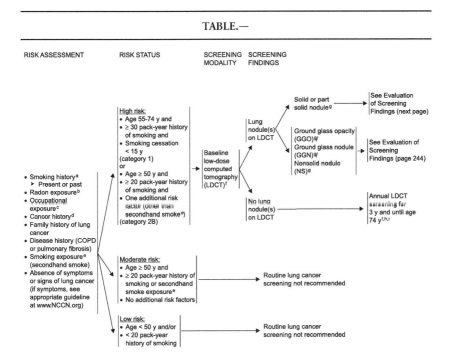

RISK ASSESSMENT	RISK STATUS	SCREENING MODALITY	SCREENING FINDINGS

- Smoking history[a]
  ➤ Present or past
- Radon exposure[b]
- Occupational exposure[c]
- Cancer history[d]
- Family history of lung cancer
- Disease history (COPD or pulmonary fibrosis)
- Smoking exposure[e] (secondhand smoke)
- Absence of symptoms or signs of lung cancer (if symptoms, see appropriate guideline at www.NCCN.org)

High risk:
- Age 55-74 y and
- ≥ 30 pack-year history of smoking and
- Smoking cessation < 15 y (category 1)
or
- Age ≥ 50 y and
- ≥ 20 pack-year history of smoking and
- One additional risk factor (other than secondhand smoke[e]) (category 2B)

Baseline low-dose computed tomography (LDCT)[f]

Lung nodule(s) on LDCT → Solid or part solid nodule[g] → See Evaluation of Screening Findings (next page)

Ground glass opacity (GGO)[g]/ Ground glass nodule (GGN)[g]/ Nonsolid nodule (NS)[g] → See Evaluation of Screening Findings (page 244)

No lung nodule(s) on LDCT → Annual LDCT screening for 3 y and until age 74 y[f,h,i]

Moderate risk:
- Age ≥ 50 y and
- ≥ 20 pack-year history of smoking or secondhand smoke exposure[e]
- No additional risk factors

→ Routine lung cancer screening not recommended

Low risk:
- Age < 50 y and/or
- < 20 pack-year history of smoking

→ Routine lung cancer screening not recommended

[a]Smokers should always be encouraged to quit smoking (http://www.smokefree.gov/).
[b]Documented high radon exposure.
[c]Agents that are identified specifically as carcinogens targeting the lungs: silica, cadmium, asbestos, arsenic, beryllium, chromium, diesel fumes, and nickel.
[d]There is increased risk of developing new primary lung cancer among survivors of lung cancer, lymphomas, cancers of the head and neck, or smoking-related cancers.
[e]Individuals exposed to secondhand smoke have a highly variable exposure to the carcinogens, with varying evidence for increased risk after this variable exposure. Therefore, secondhand smoke is not independently considered a risk factor for lung cancer screening.
[f]All screening and follow-up CT scans should be performed at low dose (100-120 kVp and 40-60 mAs or less), unless evaluating mediastinal abnormalities or lymph nodes, for which standard-dose CT with IV contrast might be appropriate.
[g]Without benign pattern of calcification, fat in nodule as in hamartoma, or features suggesting inflammatory etiology. When multiple nodules are present and occult infection or inflammation is a possibility, an added option is a course of a broad-spectrum antibiotic with anaerobic coverage, followed by low-dose CT 1-2 mo later.
[h]If new nodule at annual or follow-up LDCT, see page 245. New nodule is defined as ≥ 3 mm in mean diameter
[i]There is uncertainty about the appropriate duration of screening and the age at which screening is no longer appropriate.

(Continued)

---

disease. Ideally a screening test will improve outcomes, be scientifically validated, and be low-risk, reproducible, accessible, and cost-effective. Recent data support the use of spiral (helical) low-dose computed tomography (LDCT) of the chest to screen high-risk patients. The National Comprehensive Cancer Network (NCCN) Lung Cancer Screening Panel 2011 screening guidelines describe risk factors for lung cancer, recommend criteria for selecting patients to screen, recommend how to evaluate and follow up on findings, describe the accuracy of LDCT protocols and imaging modalities, and outline the benefits and risks of screening.

Table.—(*Continued*)

EVALUATION OF
SCREENING FINDINGS

FOLLOW-UP OF SCREENING FINDINGS

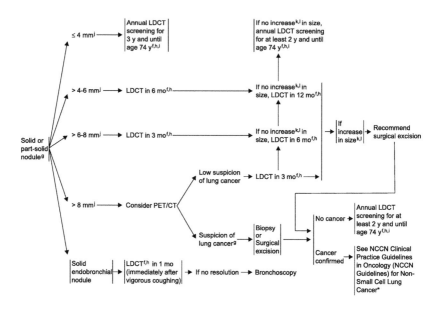

*To view the most recent version of these guidelines, visit the NCCN Web site at www.NCCN.org.

fAll screening and follow-up CT scans should be performed at low dose (100-120 kVp and 40-60 mAs or less), unless evaluating mediastinal abnormalities or lymph nodes, where standard-dose CT with IV contrast might be appropriate.

gWithout benign pattern of calcification, fat in nodule as in hamartoma, or features suggesting inflammatory etiology. When multiple nodules are present and occult infection or inflammation is a possibility, an added option is a course of a broad-spectrum antibiotic with anaerobic coverage, followed by low-dose CT 1-2 mo later.

hIf new nodule at annual or follow-up LDCT, see page 245. New nodule is defined as ≥ 3 mm in mean diameter

iThere is uncertainty about the appropriate duration of screening and the age at which screening is no longer appropriate.

jMean diameter is the mean of the longest diameter of the nodule and its perpendicular diameter when compared with the baseline scan.

kFor nodules ≤ 15 mm: increase in mean diameter ≥ 2 mm in any node or in the solid portion of a part solid nodule compared with baseline scan. For nodules ≥ 15 mm: increase in mean diameter of ≥ 15% compared with baseline scan.

lRapid increase in size should raise suspicion of inflammatory etiology or malignancy other than NSCLC.

(*Continued*)

Guidelines.—The guidelines focus mainly on detecting non-n-small cell lung cancer. Lung cancer screening with CT should be done as part of a program of care and not performed in isolation as a free-standing test. The risks and benefits of screening should be discussed with the patient before performing the LDCT scan. Optimally a multidisciplinary approach, including specialists in radiology, pulmonary medicine, internal medicine, thoracic oncology, and thoracic surgery, should be used. Processes to ensure adequate follow-up of any downstream testing and evaluation of small nodules may also be needed. The lead time in diagnosis offers the benefit of greater survival. Drawbacks include the possibility of overdiagnosis and

Table.—(*Continued*)

EVALUATION OF
SCREENING FINDINGS

FOLLOW-UP OF SCREENING FINDINGS

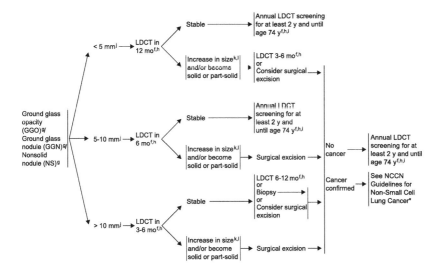

*To view the most recent version of these guidelines, visit the NCCN Web site at www.NCCN.org.

---

[f] All screening and follow-up CT scans should be performed at low dose (100-120 kVp and 40-60 mAs or less), unless evaluating mediastinal abnormalities or lymph nodes, where standard-dose CT with IV contrast might be appropriate.
[g] Without benign pattern of calcification, fat in nodule as in hamartoma, or features suggesting inflammatory etiology. When multiple nodules are present and occult infection or inflammation is a possibility, an added option is a course of a broad-spectrum antibiotic with anaerobic coverage, followed by low-dose CT 1-2 mo later.
[h] If new nodule at annual or follow-up LDCT, see page 245. New nodule is defined as ≥ 3 mm in mean diameter
[i] There is uncertainty about the appropriate duration of screening and the age at which screening is no longer appropriate.
[j] Mean diameter is the mean of the longest diameter of the nodule and its perpendicular diameter when compared with the baseline scan.
[k] For nodules ≤ 15 mm: increase in mean diameter ≥ 2 mm in any nodule or in the solid portion of a part-solid nodule compared with baseline scan. For nodules ≥ 15 mm: increase in mean diameter of ≥ 15% compared with baseline scan.
[l] Rapid increase in size should raise suspicion of inflammatory etiology or malignancy other than NSCLC.

(*Continued*)

false-positive screening tests. Currently LDCT screening diminishes disease-specific mortality by 20% and all-cause mortality by 7% compared to the use of chest radiographs alone.

Populations that benefit most are those at high risk for disease. Smoking, whether active or passive, is a well-established risk factor, but other factors that contribute to the risk profile include occupational exposure, residential exposure to radon, a history of cancer, a family history of lung cancer, a patient history of lung disease such as chronic obstructive pulmonary disease or pulmonary fibrosis, and hormone replacement therapy. The NCCN guidelines recommend that high-risk individuals be screened, but

Table.—(*Continued*)

EVALUATION OF
SCREENING FINDINGS

FOLLOW-UP OF SCREENING FINDINGS

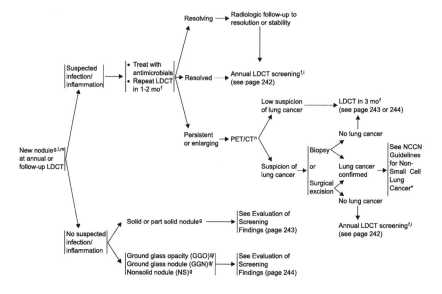

*To view the most recent version of these guidelines, visit the NCCN Web site at www.NCCN.org.

fAll screening and follow-up CT scans should be performed at low dose (100-120 kVp and 40-60 mAs or less), unless evaluating mediastinal abnormalities or lymph nodes, where standard-dose CT with IV contrast might be appropriate.
gWithout benign pattern of calcification, fat in nodule as in hamartoma, or features suggesting inflammatory etiology. When multiple nodules are present and occult infection or inflammation is a possibility, an added option is a course of a broad-spectrum antibiotic with anaerobic coverage, followed by low-dose CT 1-2 mo later.
iThere is uncertainty about the appropriate duration of screening and the age at which screening is no longer appropriate.
lRapid increase in size should raise suspicion of inflammatory etiology or malignancy other than NSCLC.
mNew nodule is defined as ≥ 3 mm in mean diameter.
nPET-CT for lesions > 8 mm.

RISKS/BENEFITS OF LUNG CANCER SCREENING

RISKS
• Futile detection of small aggressive tumors or indolent disease
• Quality of life
  ➤ Anxiety of test findings
• Physical complications from diagnostic workup
• False-positive results
• False-negative results
• Unnecessary testing
• Radiation exposure
• Cost

BENEFITS
• Decreased lung cancer mortality
• Quality of life
  ➤ Reduction in disease-related morbidity
  ➤ Reduction in treatment-related morbidity
  ➤ Improvement in healthy lifestyles
  ➤ Reduction in anxiety/psychosocial burden
• Cost-effectiveness

moderate- and low-risk individuals should not. High-risk patients are those age 55 to 74 years with 30 or more pack-years of smoking tobacco, and, for former smokers, who quit within 15 years. Another high-risk category is for persons age 50 years or older with 20 or more pack-years of smoking and one additional risk factor. Moderate-risk persons are those age 50 years or older with 20 or more pack-years of smoking or second-hand smoke exposure but no additional risk factors. Low-risk persons are those younger than age 50 years and/or a smoking history of less than 20 pack-years.

Protocols and Imaging Factors.—LDCT is recommended for identifying noncalcified nodules suspicious for lung cancer depending on type and size. Helical multidetector CT (MDCT) allows one to detect very small lung nodules, both benign and malignant. LDCT without intravenous contrast injection is recommended rather than standard-dose CT to diminish radiation dose. Usually it is as accurate as standard-dose CT for solid pulmonary nodules, except possibly in larger persons. It may be less sensitive in identifying very low-density non-solid nodules or ground glass opacities. Patient population, methodology used, length of follow-up, and statistical analyses of various studies have not revealed which is the most accurate protocol for lung cancer detection using LDCT. New LDCT technologies may make it possible to significantly diminish radiation dose without compromising the ability to detect and assess nodules.

Benefits and Risks.—The possible benefits of screening for lung cancer using helical LDCT scans include decreased lung cancer mortality or improvement in other oncologic outcomes, quality of life benefits associated with early detection and screening, cost-effectiveness of screening, and the detection of diseases other than lung cancer that can be addressed with interventions. The risks associated with screening include false-positive results, which can lead to unneeded testing, invasive procedures, cost, and diminished quality of life related to mental anguish; false-negative results that can delay or prevent diagnosis and treatment; futile detection of small aggressive tumors related to the lack of any meaningful survival benefit from screening; indeterminate results that lead to further testing; radiation exposure; and physical complications related to the diagnostic work-up. Patients who have several comorbid conditions may be at greater risk for adverse outcomes than those who have fewer or no comorbidity concerns.

Conclusions.—Screening for lung cancer using LDCT has inherent risks and benefits, but the NCCN recommends helical LDCT for select patients at high risk for this disease. Patients should be adequately informed of the risks and benefits and should be managed through a multidisciplinary approach to optimize decision-making and minimize interventions for benign lung disease (Table).

▶ This report outlines the National Comprehensive Cancer Network (NCCN) Clinical Practice Guidelines in Oncology for Lung Cancer Screening. Lung cancer screening remains a controversial topic. The National Lung Screening Trial (NLST) provided a strong evidence base supporting screening with low-dose chest computed tomograph (CT) in individuals matching its subject entry criteria: age 55-74 years, > 30 pack-year smoking history, and currently smoking or with smoking cessation duration < 15 years.[1] The NCCN practice guidelines recommend screening, not just for the NLST population, but for a broader population. In the algorithm demonstrated in the Table, the NCCN also recommends screening for individuals who would have qualified for the NLST as well as another broader group meeting the following criteria: age > 50 years, > 20 pack-years smoking without specification of cessation duration (if any), and 1 additional risk factor (personal cancer history, history of lung disease, family history of lung cancer, documented radon exposure, or occupational exposure to lung carcinogens). This second recommendation is quite controversial. The NCCN acknowledges that the evidence base for this recommendation is not strong, as it is based on observational studies and expert opinion, stating, "Based upon lower-level evidence, there is NCCN consensus that the intervention is appropriate." It seems very unlikely that an evidence base supporting or arguing against screening with low-dose CT scan in these broader and more varied population groups will be forthcoming, given the sheer magnitude and cost of the types of studies that would be required. The NCCN recommendation will likely remain a topic of considerable debate, as demonstrated by the multisociety statement from the American Cancer Society, the American College of Chest Physicians, the Society of Thoracic Surgeons, and the American Thoracic Society, which does not support lung cancer screening with low-dose chest CT scan for individuals not meeting NLST criteria.[2]

L. T. Tanoue, MD

References

1. Aberle DR, Adams AM, Berg CD, et al. Reduced lung-cancer mortality with low-dose computed tomographic screening. *N Engl J Med.* 2011;365:395-409.
2. Bach PB, Mirkin JN, Oliver TK, et al. Benefits and harms of CT screening for lung cancer: a systematic review. *JAMA.* 2012;307:2418-2429.

Predicting and managing the risk of pulmonary haemorrhage in patients with NSCLC treated with bevacizumab: a consensus report from a panel of experts
Reck M, Barlesi F, Crinò L, et al (Hosp Grosshansdorf, Germany; Hôpitaux de Marseille, France; Hosp Santa Maria della Misericordia, Perugia, Italy; et al)
Ann Oncol 23:1111-1120, 2012

Background.—Bevacizumab is a monoclonal antibody against vascular endothelial growth factor. Severe pulmonary haemorrhage (PH) is a rare but serious potential adverse event associated with bevacizumab therapy for advanced non-squamous non-small-cell lung cancer (NSCLC).

Methods.—A panel of expert oncologists, pulmonologists and radiologists reviewed the available data to identify predictive factors for PH in order to help guide physicians using bevacizumab in patients with NSCLC.

Results.—Patients with NSCLC are at an increased risk of PH owing to the underlying disease process. Patients with squamous histology and/or a history of grade ≥ 2 haemoptysis (≥ 2.5 mL per event) should not receive bevacizumab. No clinical or radiological features (including cavitation and central tumour location) reliably predict severe PH in bevacizumab-treated patients. Major blood vessel infiltration and bronchial vessel infiltration, encasement and abutting may predict PH; however, standardised radiological criteria for defining infiltration have not been established. Eligibility for bevacizumab is not affected by patient age, performance status or anticoagulation or antiplatelet therapy.

Conclusions.—An individualised risk—benefit assessment should be undertaken in all patients with NSCLC in whom bevacizumab is being considered. Further research is required to elucidate the mechanisms underlying PH and the clinical risk factors.

▶ Bevacizumab is a recombinant, humanized monoclonal antibody directed against vascular endothelial growth factor (VEGF). Bevacizumab in combination with platinum-based chemotherapy is standard first-line treatment for patients with advanced nonsquamous non—small-cell lung cancer (NSCLC). In early-phase trials evaluating bevacizumab for NSCLC, a small but significantly increased risk of hemoptysis and potentially fatal pulmonary hemorrhage was observed.[1-3] However, the numbers of cases of severe pulmonary hemorrhage in clinical trials were few, and the incidence of fatal hemorrhage was low. Given the survival benefit observed with the addition of bevacizumab to platinum-based therapy in patients with advanced NSCLC, appropriate patients should, if possible, receive the drug.[4] The authors reviewed the clinical trials as well as meta-analyses relating to bevacizumab and the risk of pulmonary hemorrhage. Acknowledging that the pathophysiologic mechanisms relating to pulmonary hemorrhage with anti-VEGF agents are unknown, several consensus conclusions were drawn relating to predicting and managing pulmonary hemorrhage, including the following:

- Patients with advanced NSCLC of predominantly squamous histology and/ or a history of > 2.5 mL of hemoptysis (bright red blood) within 3 months of treatment should not receive bevacizumab, because these patients were excluded from clinical trials.

- No clinical or radiological features of the tumor, including cavitation and central location, are reliable predictive factors for severe pulmonary hemorrhage. Major blood vessel infiltration and bronchial vessel infiltration, encasement and abutting may predict pulmonary hemorrhage, but no standardized radiological criteria for defining infiltration are yet established.

- Eligibility for bevacizumab should not be affected by age, performance status, anticoagulation, or antiplatelet therapy.

- The optimal management of clinically significant pulmonary hemorrhage in patients with advanced nonsquamous NSCLC has not been established, but localized bronchoscopic, radiotherapy, and surgical approaches may have roles on an individualized basis.

L. T. Tanoue, MD

References

1. Johnson DH, Fehrenbacher L, Novotny WF, et al. Randomized phase II trial comparing bevacizumab plus carboplatin and paclitaxel with carboplatin and paclitaxel alone in previously untreated locally advanced or metastatic non-small-cell lung cancer. *J Clin Oncol.* 2004;22:2184-2191.
2. Hapani S, Sher A, Chu D, Wu S. Increased risk of serious hemorrhage with bevacizumab in cancer patients: a meta-analysis. *Oncology.* 2010;79:27-38.
3. Ranpura V, Hapani S, Wu S. Treatment-related mortality with bevacizumab in cancer patients: a meta-analysis. *JAMA.* 2011;305:487-494.
4. Sandler A, Gray R, Perry MC, et al. Paclitaxel-carboplatin alone or with bevacizumab for non-small-cell lung cancer. *N Engl J Med.* 2006;355:2542-2550.

Lung Cancer Risk Prediction: Prostate, Lung, Colorectal and Ovarian Cancer Screening Trial Models and Validation
Tammemagi CM, Pinsky PF, Caporaso NE, et al (Brock Univ, Ontario, Canada; Natl Cancer Inst, Bethesda, MD; et al)
J Natl Cancer Inst 103:1058-1068, 2011

Introduction.—Identification of individuals at high risk for lung cancer should be of value to individuals, patients, clinicians, and researchers. Existing prediction models have only modest capabilities to classify persons at risk accurately.

Methods.—Prospective data from 70 962 control subjects in the Prostate, Lung, Colorectal, and Ovarian Cancer Screening Trial (PLCO) were used in models for the general population (model 1) and for a subcohort of ever-smokers (N = 38 254) (model 2). Both models included age, socioeconomic status (education), body mass index, family history of lung cancer, chronic obstructive pulmonary disease, recent chest x-ray, smoking status (never, former, or current), pack-years smoked, and smoking duration. Model 2 also included smoking quit-time (time in years since ever-smokers permanently quit smoking). External validation was performed with 44 223 PLCO intervention arm participants who completed a supplemental questionnaire and were subsequently followed. Known available risk factors were included in logistic regression models. Bootstrap optimism-corrected estimates of predictive performance were calculated (internal validation). Nonlinear relationships for age, pack-years smoked, smoking duration, and quit-time were modeled using restricted cubic splines. All reported *P* values are two-sided.

Results.—During follow-up (median 9.2 years) of the control arm subjects, 1040 lung cancers occurred. During follow-up of the external validation sample (median 3.0 years), 213 lung cancers occurred. For models 1 and 2, bootstrap optimism-corrected receiver operator characteristic area under the curves were 0.857 and 0.805, and calibration slopes (model-predicted probabilities vs observed probabilities) were 0.987 and 0.979, respectively. In the external validation sample, models 1 and 2 had area under the curves of 0.841 and 0.784, respectively. These models had high discrimination in women, men, whites, and nonwhites.

Conclusion.—The PLCO lung cancer risk models demonstrate high discrimination and calibration.

▶ The Prostate, Lung, Colorectal, and Ovarian (PLCO) Cancer Screening Trial is still ongoing. Initiated in 1993, it has enrolled > 154 000 subjects in the United States aged 55 to 74 years and is designed to assess the effect of screening interventions on prevention of death from 4 different cancers, including lung cancer. Smoking was not a required entry criterion. The PLCO trial confirmed that lung cancer screening with chest radiography is not effective in reducing mortality from lung cancer.[1] This in itself was an important finding because it provided information vital to the interpretation of the National Lung Screening Trial.[2] From a thoracic oncology perspective, the PLCO has enormous potential to develop risk predictive tools for lung cancer, given its large and robust prospective database.

This article describes 2 risk predictive models developed from the PLCO database. Data from > 70 000 control arm subjects informed 1 logistic regression model; a subcohort of > 38 000 ever-smokers informed the second model. As is the case with all models developed for this purpose, the variables available for building the models were limited to the data collected. The available potential predictor variables in the PLCO database included sociodemographic factors (age, educational/socioeconomic status, race/ethnicity, sex, family history of lung cancer) and medical history (body mass index, history of chronic obstructive pulmonary disease, history of chest radiograph in the 3 years before baseline, smoking history). Data were not available for exposures such as asbestos, radon, or environmental tobacco.

The first model developed using the control arm subject cohort is potentially applicable to the general population. This is an important strength of this model; some lung cancer risk predictive models have been developed in cohorts of individuals at increased risk of lung cancer risk specifically because of smoking, and, therefore, would not be relevant in a population of never-smokers. The second model was developed in a smoking cohort. Both models performed well when applied to external validation samples. The authors provide a nomogram designed to facilitate interpretation and use of the second model, which estimates the 9-year probability of lung cancer based on an individual's specific risk factors. Supplementary, Fig 1 in the original article shows the nomogram, which allows the conversion of the individual variables into points, the sum of which is then converted to the probability of lung cancer. The power of the nomogram is that it is usable on a practical level, as opposed to some of the other lung cancer predictive models that, although robust and validated, have complicated multivariable mathematical equations not readily accessible to a clinician in practice.[3-5]

The prospective design of the PLCO, the very large number of subjects it enrolled and is following, and the high quality of the intake and follow-up information being collected all render the PLCO an important resource. As time passes and more outcome events occur, there will be more opportunity for refining these and other predictive models. Moreover, because the PLCO trial was not restricted to high-risk individuals, modeling applicable to the general population is possible, in contrast to other models developed only in smoking subjects. Although the PLCO does lack data relating to some potentially significant exposures, improvement of the lung cancer predictive models is likely still to be gained by the incorporation in the future of physiologic, blood, and molecular biomarkers. There is great potential for such improved models to guide clinical practice in decisions about whom to screen for lung cancer.

L. T. Tanoue, MD

References

1. Oken MM, Hocking WG, Kvale PA, et al. Screening by chest radiograph and lung cancer mortality: the Prostate, Lung, Colorectal, and Ovarian (PLCO) randomized trial. *JAMA.* 2011;306:1865-1873.
2. Aberle DR, Adams AM, Berg CD, et al. Reduced lung-cancer mortality with low-dose computed tomographic screening. *N Engl J Med.* 2011;365:395-409.
3. Spitz MR, Etzel CJ, Dong Q, et al. An expanded risk prediction model for lung cancer. *Cancer Prev Res (Phila).* 2008;1:250-254.
4. Raji OY, Duffy SW, Agbaje OF, et al. Predictive accuracy of the Liverpool Lung Project risk model for stratifying patients for computed tomography screening for lung cancer: a case-control and cohort validation study. *Ann Intern Med.* 2012;157:242-250.
5. Bach PB, Kattan MW, Thornquist MD, et al. Variations in lung cancer risk among smokers. *J Natl Cancer Inst.* 2003;95:470-478.

Predictive Accuracy of the Liverpool Lung Project Risk Model for Stratifying Patients for Computed Tomography Screening for Lung Cancer: A Case–Control and Cohort Validation Study

Raji OY, Duffy SW, Agbaje OF, et al (The Univ of Liverpool, UK; Queen Mary Univ of London, UK; Natl Cancer Inst, Bethesda, MD; et al)

Ann Intern Med 157:242-250, 2012

Background.—External validation of existing lung cancer risk prediction models is limited. Using such models in clinical practice to guide the referral of patients for computed tomography (CT) screening for lung cancer depends on external validation and evidence of predicted clinical benefit.

Objective.—To evaluate the discrimination of the Liverpool Lung Project (LLP) risk model and demonstrate its predicted benefit for stratifying patients for CT screening by using data from 3 independent studies from Europe and North America.

Design.—Case–control and prospective cohort study.

Setting.—Europe and North America.

Patients.—Participants in the European Early Lung Cancer (EUELC) and Harvard case–control studies and the LLP population-based prospective cohort (LLPC) study.

Measurements.—5-year absolute risks for lung cancer predicted by the LLP model.

Results.—The LLP risk model had good discrimination in both the Harvard (area under the receiver-operating characteristic curve [AUC], 0.76 [95% CI, 0.75 to 0.78]) and the LLPC (AUC, 0.82 [CI, 0.80 to 0.85]) studies and modest discrimination in the EUELC (AUC, 0.67 [CI, 0.64 to 0.69]) study. The decision utility analysis, which incorporates the harms and benefit of using a risk model to make clinical decisions, indicates that the LLP risk model performed better than smoking duration or family history alone in stratifying high-risk patients for lung cancer CT screening.

Limitations.—The model cannot assess whether including other risk factors, such as lung function or genetic markers, would improve accuracy. Lack of information on asbestos exposure in the LLPC limited the ability to validate the complete LLP risk model.

Conclusion.—Validation of the LLP risk model in 3 independent external data sets demonstrated good discrimination and evidence of predicted benefits for stratifying patients for lung cancer CT screening. Further studies are needed to prospectively evaluate model performance and evaluate the optimal population risk thresholds for initiating lung cancer screening.

▶ There are several published lung cancer risk predictive models, the most robust of which are those by Bach and colleagues,[1] Tammemagi and colleagues,[2] Spitz and colleagues,[3] and the Liverpool Lung Project (LLP).[4] The LLP is the largest prospective population based study on lung cancer in Europe.[5] Initiated in 1998, more than 11 500 lung cancer patients and controls have been recruited into the LLP biorepository. The original LLP lung cancer risk predictive model was based on 579 lung cancer cases and 1157 age- and sex-matched controls.[4]

The published models use different sets of overlapping variables. The Bach model is applicable only to smokers, whereas the Tammemagi, Spitz, and LLP models all have the ability to be applied to a general population (ie, including nonsmokers). This article by Raji and colleagues externally validated the LLP risk predictive model in 3 independent datasets from case-control studies in Europe, the United States, and a prospective LLP cohort. The LLP model predicts an individual's 5-year risk of lung cancer based on the following variables: smoking duration (including never smoking), history of pneumonia, asbestos exposure, history of personal cancer, and family history of lung cancer. The model performed with good discrimination in the validation sets. In comparison to the Tammemagi model developed in the Prostate, Lung, Colorectal and Ovarian screening trial to which it is perhaps most similar, the LLP model uses fewer variables, incorporates information about asbestos exposure and personal history of cancer, and yields a 5-year as opposed to 9-year risk of lung cancer. The authors argue that the LLP model is simple and potentially more useful clinically because of that. Future refinement of this and other lung cancer risk predictive models will likely involve incorporation of spirometric data as well as molecular biomarkers. The discriminative ability of these models to estimate risk for lung cancer is approaching that of the Gail model for breast cancer[6] and the Framingham risk score for coronary artery disease.[7] The ability to objectively and quantitatively assess lung cancer risk to inform clinical decisions about screening will be extraordinarily useful in the care of our patients.

L. T. Tanoue, MD

References

1. Bach PB, Kattan MW, Thornquist MD, et al. Variations in lung cancer risk among smokers. *J Natl Cancer Inst.* 2003;95:470-478.
2. Tammemagi CM, Pinsky PF, Caporaso NE, et al. Lung cancer risk prediction: Prostate, Lung, Colorectal and Ovarian Cancer Screening Trial models and validation. *J Natl Cancer Inst.* 2011;103:1058-1068.
3. Spitz MR, Hong WK, Amos CI, et al. A risk model for prediction of lung cancer. *J Natl Cancer Inst.* 2007;99:715-726.
4. Cassidy A, Myles JP, van Tongeren M, et al. The LLP risk model: an individual risk prediction model for lung cancer. *Br J Cancer.* 2008;98:270-276.
5. Field JK, Smith DL, Duffy S, Cassidy A. The Liverpool Lung Project research protocol. *Int J Oncol.* 2005;27:1633-1645.
6. Barlow WE, White E, Ballard-Barbash R, et al. Prospective breast cancer risk prediction model for women undergoing screening mammography. *J Natl Cancer Inst.* 2006;98:1204-1214.
7. Brindle P, Beswick A, Fahey T, Ebrahim S. Accuracy and impact of risk assessment in the primary prevention of cardiovascular disease: a systematic review. *Heart.* 2006;92:1752-1759.

CT screening for lung cancer brings forward early disease. The randomised Danish Lung Cancer Screening Trial: status after five annual screening rounds with low-dose CT

Saghir Z, Dirksen A, Ashraf H, et al (Gentofte Univ Hosp, Hellerup, Denmark; Akershus Univ Hosp, Lørenskog, Norway; et al)
Thorax 67:296-301, 2012

Background.—The effects of low-dose CT screening on disease stage shift, mortality and overdiagnosis are unclear. Lung cancer findings and mortality rates are reported at the end of screening in the Danish Lung Cancer Screening Trial.

Methods.—4104 men and women, healthy heavy smokers/former smokers were randomised to five annual low-dose CT screenings or no screening. Two experienced chest radiologists read all CT scans and registered the location, size and morphology of nodules. Nodules between 5 and 15 mm without benign characteristics were rescanned after 3 months. Growing nodules (> 25% volume increase and/or volume doubling time < 400 days) and nodules > 15 mm were referred for diagnostic workup. In the control group, lung cancers were diagnosed and treated outside the study by the usual clinical practice.

Results.—Participation rates were high in both groups (screening: 95.5%; control: 93.0%; $p < 0.001$). Lung cancer detection rate was 0.83% at baseline and mean annual detection rate was 0.67% at incidence rounds ($p = 0.535$). More lung cancers were diagnosed in the screening group (69 vs 24, $p < 0.001$), and more were low stage (48 vs 21 stage I–IIB non-small cell lung cancer (NSCLC) and limited stage small cell lung cancer (SCLC), $p = 0.002$), whereas frequencies of high-stage lung cancer were the same (21 vs 16 stage IIIA–IV NSCLC and extensive stage SCLC, $p = 0.509$). At the end of screening, 61 patients died in the screening group and 42 in the control group ($p = 0.059$). 15 and 11 died of lung cancer, respectively ($p = 0.428$).

Conclusion.—CT screening for lung cancer brings forward early disease, and at this point no stage shift or reduction in mortality was observed. More lung cancers were diagnosed in the screening group, indicating some degree of overdiagnosis and need for longer follow-up.

▶ In 2011, the National Lung Screening Trial (NLST) reported a 20% relative reduction in lung cancer mortality related to screening with low-dose chest computed tomography scanning.[1] Several other randomized prospective lung cancer screening trials are ongoing internationally, including the Danish Lung Cancer Screening Trial (DLCST) discussed in this report by Saghir and colleagues. The enrollment in the DLCST is smaller than the NLST, 5104 compared with 53454 subjects, respectively. As with other screening studies, at 5 years of follow-up, the DLCST demonstrated that the number of early-stage lung cancers was significantly higher (6-fold) in the screened versus control group, whereas no difference was seen in the numbers of late-stage cancers. This does not support an absolute stage shift and, as has been the case with most screening trials, raises the concern for overdiagnosis. At the 5-year mark, no mortality difference was observed in lung cancer or all-cause mortality, but this is likely still explainable by the relative small subject sample size and as yet short follow-up time.

The results of the DLCST as well as other international lung cancer screening trials will be important because they are studying populations that are in some ways different than the NLST. The subject inclusion criteria for the DLSCT were ages 50 to 70 years, with a smoking history of > 20 pack-years, and currently smoking or having quit within 10 years. These differ from the NLST, whose subjects were ages 55 to 74 with > 30 pack-years of smoking, currently smoking or having quit within the past 15 years. The DLCST data may be able to be pooled with other European randomized lung cancer screening trials to obtain more statistical power. If so, these results may be able to answer lung cancer screening questions in a broader population than the NLST, specifically in individuals who are younger and have less accumulated tobacco exposure.

L. T. Tanoue, MD

Reference

1. Aberle DR, Adams AM, Berg CD, et al. Reduced lung-cancer mortality with low-dose computed tomographic screening. *N Engl J Med.* 2011;365:395-409.

Diagnostic Evaluation

Estimating Overdiagnosis in Low-Dose Computed Tomography Screening for Lung Cancer: A Cohort Study

Veronesi G, Maisonneuve P, Bellomi M, et al (Univ of Milan, Italy)
Ann Intern Med 157:776-784, 2012

Background.—Lung cancer screening may detect cancer that will never become symptomatic (overdiagnosis), leading to overtreatment. Changes in size on sequential low-dose computed tomography (LDCT) screening, expressed as volume-doubling time (VDT), may help to distinguish aggressive cancer from cases that are unlikely to become symptomatic.

Objective.—To assess VDT for screening-detected lung cancer as an indicator of overdiagnosis.

Design.—Retrospective estimation of the VDT of cancer detected in a prospective LDCT screening cohort.

Setting.—Nonrandomized, single-center screening study involving persons at high risk for lung cancer enrolled between 2004 and 2005 who received LDCT annually for 5 years.

Patients.—175 study patients diagnosed with primary lung cancer.

Measurements.—VDT was measured on LDCT and classified as fast-growing (< 400 days), slow-growing (between 400 and 599 days), or indolent (≥ 600 days).

Results.—Fifty-five cases of cancer were diagnosed at baseline, and 120 were diagnosed subsequently. Of the latter group, 19 cases (15.8%) were new (not visible on previous scans) and fast-growing (median VDT, 52 days); 101 (84.2%) were progressive, including 70 (58.3%) fast-growing and 31 (25.8%) slow-growing (15.0%) or indolent (10.8%) cases. Lung cancer–specific mortality was significantly higher (9.2% per year) in patients with new compared with slow-growing or indolent (0.9% per year) cancer. Sixty percent of fast-growing progressive cancer and 45% of new cancer were stage I, for which survival was good.

Limitations.—This is a retrospective study. Volume-doubling time can only indicate overdiagnosis and was estimated for new cancer from 1 measurement (a diameter of 2 mm assumed the previous year).

Conclusion.—Slow-growing or indolent cancer comprised approximately 25% of incident cases, many of which may have been overdiagnosed. To limit overtreatment in these cases, minimally invasive limited resection and nonsurgical treatments should be investigated.

▶ Overdiagnosis is defined as the identification by screening of indolent cancers that would not otherwise have been diagnosed or caused harm. In cancers where screening is widely practiced, including breast and prostate cancers, overdiagnosis does appear to occur.[1,2] Overdiagnosis with respect to lung cancer has been a topic of intense discussion. More than 3 decades ago, the Mayo Lung Project examined screening for lung cancer by chest radiography and sputum cytology in approximately 9000 men who had smoked.[3,4] More lung cancers were found in the screened subjects, but ultimately no difference was found in overall mortality even after more than 10 years, suggesting that the excess cancers were cases of overdiagnosis.[5] Pooling of diagnosis and outcome data from 3 more recent large screening trials also strongly suggested the presence of over-diagnosis.[6] However, the National Lung Screening Trial (NLST) demonstrated a 20% reduction in mortality rate from lung cancer related to screening with low-dose chest computed tomography (LDCT) scanning, and based on this mortality reduction, the major societies involved in chest medicine now recommend screening for the population who fit the entry criteria for the NLST.

Nonetheless, screening-related overdiagnosis of lung cancer is still widely held to exist. This study by Veronesi and colleagues attempts to address this problem by assessing volume doubling time (VDT) of lung cancers identified by LDCT screening. Nodules identified as new or increasing in size on follow-up CT screening studies had volumes and VDT calculated using CT software that is commonly available with new-generation scanners, but not necessarily widely used. Previous studies have defined cancers with VDT < 400 days as aggressive or "fast growing," VDT 400 to 599 days as "slow growing," and VDT > 600 days as "indolent."[7,8] These criteria were examined in subjects in the Italian Continuous Observation of Smoking Subjects (COSMOS) study who were diagnosed with incident lung cancers (ie, cancers diagnosed with screening but not on the base-line study). The distribution of VDTs of these lung cancers was continuous, as seen in Fig 1 in the original article, with 25% of incident cancers demonstrating VDT > 400 days. Notably, VDT appeared to correlate not only with cancer ag-gressivity but also with mortality; cancers with shorter VDT had a worse prognosis than cancers with longer VDT, as shown in Fig 2 in the original article.

Several interesting conclusions might be drawn from the findings of this study. First, 75% of the incident lung cancer cases in the COSMOS study appear to fall in the fast-growing category; if that is indeed the case, then the problem of overdiag nosis may be less concerning than previously thought. Second, VDT is not widely used in clinical practice; this study adds to a growing body of literature supporting its adoption on a more regular basis for nodules identified by screening LDCT. Third, if we are able to reliably identify slow-growing or indolent cancers, then less aggressive treatment approaches—for example, limited surgical resection or stereotactic body radiotherapy—should be considered and studied in a rigorous fashion. Finally, if conversely we are able to reliably identify cancers that are more likely to result in death, then consideration could be given to treating those patients more aggressively early on.

L. T. Tanoue, MD

References

1. Ernster VL, Barclay J. Increases in ductal carcinoma in situ (DCIS) of the breast in relation to mammography: a dilemma. *J Natl Cancer Inst Monogr.* 1997;(22): 151-156.
2. Zappa M, Ciatto S, Bonardi R, Mazzotta A. Overdiagnosis of prostate carcinoma by screening: an estimate based on the results of the Florence Screening Pilot Study. *Ann Oncol.* 1998;9:1297-1300.

3. Fontana RS, Sanderson DR, Taylor WF, et al. Early lung cancer detection: results of the initial (prevalence) radiologic and cytologic screening in the Mayo Clinic study. *Am Rev Respir Dis.* 1984;130:561-565.
4. Fontana RS, Sanderson DR, Woolner LB, et al. Screening for lung cancer. A critique of the Mayo Lung Project. *Cancer.* 1991;67:1155-1164.
5. Marcus PM, Bergstralh EJ, Zweig MH, Harris A, Offord KP, Fontana RS. Extended lung cancer incidence follow-up in the Mayo Lung Project and overdiagnosis. *J Natl Cancer Inst.* 2006;98:748-756.
6. Bach PB, Jett JR, Pastorino U, Tockman MS, Swensen SJ, Begg CB. Computed tomography screening and lung cancer outcomes. *JAMA.* 2007;297:953-961.
7. van Klaveren RJ, Oudkerk M, Prokop M, et al. Management of lung nodules detected by volume CT scanning. *N Engl J Med.* 2009;361:2221-2229.
8. Yankelevitz DF, Kostis WJ, Henschke CI, et al. Overdiagnosis in chest radiographic screening for lung carcinoma: frequency. *Cancer.* 2003;97:1271-1275.

Lung cancer detection by canine scent: will there be a lab in the lab?

McCulloch M, Turner K, Broffman M (Pine Street Foundation, San Anselmo, CA; EZ Train, El Sobrante, CA)

Eur Respir J 39:511-512, 2012

Background.—Two studies have documented the ability of trained dogs to detect lung cancer with high sensitivity and specificity. Because safe, noninvasive methods for detecting lung cancer in its early and curable stages are highly desirable, it is important to explore the possibility that the analysis of exhaled breath, which is essentially what dogs do, may be able to provide such early detection.

Exhaled Breath Analysis.—Work has been done to develop an "electronic nose" for cancer detection over the past several decades. In addition, cancer biomarkers in exhaled breath have been sought. No standards for sampling methods or detecting technology platforms have been accepted for these efforts. In addition, all of these methods have limitations that interfere with their accuracy for lung cancer screening. Dogs have higher sensitivity (reported as 90% and 99%) and specificity (reported as 72% and 99%) and are far superior to all the other methods that have been tried.

Role for Dogs in Cancer Detection.—Patients, clinicians, and researchers complain constantly about the frustrations related to the slow progress in early cancer detection and the anxieties caused by false positive results, the regrets resulting from false negatives, and the inability of current cancer screening and diagnostic methods to do better. Dogs may be able to serve an inspirational role, provide a friendly message to the public, and perhaps would even encourage patients to seek medical treatment earlier. If sufficient funding is allocated to permit other research groups to replicate and refine existing results on canine scent detection for lung cancer, they could be used as a noninvasive preliminary diagnostic screening tool or help reduce false positive and false negatives gained through existing technologies.

Conclusions.—Dogs are already serving faithfully as friends and protectors. They also help in finding cadavers, bombs, drugs, weapons and truffles; they detect diabetes and seizures; they provide search and rescue help; they serve as sight assistance, and they function as loving companions. It is possible that they could identify lung cancer or other cancers early enough to foster interventions that increase longevity and decrease morbidity, making them an even more valuable friend and protector.

▶ This engaging editorial and the 2 papers that follow in this section describe the potential of exhaled breath to be an accurate and noninvasive means of cancer diagnosis. Identifying disease by detection of smell is a practice that dates to ancient Chinese and Greek medicine; its use continues to the modern day, as we teach our students about the "fruity odor" of diabetic ketoacidosis and "fetor hepaticus" associated with liver failure. The human nose as a diagnostic instrument, though, is a crude tool. The ability of trained dogs to accurately detect lung cancer by sniffing the breath of patients has now been documented in at least 2 studies,[1,2] and there is an increasing literature supporting the concept that "smellprints" of exhaled breath analyzed by more conventional scientific instruments can do the same.[3-6] This area merits more attention. The reality is that low-dose chest computed tomography scan as a screening intervention is also a crude tool, particularly given the associated high false-positive rate. Further, analysis of exhaled breath is an attractive possibility as it potentially offers a window into effective screening for many populations, not limited necessarily to a population of intense smokers of mid- to older age. Decreasing lung cancer mortality by early detection will likely require innovative approaches, and exhaled breath analysis may well be one.

L. T. Tanoue, MD

References

1. McCulloch M, Jezierski T, Broffman M, Hubbard A, Turner K, Janecki T. Diagnostic accuracy of canine scent detection in early- and late-stage lung and breast cancers. *Integr Cancer Ther.* 2006;5:30-39.
2. Ehmann R, Boedeker E, Friedrich U, et al. Canine scent detection in the diagnosis of lung cancer: revisiting a puzzling phenomenon. *Eur Respir J.* 2012;39:669-676.
3. Phillips M, Altorki N, Austin JH, et al. Prediction of lung cancer using volatile biomarkers in breath. *Cancer Biomark.* 2007;3:95-109.
4. Mazzone PJ, Wang XF, Xu Y, et al. Exhaled breath analysis with a colorimetric sensor array for the identification and characterization of lung cancer. *J Thorac Oncol.* 2012;7:137-142.
5. Bajtarevic A, Ager C, Pienz M, et al. Noninvasive detection of lung cancer by analysis of exhaled breath. *BMC Cancer.* 2009;9:348.
6. Machado RF, Laskowski D, Deffenderfer O, et al. Detection of lung cancer by sensor array analyses of exhaled breath. *Am J Respir Crit Care Med.* 2005;171:1286-1291.

Exhaled Breath Analysis with a Colorimetric Sensor Array for the Identification and Characterization of Lung Cancer

Mazzone PJ, Wang XF, Xu Y, et al (Cleveland Clinic, OH; et al)
J Thorac Oncol 7:137-142, 2012

Introduction.—The pattern of exhaled breath volatile organic compounds represents a metabolic biosignature with the potential to identify and characterize lung cancer. Breath biosignature-based classification of homogeneous subgroups of lung cancer may be more accurate than a global breath signature. Combining breath biosignatures with clinical risk factors may improve the accuracy of the signature.

Objectives.—To develop an exhaled breath biosignature of lung cancer using a colorimetric sensor array and to determine the accuracy of breath biosignatures of lung cancer characteristics with and without the inclusion of clinical risk factors.

Methods.—The exhaled breath of 229 study subjects, 92 with lung cancer and 137 controls, was drawn across a colorimetric sensor array. Logistic

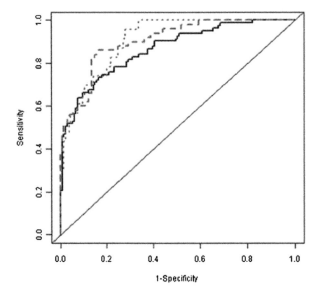

Black line = model for non-small cell vs. controls, C statistic = 0.811

Red dashed line = model for adenocarcinoma vs. controls, C statistic = 0.825

Green dotted line = model for squamous cell carcinoma vs. controls, C statistic = 0.849

FIGURE 2.—Receiver operating characteristic curves for the most accurate validated models comparing non-small cell carcinoma to controls and for the individual non-small cell carcinoma histologies to controls. (Reprinted from Mazzone PJ, Wang X-F, Xu Y, et al. Exhaled breath analysis with a colorimetric sensor array for the identification and characterization of lung cancer. *J Thorac Oncol.* 2012;7:137-142, with permission from the International Association for the Study of Lung Cancer.)

prediction models were developed and statistically validated based on the color changes of the sensor. Age, sex, smoking history, and chronic obstructive pulmonary disease were incorporated in the prediction models.

Results.—The validated prediction model of the combined breath and clinical biosignature was moderately accurate at distinguishing lung cancer from control subjects (C-statistic 0.811). The accuracy improved when the model focused on only one histology (C-statistic 0.825—0.890). Individuals with different histologies could be accurately distinguished from one another (C-statistic 0.864 for adenocarcinoma versus squamous cell carcinoma). Moderate accuracies were noted for validated breath biosignatures of stage and survival (C-statistic 0.785 and 0.693, respectively).

Conclusions.—A colorimetric sensor array is capable of identifying exhaled breath biosignatures of lung cancer. The accuracy of breath biosignatures can be optimized by evaluating specific histologies and incorporating clinical risk factors (Fig 2).

▶ Volatile organic compounds (VOCs) are present in exhaled breath in low but measurable concentrations. Cellular metabolic processes create VOCs that circulate within the blood and then are exhaled through the lungs. Prior study has suggested that lung cancer cells may have unique metabolic properties that are distinguishable from other diseases by analysis of exhaled breath VOCs.[1] The report by Ehmann and colleagues that follows in this section describing the ability of dogs to "smell" lung cancer presumably reflects the animals' ability to distinguish patterns of VOCs and perhaps other breath constituents.[2] That exhaled breath can be a noninvasive source of potential lung cancer biomarkers makes this approach particularly appealing.

In this study by Mazzone and colleagues, exhaled breath was studied by colorimetric sensor array. This technology uses a range of chemically responsive dyes, whose colors depend on their chemical environment. Exhaled breath drawn across the array yields changes in the color spectrum of the individual dyes, which are then converted to numerical values, yielding a "breath biosignature." Breath analysis was performed in subjects with biopsy-proven untreated cancer and controls at risk for developing lung cancer (individuals enrolled in a lung cancer screening study or with indeterminate pulmonary nodules felt unlikely to be cancer). Several models using breath biosignatures were developed that were able to distinguish lung cancer from controls with sensitivities ranging from 70% to 91% and specificities of 73% to 95%. Fig 2 demonstrates the receiver operating characteristic curves for predictive models developed for individual lung cancer histologies. The accuracies of these models were improved by the incorporation of patient clinical characteristics. These results suggest that breath analysis in combination with clinical variables may be useful in the diagnostic evaluation of lung cancer, with potential applicability to risk prediction and screening, nodule assessment, and prognostication.

L. T. Tanoue, MD

References

1. Machado RF, Laskowski D, Deffenderfer O, et al. Detection of lung cancer by sensor array analyses of exhaled breath. *Am J Respir Crit Care Med.* 2005;171: 1286-1291.
2. Ehmann R, Boedeker E, Friedrich U, et al. Canine scent detection in the diagnosis of lung cancer: revisiting a puzzling phenomenon. *Eur Respir J.* 2012;39:669-676.

Canine scent detection in the diagnosis of lung cancer: revisiting a puzzling phenomenon
Ehmann R, Boedeker E, Friedrich U, et al (Ambulante Pneumologie, Stuttgart, Germany; Schillerhoehe Hosp, Gerlingen, Germany; TeamCanin, Loeffingen, Germany; et al)
Eur Respir J 39:669-676, 2012

Patient prognosis in lung cancer largely depends on early diagnosis. The exhaled breath of patients may represent the ideal specimen for future lung cancer screening. However, the clinical applicability of current diagnostic sensor technologies based on signal pattern analysis remains incalculable due to their inability to identify a clear target. To test the robustness of the presence of a so far unknown volatile organic compound in the breath of patients with lung cancer, sniffer dogs were applied.

Exhalation samples of 220 volunteers (healthy individuals, confirmed lung cancer or chronic obstructive pulmonary disease (COPD)) were presented to sniffer dogs following a rigid scientific protocol. Patient history, drug administration and clinicopathological data were analysed to identify potential bias or confounders.

Lung cancer was identified with an overall sensitivity of 71% and a specificity of 93%. Lung cancer detection was independent from COPD and the presence of tobacco smoke and food odours. Logistic regression identified two drugs as potential confounders.

It must be assumed that a robust and specific volatile organic compound (or pattern) is present in the breath of patients with lung cancer. Additional research efforts are required to overcome the current technical limitations of electronic sensor technologies to engineer a clinically applicable screening tool.

▶ The ability of dogs to identify bombs, illicit drugs, people both alive and dead, and truffles is widely accepted in the modern world.[1] This study suggests that trained dogs may be more accurate in identifying lung cancer than any other current diagnostic modality, corroborating a prior report of canine scent detection of lung and breast cancers.[2] Breath samples were collected from study subjects by having them breathe into tubes containing polypropylene fleece impregnated with a silicone oil to achieve either hydrophilic- or hydrophobic-absorbing properties. Four dogs were trained to lie down with their muzzles touching the breath sample tube when they sniffed exhaled breath from patients with lung cancer. The study then had the dogs sniff breath from 110 volunteers, 84 lung cancer patients, and 50 patients with chronic obstructive pulmonary disease (COPD). The dogs correctly identified lung cancer exhaled breath with a sensitivity of 0.72 (0.51-0.88), specificity of 0.94 (0.87-0.98), positive predictive value of 0.75 (0.53-0.91), and negative predictive value of 0.93 (0.86-0.97).

It seems likely that the dogs are identifying volatile organic compounds (VOCs) or patterns of VOCs that are associated with lung cancer. What is particularly impressive about the results presented is that the dogs were able to correctly identify lung cancer, not just in general, but in patients with other conditions that could potentially confound olfactory discrimination, including cigarette smoking and COPD. Whether the use of dogs as screening tools for lung cancer detection is practical will inevitably be raised, but this study supports further investigation into more conventional instruments, such as the electronic nose, that can reliably identify VOCs.

L. T. Tanoue, MD

References

1. McCulloch M, Turner K, Broffman M. Lung cancer detection by canine scent: will there be a lab in the lab? *Eur Respir J*. 2012;39:511-512.
2. McCulloch M, Jezierski T, Broffman M, Hubbard A, Turner K, Janecki T. Diagnostic accuracy of canine scent detection in early- and late-stage lung and breast cancers. *Integr Cancer Ther*. 2006;5:30-39.

Lung Cancer Treatment

Cancer Treatment and Survivorship Statistics, 2012
Siegel R, DeSantis C, Virgo K, et al (American Cancer Society, Atlanta, GA; et al)
CA Cancer J Clin 62:220-241, 2012

Although there has been considerable progress in reducing cancer incidence in the United States, the number of cancer survivors continues to increase due to the aging and growth of the population and improvements in survival rates. As a result, it is increasingly important to understand the unique medical and psychosocial needs of survivors and be aware of resources that can assist patients, caregivers, and health care providers in navigating the various phases of cancer survivorship. To highlight the challenges and opportunities to serve these survivors, the American Cancer Society and the National Cancer Institute estimated the prevalence of cancer survivors on January 1, 2012 and January 1, 2022, by cancer site. Data from Surveillance, Epidemiology, and End Results (SEER) registries were used to describe median age and stage at diagnosis and survival; data from the National Cancer Data Base and the SEER-Medicare Database were used to describe patterns of cancer treatment. An estimated 13.7 million Americans with a history of cancer were alive on January 1, 2012, and by January 1, 2022, that number will increase to nearly 18 million. The 3 most prevalent cancers among males are prostate (43%), colorectal (9%), and melanoma of the skin (7%), and those among females are breast (41%), uterine corpus (8%), and colorectal (8%). This article summarizes common cancer treatments, survival rates, and posttreatment concerns and introduces the new National Cancer Survivorship Resource Center, which has engaged more than 100 volunteer survivorship experts nationwide to develop tools for cancer survivors, caregivers, health care professionals, advocates, and policy makers.

▶ Cancer survivorship is an area of ever-increasing interest. The cancer survivor population in the United States is currently estimated at 13.7 million, and is projected to substantially increase over time. Two general factors contribute to this. First, the population of the country is aging and growing, with half of all men and 1 in every 3 women diagnosed with cancer over their lifetimes. Second, early diagnosis and improved treatments are contributing to longer survival. Thus, the survivorship "movement" is the result of improvements in diagnosis and treatment, with resultant better longevity. The physical, psychological, and societal consequences of cancer survivorship, both positive and negative, are appropriately starting to be addressed in both clinical and research arenas. For lung cancer, long-term survival is still poor; overall 5-year survival is 17.1% for non–small-cell lung cancer and 6.1% for small-cell lung cancer. Five-year survival even for localized disease is only 52.2%. Nonetheless, approximately 412 000 persons in the United States are currently living with a history of lung cancer. For these patients, pulmonary physiologic impairment is common, related to underlying lung disease (eg, chronic obstructive pulmonary disease, interstitial lung disease) and/or surgery, risk for other tobacco-related cancers is elevated, and the societal empathy and support that are almost inherent with other cancers may be lacking because of the perception of the patient's contribution to cause (ie, smoking).[1] Further, guidelines for the appropriate medical follow-up of these patients are generally lacking an evidence base. With lung cancer screening now of demonstrated benefit, at least in the population studied in the National Lung Screening Trial,[2] and with an increasing number of new medical therapies in clinical trials, the lung cancer survivor population will surely grow, meriting focused clinical and research efforts to ensure maximal quality of their longer lives.

The American Cancer Society and the George Washington Cancer Institute, funded by the Centers for Disease Control and Prevention, has created the National Cancer Survivorship Resource Center. Educational tools for cancer survivors, caregivers, health care professionals, and policy makers are available at cancer.org/survivorshipcenter.

L. T. Tanoue, MD

References

1. Chapple A, Ziebland S, McPherson A. Stigma, shame, and blame experienced by patients with lung cancer: qualitative study. *BMJ.* 2004;328:1470.
2. Aberle DR, Adams AM, Berg CD, et al. Reduced lung-cancer mortality with low-dose computed tomographic screening. *N Engl J Med.* 2011;365:395-409.

Safety, Activity, and Immune Correlates of Anti–PD-1 Antibody in Cancer
Topalian SL, Hodi FS, Brahmer JR, et al (Johns Hopkins Univ School of Medicine and the Sidney Kimmel Comprehensive Cancer Ctr, Baltimore, MD; Dana–Farber Cancer Inst, Boston, MA; et al)
N Engl J Med 366:2443-2454, 2012

Background.—Blockade of programmed death 1 (PD-1), an inhibitory receptor expressed by T cells, can overcome immune resistance. We assessed the antitumor activity and safety of BMS-936558, an antibody that specifically blocks PD-1.

Methods.—We enrolled patients with advanced melanoma, non–small-cell lung cancer, castration-resistant prostate cancer, or renal-cell or colorectal cancer to receive anti–PD-1 antibody at a dose of 0.1 to 10.0 mg per kilogram of body weight every 2 weeks. Response was assessed after each 8-week treatment cycle. Patients received up to 12 cycles until disease progression or a complete response occurred.

Results.—A total of 296 patients received treatment through February 24, 2012. Grade 3 or 4 drug-related adverse events occurred in 14% of patients; there were three deaths from pulmonary toxicity. No maximum tolerated dose was defined. Adverse events consistent with immune-related causes were observed. Among 236 patients in whom response could be evaluated, objective responses (complete or partial responses) were observed in those with non–small-cell lung cancer, melanoma, or renal-cell cancer. Cumulative response rates (all doses) were 18% among patients with non–small-cell lung cancer (14 of 76 patients), 28% among patients with melanoma (26 of 94 patients), and 27% among patients with renal-cell cancer (9 of 33 patients). Responses were durable; 20 of 31 responses lasted 1 year or more in patients with 1 year or more of follow-up. To assess the role of intratumoral PD-1 ligand (PD-L1) expression in the modulation of the PD-1–PD-L1 pathway, immunohistochemical analysis was performed on pretreatment tumor specimens obtained from 42 patients. Of 17 patients with PD-L1–negative tumors, none had an objective response; 9 of 25 patients (36%) with PD-L1–positive tumors had an objective response ($P = 0.006$).

Conclusions.—Anti–PD-1 antibody produced objective responses in approximately one in four to one in five patients with non–small-cell lung cancer, melanoma, or renal-cell cancer; the adverse-event profile does not appear to preclude its use. Preliminary data suggest a relationship between PD-L1 expression on tumor cells and objective response. (Funded by Bristol-Myers Squibb and others; ClinicalTrials.gov number, NCT00730639.)

▶ Though the concept that the immune system can be harnessed for antitumor effects is a longstanding one in cancer treatment, solid tumors, including non–small-cell lung cancer (NSCLC), have historically been unresponsive to immunotherapy. An endogenous anticancer immune response is generally held to exist, but tumors develop resistance to this protective response by a variety of mechanisms, including local immune suppression, induction of tolerance among tumor-specific T cells, and immune dysfunction related to tumor ligands that block T-cell signaling. Tumors may evade immune destruction by exploiting immune "checkpoints" that suppress immune responses after antigen activation. Interest in therapeutic antitumor effect gained by inhibition at these immune checkpoints led to the development of the anti–CTLA-4 antibody ipilimumab, which has proved beneficial in patients with advanced melanoma, presumably by enhancing the endogenous antitumor immune response. Programed death-1 (PD-1) is another key immune checkpoint receptor expressed by activated T cells. PD-1 has 2 known ligands, PD-L1 and PD-L2. PD-L1 is expressed on many tumors, not only by tumor cells but by stromal cells within the tumor microenvironment. Blockade of the interaction between PD-1 and PD-L1 potentiates immune responses in vitro, and appears to enhance antitumor activity. This study and a companion study by Brahmer and colleagues[1] examined the safety and activity of anti–PD-1 and anti–PD-L1 antibodies in the treatment of a variety of advanced solid tumors refractory to multiple lines of chemotherapy, including NSCLC. Although this was a phase I study intended primarily to analyze safety, dose, and tolerability, anti–PD-1 antibody resulted in an objective response in 14/76 patients with NSCLC, 8 of whom had a response that lasted 24 weeks or more, and 2 of whom had a response lasting a year or more. Importantly, PD-L1 expression in tumors appeared in this study to be a potential biomarker for response because positive results were seen in 36% of patients with PD-L1–positive tumors as compared with none of the patients with PD-L1–negative tumors. These results suggest that the PD-1–PD-L1 pathway may be important mechanistically in a subpopulation of patients with NSCLC who may be identifiable by tumor expression of PD-L1.

L. T. Tanoue, MD

Reference

1. Brahmer JR, Tykodi SS, Chow LQ, et al. Safety and activity of anti-PD-L1 antibody in patients with advanced cancer. N Engl J Med. 2012;366:2455-2465.

Safety and Activity of Anti–PD-L1 Antibody in Patients with Advanced Cancer
Brahmer JR, Tykodi SS, Chow LQM, et al (Johns Hopkins Univ School of Medicine and the Sidney Kimmel Comprehensive Cancer Ctr, Baltimore, MD; Univ of Washington and Fred Hutchinson Cancer Res Ctr, Seattle; et al)
N Engl J Med 366:2455-2465, 2012

Background.—Programmed death 1 (PD-1) protein, a T-cell coinhibitory receptor, and one of its ligands, PD-L1, play a pivotal role in the ability of tumor cells to evade the host's immune system. Blockade of interactions between PD-1 and PD-L1 enhances immune function in vitro and mediates antitumor activity in preclinical models.

Methods.—In this multicenter phase 1 trial, we administered intravenous anti–PD-L1 antibody (at escalating doses ranging from 0.3 to 10 mg per kilogram of body weight) to patients with selected advanced cancers. Anti—PD-L1 antibody was administered every 14 days in 6-week cycles for up to 16 cycles or until the patient had a complete response or confirmed disease progression.

Results.—As of February 24, 2012, a total of 207 patients — 75 with non—small-cell lung cancer, 55 with melanoma, 18 with colorectal cancer, 17 with renal-cell cancer, 17 with ovarian cancer, 14 with pancreatic cancer, 7 with gastric cancer, and 4 with breast cancer — had received anti—PD-L1 antibody. The median duration of therapy was 12 weeks (range, 2 to 111). Grade 3 or 4 toxic effects that investigators considered to be related to treatment occurred in 9% of patients. Among patients with a response that could be evaluated, an objective response (a complete or partial response) was observed in 9 of 52 patients with melanoma, 2 of 17 with renal-cell cancer, 5 of 49 with non—small-cell lung cancer, and 1 of 17 with ovarian cancer. Responses lasted for 1 year or more in 8 of 16 patients with at least 1 year of follow-up.

Conclusions.—Antibody-mediated blockade of PD-L1 induced durable tumor regression (objective response rate of 6 to 17%) and prolonged stabilization of disease (rates of 12 to 41% at 24 weeks) in patients with advanced cancers, including non—small-cell lung cancer, melanoma, and renal-cell cancer. (Funded by Bristol-Myers Squibb and others; ClinicalTrials.gov number, NCT00729664.)

▶ Programmed death-1 (PD-1) is an immune checkpoint receptor with 2 known ligands, PD-L1 and PD-L2. PD-L1 is selectively expressed on many tumors, including non-small cell lung cancer (NSCLC). PD-L1 is upregulated in solid tumors and can inhibit the cytolytic activity of PD-1+, CD4+, and CD8+ T cells.[1-3] In this report by Brahmer and colleagues, an anti—PD-L1 monoclonal antibody inhibiting the binding of PD-L1 to PD-1 and CD80 was evaluated in a phase I trial in patients with a variety of refractory advanced solid tumors, including non—small-cell lung cancer (NSCLC). Although immunotherapy has generally not been therapeutically effective in patients with lung cancer, 10% of the 49 patients with NSCLC included in this study demonstrated objective response. In a companion article by Topalian and colleagues, a phase I trial evaluating antibody blockade of PD-1 resulted in objective responses in a variety of advanced solid tumors refractory to multiple lines of chemotherapy, including patients with NSCLC.[4] The demonstration of antitumor effects with both anti—PD-1 and anti—PD-L1 antibodies strongly supports the role of this pathway in tumor immune resistance and identifies it as a potentially important therapeutic target.

L. T. Tanoue, MD

References

1. Dong H, Strome SE, Salomao DR, et al. Tumor-associated B7-H1 promotes T-cell apoptosis: a potential mechanism of immune evasion. *Nat Med.* 2002;8:793-800.
2. Iwai Y, Ishida M, Tanaka Y, Okazaki T, Honjo T, Minato N. Involvement of PD-L1 on tumor cells in the escape from host immune system and tumor immunotherapy by PD-L1 blockade. *Proc Natl Acad Sci U S A.* 2002;99:12293-12297.

3. Zou W, Chen L. Inhibitory B7-family molecules in the tumour microenvironment. *Nat Rev Immunol.* 2008;8:467-477.
4. Topalian SL, Hodi FS, Brahmer JR, et al. Safety, activity, and immune correlates of anti-PD-1 antibody in cancer. *N Engl J Med.* 2012;366:2443-2454.

Patients' Expectations about Effects of Chemotherapy for Advanced Cancer

Weeks JC, Catalano PJ, Cronin A, et al (Dana-Farber Cancer Inst, Boston, MA)
N Engl J Med 367:1616-1625, 2012

Background.—Chemotherapy for metastatic lung or colorectal cancer can prolong life by weeks or months and may provide palliation, but it is not curative.

Methods.—We studied 1193 patients participating in the Cancer Care Outcomes Research and Surveillance (CanCORS) study (a national, prospective, observational cohort study) who were alive 4 months after diagnosis and received chemotherapy for newly diagnosed metastatic (stage IV) lung or colorectal cancer. We sought to characterize the prevalence of the expectation that chemotherapy might be curative and to identify the clinical, sociodemographic, and health-system factors associated with this expectation. Data were obtained from a patient survey by professional interviewers in addition to a comprehensive review of medical records.

Results.—Overall, 69% of patients with lung cancer and 81% of those with colorectal cancer did not report understanding that chemotherapy was not at all likely to cure their cancer. In multivariable logistic regression, the risk of reporting inaccurate beliefs about chemotherapy was higher among patients with colorectal cancer, as compared with those with lung cancer (odds ratio, 1.75; 95% confidence interval [CI], 1.29 to 2.37); among nonwhite and Hispanic patients, as compared with non-Hispanic white patients (odds ratio for Hispanic patients, 2.82; 95% CI, 1.51 to 5.27; odds ratio for black patients, 2.93; 95% CI, 1.80 to 4.78); and among patients who rated their communication with their physician very favorably, as compared with less favorably (odds ratio for highest third vs. lowest third, 1.90; 95% CI, 1.33 to 2.72). Educational level, functional status, and the patient's role in decision making were not associated with such inaccurate beliefs about chemotherapy.

Conclusions.—Many patients receiving chemotherapy for incurable cancers may not understand that chemotherapy is unlikely to be curative, which could compromise their ability to make informed treatment decisions that are consonant with their preferences. Physicians may be able to improve patients' understanding, but this may come at the cost of patients' satisfaction with them. (Funded by the National Cancer Institute and others.)

▶ This report by Weeks and colleagues corroborates what many of us suspect but perhaps do not usually ask: that patients with metastatic lung (or colorectal) cancer do not understand that chemotherapy is very unlikely to cure their disease. In this very large study of 1193 patients receiving chemotherapy for newly diagnosed stage IV lung or colorectal cancer, only a small minority felt that treatment was not at all likely to result in cure or life extension, as demonstrated in Fig 1 in the original article. Although it was not possible to know what physicians told patients about the expected outcomes of chemotherapy or to examine the roles of physicians in the stated expectations of patients for their treatment, many studies have demonstrated that oncologists usually do tell patients when their cancers are not curable.[1,2] Whether this translates into patients actually understanding or accepting the difficult truths is perhaps less clear.

This article is accompanied by a thoughtful editorial by Smith and Longo discussing the challenges of talking to patients about terminal illness.[3] As they point out, "These are not trivial issues." The editorial brings the findings of the study by Weeks and colleagues back to the doctor-patient relationship, emphasizing that the coping mechanisms of optimism and self-deception are not exclusive to truthful and effective conversations about palliative care and prognosis and discussions of advance directives including hospice.

L. T. Tanoue, MD

References

1. Gattellari M, Voigt KJ, Butow PN, Tattersall MH. When the treatment goal is not cure: are cancer patients equipped to make informed decisions? *J Clin Oncol.* 2002;20:503-513.
2. The AM, Hak T, Koëter G, van Der Wal G. Collusion in doctor-patient communication about imminent death: an ethnographic study. *BMJ.* 2000;321:1376-1381.
3. Smith TJ, Longo DL. Talking with patients about dying. *N Engl J Med.* 2012;367:1651-1652.

Lobectomy in Octogenarians With Non-Small Cell Lung Cancer: Ramifications of Increasing Life Expectancy and the Benefits of Minimally Invasive Surgery

Port JL, Mirza FM, Lee PC, et al (Weill Med College of Cornell Univ, NY)
Ann Thorac Surg 92:1951-1957, 2011

Background.—As the population ages, clinicians are increasingly confronted with octogenarians with resectable non-small cell lung cancer (NSCLC). We reviewed the outcomes of octogenarians who underwent lobectomy for NSCLC by video-assisted thoracic surgery (VATS) versus open thoracotomy, to determine if there was a benefit to the VATS approach in this group.

Methods.—We conducted a retrospective single-institution review of patients age 80 years or greater who underwent a lobectomy for NSCLC from 1998 to 2009. Outcomes including complication rates, length of stay, disposition, and long-term survival were analyzed.

Results.—One hundred twenty-one octogenarians underwent lobectomy: 40 VATS and 81 through open thoracotomy. Compared with thoracotomy, VATS patients had fewer complications (35.0% vs 63.0%, $p = 0.004$), shorter length of stay (5 vs 6 days, $p = 0.001$), and were less likely to require admission to the intensive care unit (2.5% vs 14.8%, $p = 0.038$) or rehabilitation after discharge (5% vs 22.5%, $p = 0.015$). In multivariate analysis, VATS was an independent predictor of reduced complications (odds ratio, 0.35; 95% confidence interval, 0.15 to 0.84; $p = 0.019$). Survival comparisons demonstrated no significant difference between the two techniques, either in univariate analysis of stage I patients (5-year VATS, 76.0%; thoracotomy, 65.3%; $p = 0.111$) or multivariate analysis of the entire cohort (adjusted hazard ratio, 0.59; 95% confidence interval, 0.27 to 1.28; $p = 0.183$).

Conclusions.—Octogenarians with NSCLC can undergo resection with low mortality and survival among stage I patients, which is comparable with the general lung cancer population. The VATS approach to resection reduces morbidity in this age demographic, resulting in shorter, less intensive hospitalization, and less frequent need for postoperative rehabilitation.

▶ Lung cancer is primarily a disease of older persons. The peak incidence of non–small-cell lung cancer (NSCLC) incidence occurs among patients ages 75 to 79. Thirty to 40% of lung cancer cases occur in patients > 70 years of age, and a substantial number of these occur in patients over the age of 80. The American College of Chest Physicians' evidence-based lung cancer guidelines recommend that fit elderly patients with early-stage NSCLC should not be denied curative intent treatment, and yet it is well-recognized that elderly patients are less likely to undergo curative resection when compared with younger patients.[1] Nonetheless, many studies have demonstrated that, when surgery is performed, survival is independent of age.[2,3] This report by Port and colleagues is a single-institution retrospective analysis of 121 octogenarians with early-stage NSCLC who underwent lobectomy either by open thoracotomy ($n = 81$) or video-assisted thoracoscopic surgery (VATS) ($n = 40$). As has been previously described, there was no difference in survival outcome between the 2 groups.[4] Notably, VATS resection was an independent predictor of reduced complications and was less likely to require admission to the intensive care unit or rehabilitation after discharge.

These results reinforce the American College of Chest Physicians' evidence-based lung cancer guidelines recommendation that fit elderly patients with early-stage NSCLC should not be denied curative intent treatment.[1] Moreover, they suggest that a VATS minimally invasive approach to surgical resection may have better outcomes in elderly patients with lung cancer than traditional open lobectomy. This should be a consideration in the evaluation of older patients with early-stage NSCLC who are fit for surgery.

L. T. Tanoue, MD

References

1. Colice GL, Shafazand S, Griffin JP, Keenan R, Bolliger CT. Physiologic evaluation of the patient with lung cancer being considered for resectional surgery: ACCP evidenced-based clinical practice guidelines (2nd edition). *Chest.* 2007;132: 161S-177S.
2. Kilic A, Schuchert MJ, Pettiford BL, et al. Anatomic segmentectomy for stage I non-small cell lung cancer in the elderly. *Ann Thorac Surg.* 2009;87:1662-1666.

3. Palma DA, Tyldesley S, Sheehan F, et al. Stage I non-small cell lung cancer (NSCLC) in patients aged 75 years and older: does age determine survival after radical treatment? *J Thorac Oncol.* 2010;5:818-824.
4. Boffa DJ, Allen MS, Grab JD, Gaissert HA, Harpole DH, Wright CD. Data from the Society of Thoracic Surgeons General Thoracic Surgery database: the surgical management of primary lung tumors. *J Thorac Cardiovasc Surg.* 2008;135:247-254.

Molecular Approach to Lung Cancer

ROS1 Rearrangements Define a Unique Molecular Class of Lung Cancers

Bergethon K, Shaw AT, Ou S-HI, et al (Massachusetts General Hosp, Boston, MA; Univ of California Irvine Med Ctr, Orange; et al)
J Clin Oncol 30:863-870, 2012

Purpose.—Chromosomal rearrangements involving the *ROS1* receptor tyrosine kinase gene have recently been described in a subset of non–small-cell lung cancers (NSCLCs). Because little is known about these tumors, we examined the clinical characteristics and treatment outcomes of patients with NSCLC with ROS1 rearrangement.

Patients and Methods.—Using a *ROS1* fluorescent in situ hybridization (FISH) assay, we screened 1,073 patients with NSCLC and correlated *ROS1* rearrangement status with clinical characteristics, overall survival, and when available, *ALK* rearrangement status. In vitro studies assessed the responsiveness of cells with *ROS1* rearrangement to the tyrosine kinase inhibitor crizotinib. The clinical response of one patient with *ROS1*-rearranged NSCLC to crizotinib was investigated as part of an expanded phase I cohort.

Results.—Of 1,073 tumors screened, 18 (1.7%) were *ROS1* rearranged by FISH, and 31 (2.9%) were *ALK* rearranged. Compared with the *ROS1*-negative group, patients with ROS1 rearrangements were significantly younger and more likely to be never-smokers (each *P* < .001). All of the *ROS1*-positive tumors were adenocarcinomas, with a tendency toward higher grade. *ROS1*-positive and-negative groups showed no difference in overall survival. The HCC78 *ROS1*-rearranged NSCLC cell line and 293 cells transfected with *CD74-ROS1* showed evidence of sensitivity to crizotinib. The patient treated with crizotinib showed tumor shrinkage, with a near complete response.

Conclusion.—*ROS1* rearrangement defines a molecular subset of NSCLC with distinct clinical characteristics that are similar to those observed in patients with *ALK*-rearranged NSCLC. Crizotinib shows in vitro activity and early evidence of clinical activity in *ROS1*-rearranged NSCLC.

▶ There is an increasing appreciation for the role of driver mutations in the pathogenesis of lung cancer, including their potential as targets for effective and specific drug development. Therapies directed against epidermal growth factor receptor (EGFR) and the EML4-ALK fusion oncogene, for example, have changed the paradigm of treatment in many lung cancer patients. ROS1, a receptor tyrosine kinase of the insulin receptor family, is a gene felt to be involved in chromosomal translocations in lung cancer. Chromosomal rearrangements involving ROS1 have been described in glioblastoma and cholangiocarcinoma, and now in lung adenocarcinoma.[1,2] Bergethon and colleagues screened 1073 lung cancer tumors and found that 1.7% demonstrated ROS1 rearrangements, which were mutually exclusive from ALK rearrangements. Patients with ROS1 rearrangements were younger and more likely to be never-smokers than those without rearrangements, characteristics similar to patients with EGFR mutations or ALK rearrangments.[3,4] Although the prevalence of ROS1 rearrangements was low, this finding nonetheless highlights the increasing number of genetic subtypes associated with non—small-cell lung cancer, and identifies another potential target for molecularly directed drug development.

L. T. Tanoue, MD

References

1. Gu TL, Deng X, Huang F, et al. Survey of tyrosine kinase signaling reveals ROS kinase fusions in human cholangiocarcinoma. *PLoS One.* 2011;6:e15640.
2. Birchmeier C, Sharma S, Wigler M. Expression and rearrangement of the ROS1 gene in human glioblastoma cells. *Proc Natl Acad Sci U S A.* 1987;84:9270-9274.
3. Pao W, Girard N. New driver mutations in non-small-cell lung cancer. *Lancet Oncol.* 2011;12:175-180.
4. Kwak EL, Bang YJ, Camidge DR, et al. Anaplastic lymphoma kinase inhibition in non-small-cell lung cancer. *N Engl J Med.* 2010;363:1693-1703.

Epigenetic Control of Gene Expression in the Lung
Yang IV, Schwartz DA (Natl Jewish Health, Denver, CO)
Am J Respir Crit Care Med 183:1295-1301, 2011

Epigenetics is traditionally defined as the study of heritable changes in gene expression caused by mechanisms other than changes in the underlying DNA sequence. There are three main classes of epigenetic marks—DNA methylation, modifications of histone tails, and noncoding RNAs—each of which may be influenced by the environment, diet, diseases, and ageing. Importantly, epigenetic marks have been shown to influence immune cell maturation and are associated with the risk of developing various forms of cancer, including lung cancer. Moreover, there is emerging evidence that these epigenetic marks affect gene expression in the lung and are associated with benign lung diseases, such as asthma, chronic obstructive pulmonary disease, and interstitial lung disease. Technological advances have made it feasible to study epigenetic marks in the lung, and it is anticipated that this knowledge will enhance our understanding of the dynamic biology in the lung and lead to the development of novel diagnostic and therapeutic approaches for our patients with lung disease.

▶ Much of the current focus in translational lung cancer research is directed to the identification of driver mutations and chromosomal translocations because these provide potentially suitable targets for therapeutic interventions. As opposed to changes in the DNA sequence, epigenetics is a field that studies heritable changes in gene expression caused by other mechanisms. The 3 main classes of epigenetic changes—DNA methylation, modifications of histone tails, and noncoding RNAs such as microRNA (miRNAs)—can be influenced by environmental exposures, diet, and aging. For example, cigarette smoke exposure appears to be associated with differential methylation of specific areas of the genome as well as with expression of miRNAs.[1-4] Epigenetic mechanisms appear to be involved in T-cell differentiation, which may play a role in diseases whose prevalence is changing, for example asthma, and in the control of gene expression in chronic lung diseases, including chronic obstructive pulmonary disease. More recently, demonstration of epigenetic regulation in lung cancer related to DNA methylation, histone methylation, and miRNA expression have been described.[5-8] Understanding these dynamic processes in the lung may help further clarify the mechanisms and influence of modifiable and nonmodifiable factors in the development of lung cancer and contribute to the development of novel therapeutic approaches.

L. T. Tanoue, MD

References

1. Breton CV, Byun HM, Wang X, Salam MT, Siegmund K, Gilliland FD. DNA methylation in the arginase-nitric oxide synthase pathway is associated with exhaled nitric oxide in children with asthma. *Am J Respir Crit Care Med.* 2011;184:191-197.
2. Liu F, Killian JK, Yang M, et al. Epigenomic alterations and gene expression profiles in respiratory epithelia exposed to cigarette smoke condensate. *Oncogene.* 2010;29: 3650-3664.
3. Schembri F, Sridhar S, Perdomo C, et al. MicroRNAs as modulators of smoking-induced gene expression changes in human airway epithelium. *Proc Natl Acad Sci U S A.* 2009;106:2319-2324.
4. Izzotti A, Calin GA, Arrigo P, Steele VE, Croce CM, De Flora S. Downregulation of microRNA expression in the lungs of rats exposed to cigarette smoke. *FASEB J.* 2009;23:806-812.
5. Heller G, Zielinski CC, Zöchbauer-Müller S. Lung cancer: from single-gene methylation to methylome profiling. *Cancer Metastasis Rev.* 2010;29:95-107.
6. Chi P, Allis CD, Wang GG. Covalent histone modifications—miswritten, misinterpreted and mis-erased in human cancers. *Nat Rev Cancer.* 2010;10:457-469.
7. Croce CM. Causes and consequences of microRNA dysregulation in cancer. *Nat Rev Genet.* 2009;10:704-714.
8. Nana-Sinkam SP, Hunter MG, Nuovo GJ, et al. Integrating the MicroRNome into the study of lung disease. *Am J Respir Crit Care Med.* 2009;179:4-10.

4 Pleural, Interstitial Lung, and Pulmonary Vascular Disease

Introduction

The broad scope of this chapter includes, yet again, a diverse group of studies. The topics range from prognostic scales to new treatment options, and the effects of air-travel to the role of genetics. We open with three articles addressing interstitial lung disease. The first two strive to improve prediction of disease trajectory in a disease state that eludes effective medical therapy short of transplant. The third describes a hopeful therapy for severe ILD associated with connective tissue disease.

Three studies involving pleural disease follow. The first looks at outcomes for patients with fibrinous pleuritis and makes a strong argument for close surveillance. The next paper compares approaches to malignant effusion and ends with a draw. The third analyzes cost of various interventions and provides differing results for differing time points.

In pulmonary vascular disease, there was a flurry of publication this year. Of interest in the diagnosis and management in venous thromboembolism, a new long-acting direct thrombin inhibitor is found non-inferior to standard care. Extracorporeal membrane oxygenation is proposed as a salvage technique for those who are not candidates for embolectomy. Defensive medicine is exposed, and a remedy is proposed. Pre-emptive anticoagulation, on the other hand, gets a thumbs up (in certain circumstances).

In PAH, a long-held belief concerning heritable disease is debunked. A real-world study looks at the effects of commercial air travel, and exercise is found to be beneficial for even the sickest patients. On the treatment front, statins fail in humans once again, and intravenous treprostinil is associated with gram negative blood stream infections. On the bright side, tadalifil is found to be a safe and effective long-term therapy, and inhaled treprostinil shows promise in pediatric patients. Additionally, the PHAROS registry describes outcomes in patients with scleroderma and "borderline" PH. The chapter concludes with long-term survival data from the REVEAL registry, which provides a strong argument that the hard work of the last 22 years has not been in vain.

Christopher D. Spradley, MD, FCCP

Interstitial Lung Disease

Predicting survival in newly diagnosed idiopathic pulmonary fibrosis: a 3-year prospective study

Mura M, Porretta MA, Bargagli E, et al (Univ of Rome "Tor Vergata", Italy; Univ of Siena, Italy; et al)
Eur Respir J 40:101-109, 2012

The natural history of idiopathic pulmonary fibrosis (IPF) is not well defined, and its clinical course is variable. We sought to investigate the survival and incidence of acute exacerbations (AEs) and their significant predictors in newly diagnosed patients.

70 patients newly diagnosed with IPF were prospectively followed for at least 3 yrs. Baseline evaluation included Medical Research Council dyspnoea score (MRCDS), 6-min walk test, pulmonary function tests, all of which were repeated at 6 months, and high-resolution computed tomography. A retrospective cohort of 68 patients was used for confirmation.

Mean survival from the time of diagnosis was 30 months, with a 3-yr mortality of 46%. A Risk stratification ScorE (ROSE) based on MRCDS > 3, 6-min walking distance $\leq$ 72% predicted and composite physiologic index > 41 predicted 3-yr mortality with high specificity. 6-month progression of ROSE predicted rapid progression. 3-yr incidence of AE was 18.6%, mostly occurring in the first 18 months; risk factors for AE were concomitant emphysema and low diffusing coefficient of the lung for carbon monoxide. Results were confirmed in an independent cohort of patients.

In newly diagnosed IPF, advanced disease at presentation, rapid progression and AEs are the determinants of 3-yr survival. The purpose of the multifactorial ROSE is to risk-stratify patients in order to predict survival and detect rapid disease progression.

▶ This Italian study was designed to develop a risk stratification score based on clinical indicators obtained at diagnosis and repeated at 6 months with the goal of optimizing timing to lung transplantation. Because transplant is the only effective therapy for this devastating disease, early determination of patients at risk is vital to select appropriate candidates for the life-saving procedure.

The study identified the Medical Research Council dyspnea score cutoff of > 3, a 6-minute walk distance less than or equal to 72% of predicted and a composite physiologic index of < 41 predictive of 3-year mortality. Six-month progression of these parameters reflected rapid progression. These findings are best summarized in Fig 4 in the original article. The findings were confirmed through utilization of a retrospective cohort of 68 patients.

The study's reliance on the retrospective cohort, its size, and exclusion of pulmonary hypertension as a prognostic factor were sited as weaknesses; still, this tool could prove useful in the future if validated in larger prospective studies of similar populations. The tool is easily reproducible in the clinical setting and thus demonstrates practical applicability.

C. D. Spradley, MD

Acute exacerbations and pulmonary hypertension in advanced idiopathic pulmonary fibrosis
Judge EP, Fabre A, Adamali HI, et al (Mater Misericordiae Univ Hosp, Dublin, Ireland)
Eur Respir J 40:93-100, 2012

The aim of this study was to evaluate the risk factors for and outcomes of acute exacerbations in patients with advanced idiopathic pulmonary fibrosis (IPF), and to examine the relationship between disease severity and neovascularisation in explanted IPF lung tissue.

55 IPF patients assessed for lung transplantation were divided into acute (n = 27) and non-acute exacerbation (n = 28) groups. Haemodynamic data was collected at baseline, at the time of acute exacerbation and at lung transplantation. Histological analysis and CD31 immunostaining to quantify microvessel density (MVD) was performed on the explanted lung tissue of 13 transplanted patients.

Acute exacerbations were associated with increased mortality ($p = 0.0015$). Pulmonary hypertension (PH) at baseline and acute exacerbations were associated with poor survival ($p < 0.01$). PH at baseline was associated with a significant risk of acute exacerbations (HR 2.217, $p = 0.041$). Neovascularisation (MVD) was significantly increased in areas of cellular fibrosis and significantly decreased in areas of honeycombing. There was a significant inverse correlation between mean pulmonary artery pressure and MVD in areas of honeycombing.

Acute exacerbations were associated with significantly increased mortality in patients with advanced IPF. PH was associated with the subsequent development of an acute exacerbation and with poor survival. Neovascularisation was significantly decreased in areas of honeycombing, and was significantly inversely correlated with mean pulmonary arterial pressure in areas of honeycombing.

▶ In this Irish study published in the *European Respiratory Journal*, Judge et al sought to identify the relationship between acute exacerbation (AE), pulmonary hypertension, and neovascularization and their impact on mortality.

AE was defined as acute onset of dyspnea or hypoxemia with progression of infiltrates in absence of heart failure, pulmonary embolism, and infection. AEs occurred at a rate of 19.11% per year and strongly correlated with mortality as demonstrated by the Kaplan—Meier curves comparing patients presenting with and without AE (Fig 1 in the original article).

Pulmonary hypertension at baseline in combination with AE was associated with highest mortality. Pulmonary hypertension at baseline also predicted likelihood of exacerbation in patients presenting without exacerbation.

The study also assessed CD31 markers on histologic samples from explanted lungs after transplant and found that microvascular density was inversely proportional to degree of pulmonary hypertension and degree of honeycombing.

This study highlights the important role as well as the interplay between pulmonary hypertension and AE in a patient population with poor outcomes. These findings may provide guidance in terms of timing for lung transplantation.

The study did read like 2 separate reports, and it was difficult to reconcile the histologic data with the hemodynamic and AE data. Also, in the conclusion, a call for investigation of pulmonary vasodilator therapy stands in stark contrast to the results of multiple industry-sponsored negative trials in this study population. Still, the findings are intriguing and warrant additional investigation.

C. D. Spradley, MD

Severe interstitial lung disease in connective tissue disease: rituximab as rescue therapy
Keir GJ, Maher TM, Hansell DM, et al (Royal Brompton Hosp, London, UK; et al)
Eur Respir J 40:641-648, 2012

In very severe interstitial lung disease associated with connective tissue disease (CTD-ILD), progressing despite maximal conventional immuno-suppression, there is no effective medical rescue therapy.

The aim of the present study was to test whether rituximab, a monoclonal antibody that depletes peripheral B lymphocytes, is effective as rescue therapy in very severe CTD-ILD, unresponsive to conventional immunosuppression.

We performed a retrospective assessment of eight patients with severe and progressive CTD-ILD treated with rituximab. In six patients, change in pulmonary function tests (PFTs) compared with pre-rituximab levels, was assessed at 9–12 months post-treatment. In two patients, who were mechanically ventilated at the time of treatment, clinical and HRCT changes were assessed.

Seven out of eight patients had a favourable treatment response to rituximab, while in one patient disease severity did not change. In contrast with previous progression, we observed a median significant improvement of 22% in diffusing capacity for carbon monoxide (from a median baseline of 25%; range 16–32%; $p = 0.04$), and a median significant improvement of 18% in forced vital capacity (from a median baseline of 45%; range 37–59%; $p = 0.03$), in the 9–12 months following treatment with rituximab.

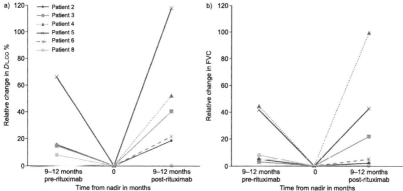

FIGURE 1.—a) Change in diffusion capacity of the lung for carbon monoxide (D_L,co) % predicted in the 9–12 months before and after rituximab administration. Following rituximab, there was a median improvement in D_L,co % pred of 22% (range 0–119%; $p = 0.04$), in contrast to a median decline of 16% (range 8–67%) prior to rituximab. b) Change in forced vital capacity (FVC) % pred in the 9–12 months before and after rituximab administration. Following rituximab, there was a median improvement in FVC % pred of 18% (range 0–100%; $p = 0.03$), in contrast to a median decline of 29% (range 3–45%) prior to rituximab. (Reprinted from Keir GJ, Maher TM, Hansell DM, et al. Severe interstitial lung disease in connective tissue disease: rituximab as rescue therapy. *Eur Respir J.* 2012;40:641-648, © 2012, European Respiratory Society.)

In very severe CTD-ILD unresponsive to conventional immunosuppression, rituximab may represent an effective, potentially life-saving, therapeutic intervention (Fig 1, Table 1).

▶ Idiopathic pulmonary fibrosis (IPF) has eluded effective medical treatment since its first description, and patients rely on appropriate and timely referral for transplantation for best outcomes. In stark contrast, connective tissue disease associated with interstitial lung disease (CTD-ILD) has demonstrated varied response to multiple medical therapies in a number of well-designed trials. Still, patients with advanced disease frequently face the same choices seen in IPF: new lungs or palliative measures.

In this article by Keir et al published in the *European Respiratory Journal*, 8 patients with severe CTD-ILD were treated with rituximab as rescue therapy. Characteristics of these patients are presented in Table 1. Fig 1 illustrates change in diffusing capacity of the lung and forced vital capacity before treatment, at time of treatment (baseline), and 9 to 12 months after therapy. Seven of 8 patients demonstrated a striking response to therapy, and these responses are summarized patient by patient in the body of the article.

This study is small and observational, but it complements earlier work[1,2] on this patient population that demonstrated favorable outcomes in patients with less severe disease.

In the appropriately selected patient, the use of rituximab as salvage therapy for severe CTD-ILD may prove an excellent choice.

C. D. Spradley, MD

TABLE 1.—Baseline Characteristics of Patients Treated with Rituximab, Including Immunosuppressive Therapy in the Previous 12 Months

Patient	Age/Sex	HRCT Pattern	Year of ILD Diagnosis	Serum Auto-Antibody/CTD Features	Pre-Rituximab Immunosuppression
Polymyositis/dermatomyositis					
1	45/M	Organising pneumonia/DAD	2009	ENA, anti-Ro positive DM on muscle biopsy	i.v. methylprednisolone
2	60/M	Fibrotic NSIP*	2003	Anti-Jo 1, myositis	MMF, prednisolone, cyclosporine i.v. cyclophosphamide
3	60/F	Fibrotic NSIP	2000	Anti-Jo 1, myositis rheumatoid factor	MMF, prednisolone i.v. cyclophosphamide
4	29/F	Fibrotic NSIP	2009	Anti-Jo 1, myositis anti-Ro	MMF, prednisolone i.v. cyclophosphamide
5	51/M	Fibrotic NSIP	2005	Anti-Jo 1, myositis	MMF, prednisolone i.v. cyclophosphamide
Undifferentiated CTD					
6	49/M	Fibrotic NSIP	2006	ANA +++ (speckled) Raynaud's, GORD	i.v. cyclophosphamide prednisolone, MMF
7	37/F	Organising pneumonia/DAD	2009	Rheumatoid factor anti-CCP, anti-Ro	i.v. methylprednisolone
Systemic sclerosis					
8	63/M	Fibrotic NSIP	1999	ATA	MMF, prednisolone

HRCT: high-resolution computed tomography; ILD: interstitial lung disease; CTD: connective tissue disease; M: male; F: female; DAD: diffuse alveolar damage; ENA: extractable nuclear antigen; DM: dermatomyositis; NSIP: non-specific interstitial pneumonia; MMF: mycophenolate mofetil; ANA: anti-nuclear antibody; GORD: gastrooesophageal reflux disease; CCP: cyclic citrullinated peptide; ATA: anti-topoisomerase antibody.
*Fibrotic NSIP confirmed on surgical lung biopsy.

References

1. Sem M, Molberg O, Lund MB, Gran JT. Rituximab treatment of the anti-synthetase syndrome: a retrospective case series. *Rheumatology (Oxford)*. 2009; 48:968-971.
2. Daoussis D, Liossis SN, Tsamandas AC, et al. Experience with rituximab in scleroderma: results from a 1-year, proof-of-principle study. *Rheumatology (Oxford)*. 2010;49:271-280.

Pleural Disease

Outcome of patients diagnosed with fibrinous pleuritis after medical thoracoscopy

Metintas M, Ak G, Cadirci O, et al (Eskisehir Osmangazi Univ, Turkey)
Respir Med 106:1177-1183, 2012

Background.—In patients with post- medical thoracoscopy histopathological diagnoses of fibrinous pleuritis, confusion can occur concerning subsequent procedures. This issue is particularly important in regions where mesothelioma is prevalent. We aimed to identify false negatives among patients where mesothelioma was common due to asbestos exposure whose histopathological diagnosis following thoracoscopy was fibrinous pleuritis. We also determined risk factors associated with patients that required additional advanced invasive procedures for diagnosis.

Methods.—Overall, 287 patients who underwent thoracoscopy were included in the study. Patients diagnosed with fibrinous pleuritis as a result of thoracoscopy were followed for 2 years regarding this condition. More invasive procedures were performed on patients who showed no recuperation or developed pleural disease again during the follow-up period.

Results.—Fibrinous pleuritis was observed in 101 (35.2%) patients. Follow-up of these patients revealed that the false negative rate was 18% for malignant pleural diseases. The thoracoscopist's opinion regarding the pleural space, computed tomography scan findings indicating malignancy, pain and female gender were determined to be risk factors for malignant pleural diseases.

Conclusions.—In regions where mesothelioma is prevalent and one of the above-stated risk factors is present, patients whose post-thoracoscopy histopathological diagnosis is fibrinous pleuritis should be treated with a more advanced invasive diagnosis procedure.

▶ Medical thoracoscopy is a powerful tool in the field of pleural disease based on its ability to obtain tissue diagnosis in the setting of negative pleural fluid studies.[1] In this study by Metintas et al, the diagnostic yield of this tool is called into question, specifically in the setting of a tissue diagnosis of fibrinous pleuritis.

The team followed patients with this "benign" diagnosis for 2 years and found a false-negative rate of 18% for their population. They identified the thoracoscopist's opinion regarding the pleural space, suspicious findings on imaging, pain, and female gender to be independent factors. The population studied demonstrated a high incidence of mesothelioma, and females tended to have higher levels of exposure to asbestos than males.

Imaging findings that increase suspicion of false-negative results included a rind-like appearance of the pleura, mediastinal involvement, thickness greater than 1 cm, and invasion of surrounding structures.

Based on the findings of this study, a tissue diagnosis of fibrinous pleuritis by medical thoracoscopy should be questioned when the described risk factors are identified, particularly if there is a high incidence of mesothelioma in the population.

C. D. Spradley, MD

Reference

1. Blanc FX, Atassi K, Bignon J, Housset B. Diagnostic value of medical thoracoscopy in pleural disease: a 6-year retrospective study. *Chest.* 2002;121:1677-1683.

Effect of an Indwelling Pleural Catheter vs Chest Tube and Talc Pleurodesis for Relieving Dyspnea in Patients With Malignant Pleural Effusion: The TIME2 Randomized Controlled Trial

Davies HE, Mishra EK, Kahan BC, et al (Univ Hosp of Wales, Cardiff; Churchill Hosp, Oxford, England; Med Res Council's Clinical Trials Unit, London; UK)
JAMA 307:2383-2389, 2012

Context.—Malignant pleural effusion causes disabling dyspnea in patients with a short life expectancy. Palliation is achieved by fluid drainage, but the most effective first-line method has not been determined.

Objective.—To determine whether indwelling pleural catheters (IPCs) are more effective than chest tube and talc slurry pleurodesis (talc) at relieving dyspnea.

Design.—Unblinded randomized controlled trial (Second Therapeutic Intervention in Malignant Effusion Trial [TIME2]) comparing IPC and talc (1:1) for which 106 patients with malignant pleural effusion who had not previously undergone pleurodesis were recruited from 143 patients who were treated at 7 UK hospitals. Patients were screened from April 2007-February 2011 and were followed up for a year.

Intervention.—Indwelling pleural catheters were inserted on an outpatient basis, followed by initial large volume drainage, education, and subsequent home drainage. The talc group were admitted for chest tube insertion and talc for slurry pleurodesis.

Main Outcome Measure.—Patients completed daily 100-mm line visual analog scale (VAS) of dyspnea over 42 days after undergoing the intervention (0 mm represents no dyspnea and 100 mm represents maximum dyspnea; 10 mm represents minimum clinically significant difference). Mean difference was analyzed using a mixed-effects linear regression model adjusted for minimization variables.

Results.—Dyspnea improved in both groups, with no significant difference in the first 42 days with a mean VAS dyspnea score of 24.7 in the IPC group (95% CI, 19.3-30.1 mm) and 24.4 mm (95% CI, 19.4–29.4 mm) in the talc group, with a difference of 0.16 mm (95% CI, −6.82 to 7.15; $P = .96$). There was a statistically significant improvement in dyspnea in the IPC group at 6 months, with a mean difference in VAS score between the IPC group and the talc group of −14.0 mm (95% CI, −25.2 to −2.8 mm; $P = .01$). Length of initial hospitalization was significantly shorter in the IPC group with a median of 0 days (interquartile range [IQR], 0-1 day) and 4 days (IQR, 2–6 days) for the talc group, with a difference of −3.5 days (95% CI, −4.8 to −1.5 days; $P < .001$). There was no significant difference in quality of life. Twelve patients (22%) in the talc group required further pleural procedures compared with 3 (6%) in the IPC group (odds ratio [OR], 0.21; 95% CI, 0.04–0.86; $P = .03$). Twenty-one of the 52 patients in the catheter group experienced adverse events vs 7 of 54 in the talc group (OR, 4.70; 95% CI, 1.75–12.60; $P = .002$).

Conclusion.—Among patients with malignant pleural effusion and no previous pleurodesis, there was no significant difference between IPCs and talc pleurodesis at relieving patient-reported dyspnea.

Trial Registration.—isrctn.org Identifier: ISRCTN87514420.

▶ In this British study, Davies et al sought to compare tunneled pleural catheters and talc pleurodesis for treatment of malignant pleural effusion by comparing patient-reported pain and dyspnea. Quality of life, adverse events, and hospital stay were secondary end points. Patient data were collected for up to 12 months.

Both procedures performed well on the primary end point of dyspnea up to 6 months with a divergence thereafter favoring the indwelling pleural catheters (IPC) group. Chest pain was statistically similar for both sets of patients at all time points (Figs 2 and 3 in the original article.)

Length of stay for IPC averaged 0 days compared with 1 days in the talc group. Including complication-related admission during the follow-up period, those numbers rose to 1 and 4.5 days, respectively. There was no significant difference in quality of life between the 2 techniques for the time period studied. A total of 40% of patients with IPC and 13% of patients with talc experienced an adverse event, demonstrating a statistically significant difference.

In the end, the primary outcomes were the same at 6 months, and the results from secondary end points were mixed.

This study was obviously not blinded and some of the data (especially length of stay) are not generalizable to the US population. In the end, the decision of treatment modality, based on the findings of this study, will need to be based on patient preferences concerning length of stay, attitudes about home drainage, expected survival, and risk of complication. Procedural cost is considered in the next study presented here.

C. D. Spradley, MD

Treatment of Malignant Pleural Effusion: A Cost-Effectiveness Analysis
Puri V, Pyrdeck TL, Crabtree TD, et al (Washington Univ at St Louis, MO)
Ann Thorac Surg 94:374-380, 2012

Background.—Patients with malignant pleural effusion (MPE) have varied expected survival and treatment options. We studied the relative cost-effectiveness of various interventions.

Methods.—Decision analysis was used to compare repeated thoracentesis (RT), tunneled pleural catheter (TPC), bedside pleurodesis (BP), and thoracoscopic pleurodesis (TP). Outcomes and utility data were obtained from institutional data and review of literature. Medicare allowable charges were used to ensure uniformity. Base case analysis was performed for two scenarios: expected survival of 3 months and expected survival of 12 months. The incremental cost-effectiveness ratio (ICER) was estimated as the cost per quality-adjusted life-year gained over the patient's remaining lifetime.

TABLE 1.—Base Case Assumptions for a Patient With Malignant Pleural Effusion With Expected Survival of 3 Months

Treatment	Incidence of Pleural Sclerosis	Source of Pleural Sclerosis Data [Ref]	Risk of Complications	Source of Complications Data [Ref]	Total Cost (2010 US$)	Source of Cost Data
Repeated thoracentesis	0%	[6, 27, 28]	2%	[29]	4,946	CMS allowable, institutional data
Tunneled pleural catheter	40%	[8–11]	5%	[8]	6,450	CMS allowable, institutional data
Bedside pleurodesis	73%	[6, 7, 30, 31]	Complications 9%, mortality 1%	[7, 30, 32, 33]	11,224	CMS allowable, institutional data
Thoracoscopic pleurodesis	87%	[2–5, 7]	Complications 14%, mortality 2%	[2–5, 7], institutional data	18,604	CMS allowable, institutional data

Editor's Note: Please refer to original journal article for full references.
CMS = Centers for Medicare and Medicaid Services.

TABLE 2.—Results of One-Way Sensitivity Analysis With Variations in Rate of Pleural Sclerosis With Tunneled Pleural Catheter

TPC Sclerosis[a]	Strategy	Cost	Incr Cost	Eff	Incr Eff	C/E	Incr C/E (ICER)
0.25	Repeated thoracentesis	$4,946		0.1123 yrs		$44,063	
	Tunneled pleural catheter	$6,652	$1,706	0.1416 yrs	0.0294 yrs	$46,969	$58,070
	Catheter pleurodesis	$11,224		0.1362 yrs		$82,391	(Dominated)
	Thoracoscopic pleurodesis	$18,604		0.1365 yrs		$136,285	(Dominated)
0.375	Repeated thoracentesis	$4,946		0.1123 yrs		$44,063	
	Tunneled pleural catheter	$6,484	$1,538	0.1422 yrs	0.0300 yrs	$45,589	$51,300
	Catheter pleurodesis	$11,224		0.1362 yrs		$82,391	(Dominated)
	Thoracoscopic pleurodesis	$18,604		0.1365 yrs		$136,285	(Dominated)
0.5	Repeated thoracentesis	$4,946		0.1123 yrs		$44,063	
	Tunneled pleural catheter	$6,315	$1,369	0.1428 yrs	0.0305 yrs	$44,220	$44,793
	Catheter pleurodesis	$11,224		0.1362 yrs		$82,391	(Dominated)
	Thoracoscopic pleurodesis	$18,604		0.1365 yrs		$136,285	(Dominated)
0.625	Repeated thoracentesis	$4,946		0.1123 yrs		$44,063	
	Tunneled pleural catheter	$6,147	$1,201	0.1434 yrs	0.0312 yrs	$42,862	$38,535
	Catheter pleurodesis	$11,224		0.1362 yrs		$82,391	(Dominated)
	Thoracoscopic pleurodesis	$18,604		0.1365 yrs		$136,285	(Dominated)
0.75	Repeated thoracentesis	$4,946		0.1123 yrs		$44,063	
	Tunneled pleural catheter	$5,978	$1,032	0.1440 yrs	0.0318 yrs	$41,516	$32,510
	Catheter pleurodesis	$11,224		0.1362 yrs		$82,391	(Dominated)
	Thoracoscopic pleurodesis	$18,604		0.1365 yrs		$136,285	(Dominated)

As the assumed rate of pleural sclerosis with tunneled pleural catheter (TPC) increases from 15% to 75% (column 1), the strategy becomes more cost effective (C/E), demonstrated by a decrease in the incremental (Incr) cost-effectiveness ratio (ICER) from $58,070 to $32,510 (column 8).

Eff = effectiveness (in quality-adjusted life-years); yrs = years.

[a]Incidence of pleural sclerosis with TPC (shown as a fraction).

Results.—Under base case analysis for 3-month survival, RT was the least expensive treatment ($4,946) and provided the fewest utilities (0.112 quality-adjusted life-years). The cost of therapy for the other options was TPC $6,450, BP $11,224, and TP $18,604. Tunneled pleural catheter dominated both pleurodesis arms, namely, TPC was both less expensive and more effective. The ICER for TPC over RT was $49,978. The ICER was sensitive to complications and ability to achieve pleural sclerosis with TPC. Under base case analysis for 12-month survival, BP was the least expensive treatment ($13,057) and provided 0.59 quality-adjusted life-years. The cost of treatment for the other options was TPC $13,224, TP $19,074, and RT $21,377. Bedside pleurodesis dominated TPC and thoracentesis. Thoracoscopic pleurodesis was more effective than BP but the ICER for TP over BP was greater than $250,000.

Conclusions.—Using decision analysis, TPC is the preferred treatment for patients with malignant pleural effusion and limited survival; BP is the most cost-effective treatment for patients with more prolonged expected survival (Tables 1 and 2).

▶ In this study, Puri et al performed a cost-effectiveness analysis comparing repeat thoracentesis, tunneled pleural catheters, bedside pleurodesis, and thoracoscopic pleurodesis for the treatment of malignant pleural effusion. The effectiveness of treatments was assessed by evaluating quality-adjusted life years (QALY)—increase in utility multiplied by the time in years that the utility is enjoyed. The incremental cost effectiveness ration (ICER) was then calculated by dividing the actual cost of the procedure by QALY.

Tunneled pleural catheters were found to have the highest ICER for patients surviving 3 months, but this was sensitive to complication level and effectiveness of pleural sclerosis. Bedside pleurodesis demonstrated higher ICER at the 12-month survival benchmark because of reduced cost despite lower QALY, performing better than tunneled pleural catheters with long-term cost, and outperforming thoracoscopic pleurodesis despite less efficacy because of the higher cost of the latter procedure (Table 2).

The analyses make a number of assumptions, including the idea that all patients are suitable for anesthesia, lung is not trapped, and the pleural space is uncomplicated; however, putting these aside, the base case assumptions (Table 1) are easily generalizable in centers with adequate expertise at performing the procedure.

Cost-effectiveness analysis will likely be a common fixture of the medical literature going forward. This particular article, given certain plausible assumptions, provides a reasonable cost-effectiveness argument for treatment choice at 2 time points. These findings complement the results of the previous article and may help in formulation of treatment decisions based on presumed survival.

C. D. Spradley, MD

Pulmonary Vascular Disease

Enoxaparin followed by once-weekly idrabiotaparinux versus enoxaparin plus warfarin for patients with acute symptomatic pulmonary embolism: a randomised, double-blind, double-dummy, non-inferiority trial
Büller HR, on behalf of the Cassiopea Investigators (Academic Med Centre, Amsterdam, Netherlands; et al)
Lancet 379:123-129, 2012

Background.—Treatment of pulmonary embolism with low-molecular-weight heparin and vitamin K antagonists, such as warfarin, is not ideal. We aimed to assess non-inferiority of idrabiotaparinux, a reversible longlasting indirect inhibitor of activated factor X, to warfarin in patients with acute symptomatic pulmonary embolism.

Methods.—In our randomised, double-blind, double-dummy, non-inferiority trial, we enrolled adults with objectively documented acute symptomatic pulmonary embolism attending 291 centres in 37 countries. We excluded patients who were pregnant, had active bleeding, kidney failure, or malignant hypertension, or were at high risk of death, bleeding, or adverse reactions to study drugs. We randomly allocated patients to receive 5—10 days' enoxaparin 1·0 mg/kg twice daily followed by subcutaneous idrabiotaparinux (starting dose 3·0 mg) or adjusted-dose warfarin (target international normalised ratio 2·0—3·0); regimens lasted 3 months or 6 months dependent on clinical presentation. Block randomisation was done with a central interactive computerised system, stratified by study centre and intended treatment duration. The primary efficacy outcome was recurrent venous thromboembolism at 99 days after randomisation. We estimated the odds ratio and 95% CI with a Mantel-Haenszel χ^2 analysis (non-inferiority margin 2·0) in the intention-to-treat population. The main safety outcome was clinically relevant bleeding (major or non-major) in all patients at day 99. This study is registered with ClinicalTrials.gov, number NCT00345618.

Findings.—Between Aug 1, 2006, and Jan 31, 2010, we enrolled 3202 patients aged 18—96 years. 34 (2%) of 1599 patients randomly allocated to receive enoxaparin-idrabiotaparinux and 43 (3%) of 1603 patients randomly allocated to receive enoxaparin-warfarin had recurrent venous thromboembolism (odds ratio 0·79, 95% CI 0·50—1·25; $P_{non-inferiority} = 0·0001$). 72 (5%) of 1599 patients in the enoxaparin-idrabiotaparinux group and 106 (7%) of 1603 patients in the enoxaparin-warfarin group had clinically relevant bleeding (0·67, 0·49—0·91; $P_{superiority} = 0·0098$). We noted similar differences in outcomes in those patients treated to 6 months.

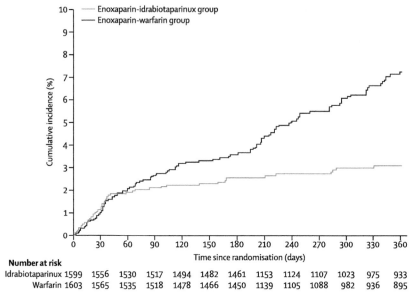

Number at risk

	0	30	60	90	120	150	180	210	240	270	300	330	360
Idrabiotaparinux	1599	1556	1530	1517	1494	1482	1461	1153	1124	1107	1023	975	933
Warfarin	1603	1565	1535	1518	1478	1466	1450	1139	1105	1088	982	936	895

FIGURE 2.—Cumulative incidence of pulmonary embolism and deep vein thrombosis (fatal or non-fatal) to study end. (Reprinted from The Lancet. Büller HR, on behalf of the Cassiopea Investigators. Enoxaparin followed by once-weekly idrabiotaparinux versus enoxaparin plus warfarin for patients with acute symptomatic pulmonary embolism: a randomised, double-blind, double-dummy, non-inferiority trial. *Lancet.* 2012;379:123-129, Copyright 2012, with permission from Elsevier.)

Interpretation.—Idrabiotaparinux could provide an attractive alternative to warfarin for the long-term treatment of pulmonary embolism, and seems to be associated with reduced bleeding (Figs 2 and 3).

▶ Heparin-based anticoagulation followed by vitamin K antagonists has been the cornerstone of therapy for deep vein thrombosis (DVT) for decades. The advent of direct thrombin inhibitors brought with it the promise of alternative therapy. For those living with the cumbersome dietary restrictions and international normalized ratio monitoring imposed by chronic warfarin therapy, these drugs were a hopeful development. Unfortunately, the new drugs are difficult to monitor and their anti-coagulant effect is irreversible, which has caused concern for clinicians, especially for patients at high bleeding risk.

Büller et al evaluated an injected thrombin inhibitor with a twist. A biotin moiety was added to idraparinux, a long-acting thrombin inhibitor formulated for weekly dosing. The addition of biotin did not change the efficacy of the drug but did allow for rapid reversal of anticoagulant effect with infusion of the readily available antidote: avidin.

This double-blind, double-dummy, randomized controlled trial was powered for noninferiority in prevention of recurrent DVT at 99 days, and the main safety outcome was clinically relevant bleeding. Interestingly, though not powered for this assessment, the study did demonstrate a trend toward reduced DVT recurrence and reduced bleeding (Figs 2 and 3).

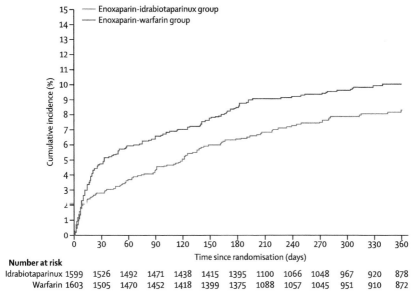

FIGURE 3.—Cumulative incidence of clinically relevant bleeding up to study end. (Reprinted from The Lancet. Büller HR, on behalf of the Cassiopea Investigators. Enoxaparin followed by once-weekly idrabiotaparinux versus enoxaparin plus warfarin for patients with acute symptomatic pulmonary embolism: a randomised, double-blind, double-dummy, non-inferiority trial. *Lancet.* 2012;379:123-129, Copyright 2012, with permission from Elsevier.)

The antidote was given 55 times in the treatment arm and was successful 3 of 4 times in reversing bleeding. It was also successful in preventing bleeding problems in 27 of 33 patients undergoing planned invasive procedures.

The authors present an attractive alternative to vitamin K antagonist therapy in patients with need for anticoagulation of 3 to 6 months' duration for the treatment of pulmonary embolus. Weekly dosing and reversibility are unique attributes that may change standard management of anticoagulation for venous thromboembolic in the near future.

C. D. Spradley, MD

Peripheral Extracorporeal Membrane Oxygenation: Comprehensive Therapy for High-Risk Massive Pulmonary Embolism
Malekan R, Saunders PC, Yu CJ, et al (New York Med College, Valhalla)
Ann Thorac Surg 94:104-108, 2012

Background.—Although commonly reserved as a last line of defense, experienced centers have reported excellent results with pulmonary embolectomy for massive and submassive pulmonary embolism (PE). We present a contemporary surgical series for PE that demonstrates the utility

TABLE.—pECMO Patient Data

Case	Sex	Age (Years)	Indication	Device	Access	PA Pre (mm Hg)	PA Post (mm Hg)	Outcome	pECMO Duration (Days)	LOS (Days)	CT Scan Resolution	CT Scan Post-PE (Weeks)
1	F	72.9	Reop/shock	Tandem	Fem-Ax	46	30	Weaned	5	15	Full	5.7
2	F	39.6	Shock/acidosis	Centrimag[a]	Fem-Ax	—	—	Weaned	5	13	Full	8
3	F	51.4	Morbid obesity	Centrimag	Fem-Ax	42	19	Weaned	6	11	Near-full	4.4
4	M	23.4	Shock/acidosis	Centrimag	RIJ-Ax	62	—	Surgery	10	23	—	—
Average		46.8				50.0	24.5		6.5	13		

CT = computed tomographic; Fem-Ax = femoral venous and right axillary arterial; LOS = length of stay; PA = pulmonary artery; PE = pulmonary embolism; pECMO = peripheral extracorporeal membrane oxygenation; Reop = reoperation; RIJ-Ax = right internal jugular axillary arterial.
[a]Centrimag (Levitronix LLC, Waltham, MA).

of peripheral extracorporeal membrane oxygenation (pECMO) for high-risk surgical candidates.

Methods.—Between June 2005 and April 2011, 29 patients were treated for massive or submassive pulmonary embolism, with surgical embolectomy performed in 26. Four high-risk patients were placed on pECMO, established by percutaneously cannulating the right atrium through a femoral vein and perfusing by a Dacron graft anastomosed to the axillary artery. A small, extracorporeal, rotary assist device was used, interposing a compact oxygenator in the circuit, and maintaining anticoagulation with heparin.

Results.—Extracorporeal membrane oxygenation was weaned in 3 of 4 patients after 5.3 days (5, 5, and 6), with normalization of right ventricular dysfunction and pulmonary artery pressure (44.0 ± 2.0 to 24.5 ± 5.5 mm Hg) by ECHO. Follow-up computed tomographies showed several peripheral, nearly resorbed emboli in 1 case and complete resolution in 2 others. The fourth patient, not improving after 10 days, underwent surgery where an embolic liposarcoma was extracted. For all 29 cases, hospital and 30-day mortality was 0% and all patients were discharged, with average postoperative length of stay of 15 days for embolectomy and 17 days for pECMO.

Conclusions.—Heparin therapy with pECMO support is a rapid, effective option for patients who might benefit from pulmonary embolectomy but are at high risk for surgery (Table).

▶ Extracorporeal membrane oxygenation (ECMO) used to be a tool reserved for use in the pediatric population. Recent studies[1,2] in adult patients suffering severe adult respiratory distress syndrome and in-hospital cardiac arrest have revived interest in this technology for the adult patient population.

Despite advances in treatment, massive pulmonary embolism (PE) still results in significant morbidity and mortality. Measures aimed at reducing current clot burden and restoring pulmonary circulation (thrombolysis, catheter extraction, and surgical embolectomy) have produced mixed results.

Recently published series[3] from experienced surgical centers have shown promise in terms of treatment of massive PE. Unfortunately, not all centers have experience in this procedure, and many patients are poor surgical candidates.

Venoatrial ECMO in combination with heparin may prove an attractive alternative choice in this patient population. Malekan et al present a series of 4 patients treated for massive PE with this approach (Table). The technique was successful in sustaining circulation and treating acidosis in all patients. ECMO was successfully weaned in 3 patients and provided a bridge to surgical resection of an embolized liposarcoma in the fourth. All 4 patients survived and were discharged home.

Indeed, ECMO may prove to be a useful alternative in patients too unstable to undergo surgical thrombectomy. The technique is time- and resource-intensive, but it does have the potential to save lives.

C. D. Spradley, MD

References

1. Davies A, Jones D, Bailey M, et al. Extracorporeal membrane oxygenation for 2009 influenza A(H1N1) acute respiratory distress syndrome. *JAMA.* 2009;302: 1888-1895.
2. Sakamoto S, Taniguchi N, Nakajima S, Takahashi A. Extracorporeal life support for cardiogenic shock or cardiac arrest due to acute coronary syndrome. *Ann Thorac Surg.* 2012;94:1-7.
3. Leacche M, Unic D, Goldhaber SZ, et al. Modern surgical treatment of massive pulmonary embolism: results in 47 consecutive patients after rapid diagnosis and aggressive surgical approach. *J Thorac Cardiovasc Surg.* 2005;129:1018-1023.

Ordering CT pulmonary angiography to exclude pulmonary embolism: defense versus evidence in the emergency room
Rohacek M, Buatsi J, Szucs-Farkas Z, et al (Univ Hosp Bern, Switzerland; et al)
Intensive Care Med 38:1345-1351, 2012

Purpose.—To identify reasons for ordering computed tomography pulmonary angiography (CTPA), to identify the frequency of reasons for CTPA reflecting defensive behavior and evidence-based behavior, and to identify the impact of defensive medicine and of training about diagnosing pulmonary embolism (PE) on positive results of CTPA.

Methods.—Physicians in the emergency department of a tertiary care hospital completed a questionnaire before CTPA after being trained about diagnosing PE and completing questionnaires.

Results.—Nine hundred patients received a CTPA during 3 years. For 328 CTPAs performed during the 1-year study period, 140 (43%) questionnaires were completed. The most frequent reasons for ordering a CTPA were to confirm/rule out PE (93%), elevated D-dimers (66%), fear of missing PE (55%), and Wells/simplified revised Geneva score (53%). A positive answer for "fear of missing PE" was inversely associated with positive CTPA (OR 0.36, 95% CI 0.14–0.92, $p = 0.033$), and "Wells/simplified revised Geneva score" was associated with positive CTPA (OR 3.28, 95% CI 1.24–8.68, $p = 0.017$). The proportion of positive CTPA was higher if a questionnaire was completed, compared to the 2-year comparison period (26.4 vs. 14.5%, OR 2.12, 95% CI 1.36–3.29, $p > 0.001$). The proportion of positive CTPA was non-significantly higher during the study period than during the comparison period (19.2 vs. 14.5%, OR 1.40, 95% CI 0.98–2.0, $p = 0.067$).

Conclusion.—Reasons for CTPA reflecting defensive behavior—such as "fear of missing PE"—were frequent, and were associated with a decreased odds of positive CTPA. Defensive behavior might be modifiable by training in using guidelines (Fig 2).

▶ I have occasionally joked with the house staff I work with that a computed tomography (CT) scanner should be installed at the entrance of the emergency department (ED) so that patients will be forced to crawl through on their way

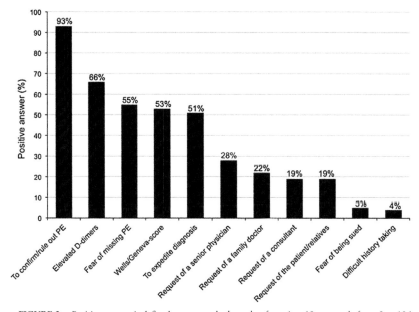

FIGURE 2.—Positive answer is defined as any marked number from 1 to 10 on a scale from 0 to 10 in the questionnaire. (With kind permission from Springer Science+Business Media: Rohacek M, Buatsi J, Szucs-Farkas Z, et al. Ordering CT pulmonary angiography to exclude pulmonary embolism: defense versus evidence in the emergency room. *Intensive Care Med.* 2012;38:1345-1351, with permission from Springer and ESICM.)

into the hospital. This way, time will be saved ordering and waiting on CT of the head and CT pulmonary angiography (CTPA).

The fact is that fear of missing a fatal diagnosis has driven a trend toward putting any patient with respiratory complaints through a CT scanner to "rule out" pulmonary embolism (PE) despite decent screening tests to rule out significant PE (D-dimer) and robust tools, such as the PE rule-out criteria (PERC), Wells, and Geneva scores.

Rohacek et al provided questionnaires to ED physicians to be completed when ordering CTPA for a 1-year period after receiving education concerning the use of Wells or Geneva scoring, as well as the utility of a normal D-dimer in ruling out significant PE.

The survey asked the physician to assign a pretest probability of PE, evidence-based or not, as well as reason for ordering. Surveys returned included responses shown in Fig 2. The authors divided responses between "evidence-based" and "defensive." Ordering practices were also compared with the prior 3 years.

The authors found that fear of missing PE as a reason for ordering was inversely related to positive CTPA, and the evidence-based approach demonstrated a positive correlation. Also, the simple act of filling out the questionnaire correlated with a positive study compared with studies that were not associated with a completed survey and the pretest period. Interestingly, for studies without a survey, there was no significant difference in rate of PE compared to the prestudy data. The proportion of positive PEs went up significantly in the completed questionnaire group.

This study suffers from low survey compliance. It was also performed at a single center in Switzerland. The litigious nature of health care in the United States would likely exaggerate the role of defensive medicine. Still, the authors have shown that defensive medicine is a problem and that through education unnecessary testing can be reduced.

C. D. Spradley, MD

Usefulness of Preemptive Anticoagulation in Patients With Suspected Pulmonary Embolism: A Decision Analysis

Blondon M, Righini M, Aujesky D, et al (Univ Hosps of Geneva, Switzerland; Bern Univ Hosp, Switzerland; et al)
Chest 142:697-703, 2012

Background.—The diagnostic workup of pulmonary embolism (PE) may take several hours. The usefulness of anticoagulant treatment while awaiting the results of diagnostic tests has not been assessed. The objective of this study was to compare the risks and benefits of bid low-molecular-weight heparin vs no treatment in patients with suspected PE.

Methods.—We developed a decision tree with the following outcomes: mortality related to untreated and treated PE, mortality due to major hemorrhage, and intracranial bleeding. The timeframe extended from the suspicion of PE to its confirmation or exclusion. Most probabilities were derived from data from the Computerized Registry of Patients with VTE (RIETE). We estimated the incidence of bleeding by categories of clinical prediction rules of PE from a recent diagnostic management study of PE. Uncertainty was assessed through one-way and probabilistic sensitivity analyses.

Results.—The model favored preemptive anticoagulation if the diagnostic delay was >6.3 h, >2.3 h, and >0.3 h (Revised Geneva low, intermediate, and high probability) and >8.1 h and >1.7 h (Wells unlikely and likely). With a diagnostic delay of 6 h, the absolute mortality reduction with anticoagulation was 0%, 0.02%, and 0.1% for low, intermediate, and high clinical

---

TABLE 2.—Preferred Strategy According to Diagnostic Delay

| | Time to Definite Diagnosis | |
Category of PE Probability	No Treatment Superior	Preemptive Anticoagulation Superior
Low RGS	<6.3 h	>6.3 h
Intermediate RGS	<2.3 h	>2.3 h
High RGS	<20 min	>20 min
Unlikely Wells Score	<8.1 h	>8.1 h
Likely Wells Score	<1.7 h	>1.7 h

See Table 1 legend for expansion of abbreviations.

probability, respectively. In one-way sensitivity analyses, the mortality of untreated PE was the most critical variable. Probabilistic analyses reinforced the superiority of anticoagulation in intermediate-and high-probability patients and suggested that low-probability patients might not benefit from treatment after diagnostic delays of <6 to 8 h.

Conclusions.—Our model suggests that patients with intermediate and high/likely probabilities of PE benefit from preemptive anticoagulation. With a low probability, the decision to treat may rely on the expected diagnostic delay (Table 2).

▶ I remember being taught in medical school that, if a pulmonary embolism (PE) is suspected, anticoagulation should be started while confirmatory testing is being arranged. The most recent American College of Chest Physicians evidence-based guideline on anticoagulation recommends treatment of patients with high clinical suspicion.[1]

The authors of this study published in *CHEST* sought to define the role of pre-emptive anticoagulation based on time to confirmative study. Their model relied on data from a venous thromboembolism registry and calculated risk of fatality due to untreated PE versus risk of bleeding. The study findings supported pre-emptive anticoagulation in patients with intermediate-to-high likelihood of PE and concluded that decision to treat low probability was dependent on the delay to confirmatory testing (Table 2 and Fig 2 in the original article). Composite probability that pre-emptive anticoagulation is the preferred approach was illustrated in Fig 3 in the original article.

The study made a number of assumptions, including constant rate of death or bleeding over time for the diagnostic delay window. The study was also retrospective in that the model was based on registry data.

The results of the study agree with the current guideline and support treatment in intermediate-risk patients. The study, when combined with evidence-based usage prediction tools,[2] provides a little more clarity for the clinician who is trying to decide to treat or not to treat.

C. D. Spradley, MD

References

1. Kearon C, Kahn SR, Agnelli G, Goldhaber S, Raskob GE, Comerota AJ; American College of Chest Physicians. Antithrombotic therapy for venous thromboembolic disease: American College of Chest Physicians evidence-based clinical practice Guidelines (8th Edition). *Chest.* 2008;133:454S-545S.
2. Laporte S, Mismetti P, Décousus H, et al; RIETE Investigators. Clinical predictors for fatal pulmonary embolism in 15,520 patients with venous thromboembolism: findings from the Registro Informatizado de la Enfermedad TromboEmbolica venosa (RIETE) Registry. *Circulation.* 2008;117:1711-1716.

Longitudinal Analysis Casts Doubt on the Presence of Genetic Anticipation in Heritable Pulmonary Arterial Hypertension

Larkin EK, Newman JH, Austin ED, et al (Vanderbilt Univ Inst for Medicine and Public Health, Nashville, TN; Vanderbilt Univ School of Medicine, Nashville, TN)
Am J Respir Crit Care Med 186:892-896, 2012

Rationale.—Analysis of the age of onset in heritable pulmonary arterial hypertension (HPAH) has led to the hypothesis that genetic anticipation causes younger age of onset and death in subsequent generations. With accrual of pedigree data over multiple decades, we retested this hypothesis using analyses that eliminate the truncation of data that exists with shorter duration of follow-up.

Objectives.—To analyze the pedigrees of families with mutations in bone morphogenetic protein receptor type 2 (BMPR2), afflicted in two or more generations with HPAH, eliminating time truncation bias by including families for whom we have at least 57 years of data.

Methods.—We analyzed 355 individuals with BMPR2 mutations from 53 families in the Vanderbilt Pulmonary Hypertension Registry. We compared age at diagnosis or death in affected individuals (n = 249) by generation within families with multi generational disease. We performed linear mixed effects models and we limited time-truncation bias by restricting date of birth to before 1955. This allowed for 57 years of follow-up (1955–2012) for mutation carriers to develop disease. We also conducted Kaplan-Meier analysis to include currently unaffected mutation carriers (n = 106).

Measurements and Main Results.—Differences in age at diagnosis by generation were found in a biased analysis that included all birth years to the present, but this finding was eliminated when the 57-year observation limit was imposed. By Kaplan-Meier analysis, inclusion of currently unaffected mutation carriers strengthens the observation that bias of ascertainment exists when recent generations are included.

Conclusions.—Genetic anticipation is likely an artifact of incomplete time of observation of kindreds with HPAH due to BMPR2 mutations.

▶ It has long been assumed that heritable pulmonary arterial hypertension (HPAH) associated with bone morphogenetic protein receptor type 2 (BMPR-2) mutation exhibits generational anticipation. This phenomenon has been identified in Huntington's disease and Fragile X,[1] and it has been found to be associated with meiotic expansion of trinucleotide repeats. This results in successive generations developing more severe disease at an earlier time. Such repeats have not been identified in BMPR-2 mutations.

The authors of this study utilized a registry of patients, including an HPAH cohort with pedigrees reaching back to before 1900. Their assumption was that the current data supporting anticipation in HPAH is biased secondary to inadequate follow-up of susceptible family members given the frequently late onset of symptomatic pulmonary arterial hypertension (PAH).

Data from their registry showed that 90% of affected individuals had PAH by age 55. As such, they limited their analysis to subjects born before 1955. With this limitation imposed, evidence of anticipation disappeared, supporting their hypothesis (Fig 1 in the original article). This finding has implications in other disease states with presumed anticipation but no evidence of trinucleotide repeats like Crohn's disease and rheumatoid arthritis.

Undoubtedly, patients with newly diagnosed HPAH will be reassured with the knowledge that their offspring will not be victims of genetic anticipation.

C. D. Spradley, MD

Reference

1. Loyd JE, Slovis B, Phillips JA 3rd, et al. The presence of genetic anticipation suggests that the molecular basis of familial primary pulmonary hypertension may be trinucleotide repeat expansion. *Chest.* 1997;111:825-835.

Effects of Commercial Air Travel on Patients With Pulmonary Hypertension

Roubinian N, Elliott CG, Barnett CF, et al (Univ of California-San Francisco; Univ of Utah, Salt Lake City)
Chest 142:885-892, 2012

Background.—Limited data are available on the effects of air travel in patients with pulmonary hypertension (PH), despite their risk of physiologic compromise. We sought to quantify the incidence and severity of hypoxemia experienced by people with PH during commercial air travel.

Methods.—We recruited 34 participants for a prospective observational study during which cabin pressure, oxygen saturation (SpO_2), heart rate, and symptoms were documented serially at multiple predefined time points throughout commercial flights. Oxygen desaturation was defined as $SpO_2 < 85\%$.

Results.—Median flight duration was 3.6 h (range, 1.0–7.3 h). Mean ± SD cabin pressure at cruising altitude was equivalent to the pressure 1,968 ± 371 m (6,456 ± 1,218 ft) above sea level (ASL) (maximum altitude = 2,621 m [8,600 ft] ASL). Median change in SpO_2 from sea level to cruising altitude was −4.9% (range, 2.0% to −15.8%). Nine subjects (26% [95% CI, 12%−38%]) experienced oxygen desaturation during flight (minimum $SpO_2 = 74\%$). Thirteen subjects (38%) reported symptoms during flight, of whom five also experienced desaturations. Oxygen desaturation was associated with cabin pressures equivalent to > 1,829 m (6,000 ft) ASL, ambulation, and flight duration (all P values < .05).

Conclusions.—Hypoxemia is common among people with PH traveling by air, occurring in one in four people studied. Hypoxemia was associated with lower cabin pressures, ambulation during flight, and longer flight duration. Patients with PH who will be traveling on flights of longer duration or

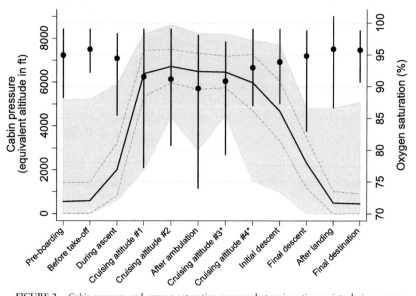

FIGURE 2.—Cabin pressure and oxygen saturation measured at various time points during commercial air travel. Solid black line 5 mean cabin pressure (dashed gray line represents ± 1.0 SD and light gray shading represents range); ● = mean oxygen saturation (vertical bars represent range). *Optional readings. (Reprinted from Roubinian N, Elliott CG, Barnett CF, et al. Effects of commercial air travel on patients with pulmonary hypertension. *Chest*. 2012;142:885-892, © 2012, American College of Chest Physicians.)

who have a history of oxygen use, including nocturnal use only, should be evaluated for supplemental in-flight oxygen (Fig 2).

▶ A pulmonary hypertension patient comes to the clinic for routine monitoring; just before the conclusion of the visit, she asks if she will need oxygen on her upcoming planned flight. In this article published in *Chest*, the authors set out to help answer that question.

They provided patients with prearranged flights with altimeters and pulse oximeters and asked them to collect data at various points during the flight. They found that on average saturations dropped 4.9% at altitude (Fig 2). Walking at altitude presented the greatest drop in saturation, to a minimum of 74% and all desaturations occurred at cabin equivalent elevation of greater than 6000 feet. The Federal Aviation Administration mandates maintaining cabin pressure at or below 8000 feet. This ceiling was violated in 1 flight from the study.

Longer flight duration was also associated with desaturation. Interestingly, resting oxygen saturation did not correlate with risk of desaturation in this population, unlike prior studies in the chronic obstructive pulmonary disease population.

Most prior studies in lung disease were performed using decreased fraction of inspired oxygen or hypobaric chambers for limited durations. The authors argue that the "real-world" scenario in this trial more realistically reflected the target environment.

Hypoxemia occurred in 26% of the study participants. Though all patients completed their flight without significant complication, this does expose a potential risk to patients. Only 1 in 10 patients from the study reported undergoing high-altitude simulation tests before the study.

Based on these findings, the authors recommend formally assessing patients with any history of oxygen supplementation, including supplemental in-flight oxygen. They also recommend assessment in patients flying longer than 2.5 hours. This is a reasonable and easy-to-follow recommendation.

C. D. Spradley, MD

Safety and efficacy of exercise training in various forms of pulmonary hypertension
Grünig F Lichtblau M, Ehlken N, et al (Univ Hosp Heidelberg, Germany; et al)
Eur Respir J 40:84-92, 2012

The objective of this prospective study was to assess safety and efficacy of exercise training in a large cohort of patients with different forms and World Health Organization (WHO) functional classes of chronic pulmonary hypertension (PH).

183 patients with PH (pulmonary arterial hypertension (PAH), chronic thromboembolic PH and PH due to respiratory or left heart diseases received exercise training in hospital for 3 weeks and continued at home. Adverse events have been monitored during the in-hospital training programme. Efficacy parameters were evaluated at baseline, and after 3 and 15 weeks.

After 3 and 15 weeks, patients significantly improved the distance walked in 6 min (6MWD) compared to baseline, scores of quality of life, WHO functional class, peak oxygen consumption, oxygen pulse, heart rate and systolic pulmonary artery pressure at rest and maximal workload. The improvement in 6MWD was similar in patients with different PH forms and functional classes. Even in severely affected patients (WHO functional class IV), exercise training was highly effective. Adverse events, such as respiratory infections, syncope or presyncope, occurred in 13% of patients.

Exercise training in PH is an effective but not a completely harmless add-on therapy, even in severely diseased patients, and should be closely monitored.

▶ In this prospective study published in the *European Respiratory Journal*, Grünig et al take a diverse group of patients with multiple forms of pulmonary hypertension (groups 1, 3, and 4) to the gym. Patients were included from all functional classes. The end result, as is the case for many disease states, is that exercise is beneficial. This even held true for the sickest patients who actually garnered the greatest proportional improvement.

As expected, this endeavor was not without risk, and there were complications. Still, the study demonstrated improvements in walk distance, quality of life, functional class, and maximum volume of oxygen, among other physiologic parameters, rivaling or surpassing landmark industry-sponsored drug treatment trials in the same population (Figs 1 and 4 in the original article). There were similar improvements across all groups and classes. The majority of patients who failed to respond were functional class I patients who entered the study with a reasonable level of fitness. The findings prompted Lewis Rubin to advocate writing an exercise prescription for pulmonary hypertension patients in the accompanying editorial.[1]

This single-center study did have limitations. It was obviously unblinded and there was no comparison group. Also, the study included a 3-week, in-hospital exercise program, which would not translate to American practice. The same level of monitoring, however, could be applied through the existing network of pulmonary and cardiac rehabilitation centers. The next challenge, unfortunately, would be getting it paid for.

C. D. Spradley, MD

Reference

1. Rubin LJ. Exercise training for pulmonary hypertension: another prescription to write? *Eur Respir J.* 2012;40:7-8.

The Minimal Important Difference in the 6-Minute Walk Test for Patients with Pulmonary Arterial Hypertension

Mathai SC, Puhan MA, Lam D, et al (Johns Hopkins Univ School of Medicine, Baltimore, MD; Johns Hopkins Bloomberg School of Public Health, Baltimore, MD; United Therapeutics Corporation, Research Triangle Park, NC)
Am J Respir Crit Care Med 186:428-433, 2012

Rationale.—Although commonly used as the primary outcome measure of clinical trials in pulmonary arterial hypertension (PAH), the minimal important difference (MID) of the 6-minute walk test (6MWT) has not been well defined for this population of patients.

Objectives.—To estimate the MID in the 6MWT in patients with PAH.

Methods.—Study subjects from the clinical trial of tadalafil in PAH, a 16-week, parallel-group, randomized clinical trial of patients who were treatment naive or on background therapy with an endothelin receptor antagonist, were eligible. 6MWT was performed using a standardized protocol. Distributional and anchor-based methods were used to estimate the MID; the latter method used the Physical Component Summary Score (PCS) of the Medical Outcomes Study 36-item short form (SF-36).

Measurements and Main Results.—Four hundred five subjects were analyzed. Domains of the SF-36 were weakly to modestly associated with 6MWT. Change in the PCS of the SF-36 was most strongly associated with change in 6MWT ($r = 0.40$, $P < 0.001$) and thus was selected as the anchor for subsequent anchor-based analyses. Distributional analyses yielded estimates of the MID ranging from 25.1 to 38.5 m, whereas anchor-based analyses yielded an estimate of 38.6 m.

TABLE 1.—Characteristics of Study Population

	Placebo	Tadalafil 2.5 mg	Tadalafil 10 mg	Tadalafil 20 mg	Tadalafil 40 mg	Overall
Age, yr	55 (15)	54 (16)	53 (15)	52 (15)	53 (15)	54 (15)
Women, n (%)	65 (79)	64 (78)	68 (84)	62 (76)	59 (75)	318 (78)
White, n (%)	73 (88)	65 (30)	65 (80)	61 (76)	64 (82)	327 (81)
PAH etiology, n (%)						
Idiopathic	54 (66)	45 (55)	52 (64)	50 (61)	46 (58)	247 (61)
Collagen vascular	16 (20)	16 (20)	24 (30)	21 (26)	19 (24)	96 (24)
Anorexigen	2 (2)	5 (6)	1 (1)	4 (5)	4 (5)	16 (4)
ASD/surgical	10 (12)	16 (20)	4 (5)	7 (8)	10 (13)	47 (11)
WHO FC baseline, n (%)						
I	1 (1)	1 (1)	0 (0)	0 (0)	2 (3)	4 (1)
II	23 (28)	29 (35)	24 (30)	28 (34)	26 (33)	130 (32)
III	56 (68)	49 (60)	55 (68)	54 (66)	51 (65)	265 (65)
IV	2 (2)	3 (4)	2 (2)	0 (0)	0 (0)	7 (2)
6MWT baseline, m	343 (84)	347 (71)	336 (77)	337 (74)	352 (78)	343 (77)
Mean Δ 6MWT, m	8.7 (60.2)	24.6 (61.6)	29.9 (63.0)	37.1 (47.8)	41.9 (49.3)	28.5 (57.5)
RAP, mm Hg	7 (4)	8 (4)	9 (6)	7 (4)	8 (4)	8 (4)
Mean PAP, mm Hg	49 (12)	55 (14)	51 (16)	58 (12)	54 (8)	54 (13)
Cardiac index, L/min/m^2	2.3 (0.6)	2.4 (0.7)	2.5 (0.8)	2.7 (0.6)	2.7 (1.0)	2.5 (0.7)
PCWP, mm Hg	9 (3)	11 (5)	10 (5)	9 (4)	9 (4)	10 (5)
PVR, Wood units	11 (5)	11 (5)	11 (6)	12 (5)	11 (6)	11 (5)
Concomitant bosentan use, n (%)	45 (55)	43 (52)	41 (51)	45 (55)	42 (53)	216 (53)

Definition of abbreviations: 6MWT = 6-min walk test; ASD = atrial septal defect; PAH = pulmonary arterial hypertension; PAP = pulmonary artery pressure; PCWP = pulmonary capillary wedge pressure; PVR = pulmonary vascular resistance; RAP = right atrial pressure; surgical = PAH after surgical repair of congenital systemic to pulmonary shunts; WHO FC = World Health Organization functional class.

All values presented are mean (SD) unless otherwise specified.

Conclusions.—Using both distributional and anchor-based methods, the estimated consensus MID in the 6MWT for PAH is approximately 33 m. These results have important implications for (1) assessing treatment responses from clinical trials and metaanalyses of specific PAH therapy, and (2) sample size calculations for future study design (Table 1).

▶ In my pulmonary hypertension clinic, I am confronted daily with 6-minute walk distance data. Some patients are walking farther. Some are doing less well. Regardless, the question always comes up: How much of a change in distance is truly important? The same goes for clinical trials. Yes, the change in walk distance is statistically significant, but is it clinically significant? Stephen Mathai and colleagues set out to find the answer in this recent article published in the blue journal.

The team used data from the Pulmonary Arterial Hypertension and Response to Tadalafil (PHIRST) trial referenced in the article here to determine the distance. To determine minimally important difference (MID), they employed an anchor-based analysis using the Physical Component Summary Score aspect of the Medical Outcomes Study 36-item short form as the anchor (Fig 1 in the original article). Distributional analysis was also performed. Results for subgroups were detailed in Table 1.

Based on their data, the MID for the 6-minute walk distance in pulmonary arterial hypertension was estimated at 33 m. This is similar to the 26-m MID identified in emphysema and the 25- to 45-m MID described in idiopathic pulmonary fibrosis.

The use of 6-minute walk test in clinical trials and follow-up has recently been questioned[1,2]; however, until the dust settles on that debate, thanks to this study, I will take comfort in the number 33.

C. D. Spradley, MD

References

1. Holland AE, Hill CJ, Rasekaba T, Lee A, Naughton MT, McDonald CF. Updating the minimal important difference for six-minute walk distance in patients with chronic obstructive pulmonary disease. *Arch Phys Med Rehabil.* 2010;91: 221-225.
2. du Bois RM, Weycker D, Albera C, et al. Six-minute-walk test in idiopathic pulmonary fibrosis: test validation and minimal clinically important difference. *Am J Respir Crit Care Med.* 2011;183:1231-1237.

Atorvastatin in Pulmonary Arterial Hypertension (APATH) study
Zeng W-J, on behalf of the Atorvastatin in Pulmonary Arterial Hypertension (APATH) Study Group (Fuwai Hosp, Beijing, China; et al)
Eur Respir J 40:67-74, 2012

Statins have been shown to both prevent and attenuate pulmonary hypertension in animal models. This study investigates the potential therapeutic benefits of atorvastatin as an affordable treatment for pulmonary hypertension patients.

220 patients with pulmonary arterial hypertension (PAH) or chronic thromboembolic pulmonary hypertension (CTEPH) were randomised, double-blind, to receive atrovastatin 10 mg daily or matching placebo in addition to supportive care.

At 6 months, 6-min walk distance decreased by 16.6 m in the atorvastatin group and 14.1 m in the placebo group. The mean placebo-corrected treatment effect was -2.5 m (95% CI: -38−33; $p = 0.96$), based on intention to treat. A small nonsignificant increase in pulmonary vascular resistance and fall in cardiac output was seen in both treatment groups. There was no significant difference in the proportion of patients who improved, remained stable or showed a deterioration in World Health Organization functional class between atorvastatin and placebo treatments. Nine patients died in the atorvastatin group and 11 in the placebo group. Serum cholesterol levels fell significantly on atorvastatin treatment. Discontinuation rates were 23.2% and 26.9% on atorvastatin and placebo, respectively.

Atorvastatin 10 mg daily has no beneficial effect on the natural history of PAH or CTEPH over 6 months.

▶ My friends in cardiology have frequently joked that statins should be added to the water supply, given their myriad clinical benefits. Animal models of pulmonary arterial hypertension (PAH) have created interest in this class of medications for the treatment of PAH. The authors of this study published in the *European Respiratory Journal* designed this excellent randomized, double-blind placebo controlled multicenter study to address this question.

Prior investigations[1,2] into the use of simvastatin in humans have proven disappointing. Still, in China, where only bosentan and iloprost are approved for therapy and access to directed therapy is estimated at 31%, investigation of an inexpensive, scientifically sound therapeutic option is warranted.

Unfortunately, in this case, like the smaller simvastatin studies before it, the Atorvastatin in Pulmonary Arterial Hypertension study was a negative study. Ten milligrams of atorvastatin did not impact walk distance (placebo corrected treatment effect −2.5 m; Fig 2 in the original article). Both placebo and study arms demonstrated an increase in pulmonary vascular resistance and cardiac output. The treatment arm did demonstrate the expected on-label treatment effect of decreased serum cholesterol levels.

The authors discuss the possibility that the dosing may not be adequate for treatment effect in PAH. They also postulate that the effect seen in animal models may be due to prevention of the changes that are already present in patients diagnosed with PAH. I tend to lean toward the second rationale.

Should we study the population of patients on chronic therapy with statins compared with the population of statin-naive patients for incidence of PAH? Possibly. It would require large numbers. Should we continue to study statins as a directed treatment modality for PAH? In light of the findings of this excellent study, probably not.

C. D. Spradley, MD

References

1. Wilkins MR, Ali O, Bradlow W, et al. Simvastatin as a treatment for pulmonary hypertension trial. *Am J Respir Crit Care Med.* 2010;181:1106-1113.
2. Kawut SM, Bagiella E, Lederer DJ, et al. Randomized clinical trial of aspirin and simvastatin for pulmonary arterial hypertension: ASA-STAT. *Circulation.* 2011; 123:2985-2993.

Bloodstream Infections in Patients With Pulmonary Arterial Hypertension Treated With Intravenous Prostanoids: Insights From the REVEAL REGISTRY®

Kitterman N, Poms A, Miller DP, et al (Intermountain Med Ctr, Salt Lake City, UT; Duke Univ School of Medicine, Durham, NC; ICON Late Phase & Outcomes Res, San Francisco, CA; et al)

Mayo Clin Proc 87:825-834, 2012

Objective.—To evaluate the rate of and potential risk factors for bloodstream infections (BSIs) using data from the REVEAL (Registry to Evaluate Early and Long-term Pulmonary Arterial Hypertension [PAH] Disease Management) REGISTRY®, which provides current information about patients with PAH.

Patients and Methods.—Patients were enrolled from March 30, 2006, through December 8, 2009, and data on reported BSIs were collected through the third quarter of 2010. Bloodstream infection rates were calculated per 1000 patient-days of risk.

Results.—Of 3518 patients enrolled, 1146 patients received intravenous (IV) prostanoid therapy for more than 1 day (no BSI, n = 1023; ≥1 BSI, n = 123; total BSI episodes, n = 166). Bloodstream infections rates were significantly increased in patients receiving IV treprostinil vs IV epoprostenol (0.36 vs 0.12 per 1000 treatment days; $P < .001$), primarily due to gram-negative organisms (0.20 vs 0.03 per 1000 treatment days; $P < .001$). Multivariate analysis adjusting for age, causes of PAH, and year of BSI found that treatment with IV treprostinil was associated with a 3.08-fold increase (95% confidence interval, 2.05-4.62; $P < .001$) in BSIs of any type and a 6.86-fold increase (95% confidence interval, 3.60-13.07; $P < .001$) in gram-negative BSIs compared with treatment with IV epoprostenol.

Conclusion.—Compared with IV epoprostenol therapy, treatment with IV treprostinil is associated with a significantly higher rate of gram-negative BSIs; observed differences in BSI rate did not seem to be due to any other analyzed factors.

Trial Registration.—clinicaltrials.gov Identifier: NCT00370214.

▶ Central line-associated blood stream infections are a risk for any parenteral therapy delivered via catheter. In pulmonary arterial hypertension, patients are frequently on continuous therapy essentially for life or until transplant. Additionally, their physiology puts them at higher risk of sepsis caused by diminished reserves.

In 2007, the Centers for Disease Control (CDC) published findings in *Morbidity and Mortality Weekly* that showed significantly increased risk of blood stream infection from intravenous treprostinil compared with epoprostenol based on retrospective data.[1] Kitterman and colleagues looked at data from the REVEAL (Registry to Evaluate Early and Long-term Pulmonary Arterial Hypertension [PAH] Disease Management) Registry to evaluate this risk and published their findings in the Mayo Clinic Proceedings.

The REVEAL Registry included 1146 patients who had received at least 1 day of parenteral prostanoid therapy. In this population, bloodstream infections were 3 times as likely in patients receiving treprostinil versus epoprostenol. Most of the difference was made up of gram-negative infections, which are uncommon in patients receiving epoprostenol.

The study population included patients receiving room-temperature stable epoprostenol, as the drug was approved 6 months before closure of the registry. No correlation was found between dosage, pump rate, or concentration. Overall improvement in bloodstream infection (BSI) rates compared with the CDC data were attributed to change in catheter care practices and use of a closed hub system, as well as recommendations for usage of Flolan diluent with treprostinil. The REVEAL Registry did not capture diluent type, so this was not assessed. There was also insufficient numbers of patients to allow for subgroup analysis.

Based on these data, individualized treatment choices should weigh risk of BSIs against the greater convenience and potential safety window afforded by the higher stability and longer half-life of treprostinil.[2] Additionally, patients presenting with BSIs who are receiving parenteral treprostinil should be empirically covered with broad-spectrum agents to cover both gram-positive and gram-negative organisms. It will be important to monitor patients receiving the new epoprostenol formulation (currently under way) for gram-negative BSIs, as this agent is reconstituted in sterile water or saline, not Flolan diluent.

C. D. Spradley, MD

References

1. Centers for Disease Control and Prevention (CDC). Bloodstream infections among patients treated with intravenous epoprostenol or intravenous treprostinil for pulmonary arterial hypertension—seven sites, United States, 2003-2006. *MMWR Morb Mortal Wkly Rep.* 2007;56:170-172.
2. Rich JD, Glassner C, Wade M, et al. The effect of diluent pH on bloodstream infection rates in patients receiving IV treprostinil for pulmonary arterial hypertension. *Chest.* 2012;141:36-42.

Tadalafil for the Treatment of Pulmonary Arterial Hypertension: A Double-Blind 52-Week Uncontrolled Extension Study

Oudiz RJ, for the PHIRST Study Group (Los Angeles Biomedical Res Inst at Harbor-UCLA Med Ctr, Torrance, CA; et al)
J Am Coll Cardiol 60:768-774, 2012

Objectives.—The aim of this study was to evaluate the long-term safety and durability of efficacy of tadalafil for pulmonary arterial hypertension.

Background.—Tadalafil is an oral phosphodiesterase-5 inhibitor approved for PAH treatment. In the multicenter, placebo-controlled, randomized, 16-week PHIRST (Pulmonary Arterial Hypertension and Response to Tadalafil) study, tadalafil 40 mg improved exercise capacity and delayed clinical worsening.

Methods.—Eligible patients from PHIRST received once-daily tadalafil 20 mg (T20 mg) or 40 mg (T40 mg) (n = 357) in the double-blind, 52-week, uncontrolled extension study (PHIRST-2); 293 patients completed PHIRST-2. Durability of efficacy was explored using the 6-min walk distance (6MWD) test. Clinical worsening and changes in World Health Organization functional class were evaluated.

Results.—The safety profile of tadalafil in PHIRST-2 was similar to that in PHIRST, with typical phosphodiesterase-5 inhibitor adverse events. The

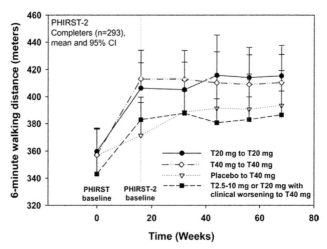

FIGURE 2.—6-Min Walk Distance for Patients Who Completed PHIRST-2 (n = 293). Data are presented for PHIRST (16 weeks) and PHIRST-2 (52 weeks). T20 mg to T20 mg: patients who received tadalafil 20 mg in both studies (n = 52). Placebo to T40 mg: patients who received placebo in PHIRST and switched to tadalafil 40 mg in PHIRST-2 (n = 62). T2.5−10 mg or T20 mg with clinical worsening to T40 mg: patients who previously received tadalafil 2.5 mg, tadalafil 10 mg, or T20 mg (with clinical worsening) in PHIRST and switched to T40 mg in PHIRST-2 (n = 120). T40 mg to T40 mg: patients who received T40 mg in PHIRST and continued to receive T40 mg in PHIRST-2 (n = 59). CI = confidence interval. (Reprinted from the Journal of the American College of Cardiology. Oudiz RJ, for the PHIRST Study Group. Tadalafil for the treatment of pulmonary arterial hypertension: a double-blind 52-week uncontrolled extension study. *J Am Coll Cardiol.* 2012;60:768-774, Copyright 2012, with permission from the American College of Cardiology.)

6MWDs achieved in PHIRST for the subset of patients receiving T20 mg and T40 mg in both PHIRST and PHIRST-2 (406 ± 67 m [n = 52] and 413 ± 81 m [n = 59] at PHIRST-2 enrollment, respectively) were maintained at PHIRST-2 completion (415 ± 80 m [n = 51] and 410 ± 78 m [n = 59], respectively). Numerically fewer patients who were on T40 mg in PHIRST and PHIRST-2 experienced World Health Organization functional class deterioration (6% [n = 5]) compared with those randomized to T20 mg (9% [n = 7]) across both studies. Post hoc analyses showed that background bosentan use and higher 6MWD at PHIRST baseline were associated with fewer clinical worsening events.

Conclusions.—Long-term treatment with tadalafil was well tolerated in patients with pulmonary arterial hypertension. In patients receiving either T20 mg or T40 mg, the improvements in 6MWD demonstrated in the 16-week PHIRST study appeared sustained for up to 52 additional weeks of treatment in PHIRST-2. (Pulmonary Arterial Hypertension and Response to Tadalafil Study; NCT00549302) (Fig 2).

▶ Based on the results of the original Pulmonary Arterial Hypertension and Response to Tadalafil (PHIRST) trial, tadalafil was approved by the US Food and Drug Administration (FDA) for the treatment of pulmonary hypertension.[1] The study found improvement in 6-minute walk distance and delay to clinical worsening in a group of treatment naïve patients as well as patients on stable bosentan monotherapy.

In this study, patients were treated with 20- and 40-mg doses for a total of 52 weeks. Patients sustained improvement in 6-minute walk distance (Fig 2), and they tolerated therapy well. Although still common, frequency of headache declined.

Unlike this study, the long-term extension study[2] of the safety and efficacy of sildenafil included treatment dosages as much as 4 times higher than currently approved by the FDA. Although clinically appropriate, dosage escalation is frequently cumbersome because the practice is off label.

This study was not placebo controlled. Additionally, patients who worsened in the PHIRST trial and those who exited the study prematurely were not included. Still, on the basis of this study, long-term therapy with tadalafil is safe, and patients who show early clinical response sustain those gains.

C. D. Spradley, MD

References

1. Galiè N, Brundage BH, Ghofrani HA, et al. Tadalafil therapy for pulmonary arterial hypertension. *Circulation.* 2009;119:2894-2903.
2. Rubin LJ, Badesch DB, Fleming TR, et al. Long-term treatment with sildenafil citrate in pulmonary arterial hypertension: the SUPER-2 study. *Chest.* 2011;140:1274-1283.

Effectiveness and Safety of Inhaled *Treprostinil* for the Treatment of Pulmonary Arterial Hypertension in Children

Krishnan U, Takatsuki S, Ivy DD, et al (College of Physicians and Surgeons of Columbia Univ Med Ctr, NY; Children's Hosp Colorado, Denver)

Am J Cardiol 110:1704-1709, 2012

The introduction of prostanoid therapy has revolutionized the treatment of pulmonary arterial hypertension (PAH). However, continuous intravenous prostacyclin infusion poses significant risks and challenges, particularly in children. Inhaled treprostinil has been shown to be safe and efficacious in adults. This study describes the safety and efficacy of inhaled treprostinil in children with PAH. A retrospective analysis of 29 children treated with inhaled treprostinil for ≥ 6 weeks was performed. Effects of inhaled treprostinil on exercise capacity, functional class, and echocardiographic and hemodynamic data were evaluated. Adverse events were documented. Patients received 3 to 9 breaths (6 μg/breath) of inhaled treprostinil 4 times/day. All were receiving background PAH therapy; 12 had previously received parenteral prostanoid. Inhaled treprostinil was

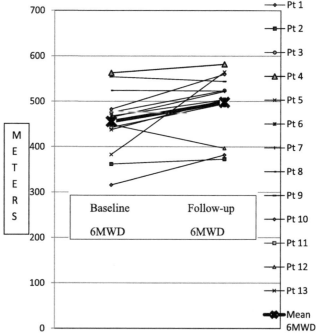

FIGURE 2.—Change in 6-minute walk distance from baseline to latest follow-up. The mean value for the group *(thick line)* is depicted. Baseline and follow-up values for each patient (Pt) *(x axis)* and meters walked in 6 minutes *(y axis)* are shown. (Reprinted from the American Journal of Cardiology. Krishnan U, Takatsuki S, Ivy DD, et al. Effectiveness and safety of inhaled *treprostinil* for the treatment of pulmonary arterial hypertension in children. *Am J Cardiol.* 2012;110:1704-1709, Copyright 2012, with permission from Elsevier.)

discontinued in 4 patients because of symptoms including cough and bronchospasm (n = 3) and progression of PAH (n = 1). Mild side effects including cough (n = 9) and sore throat (n = 6) did not require discontinuation of therapy. World Health Organization functional class improved in 19 and was unchanged in 10; exercise capacity significantly improved with the 6-minute walk distance, improving on follow-up from 455.7 ± 71.5 to 498 ± 70 m ($p = 0.01$) and peak oxygen consumption increasing from 25.5 ± 10.2 to 27.4 ± 10 ($p = 0.04$). In conclusion, inhaled treprostinil was associated with improvement in exercise capacity and World Health Organization functional class when added to background targeted PAH therapy in children and had an acceptable safety profile. Based on these early data, further study of inhaled treprostinil appears warranted in pediatric patients with PAH (Fig 2).

▶ In patients with pulmonary arterial hypertension (PAH) who fail to respond to oral therapy or who are diagnosed functional Class IV, prostacyclin-based therapy requires a considerable adjustment. Choices include continuous intravenous delivery, continuous subcutaneous delivery, and inhalation. In the pediatric PAH population, this change in therapy can prove even more of a challenge. Though it provides decreased risk of treatment-associated adverse events, inhaled iloprost requires frequent dosing and a level of technical skill on the part of the patient to efficiently receive adequate therapy. Recent concerns over phosphodiesterase 5 inhibitor therapy in children threaten to further limit treatment options in this population.[1]

Inhaled treprostinil has been approved for the treatment of PAH in adults. The frequency of therapy is less (4 times daily) and the delivery device requires less technical skill. In this study, given the above information, the authors set out to study inhaled treprostinil in pediatric patients with PAH.

This retrospective study evaluated 29 patients treated with inhaled treprostinil for longer than 6 weeks when added to background therapy. It was well tolerated and was associated with improved exercise capacity (Fig 2.)

Prospective evaluation is indicated, but these findings are promising, potentially providing a safe and less cumbersome prostacyclin-based treatment option for children with PAH.

C. D. Spradley, MD

Reference

1. Abman SH, Kinsella JP, Rosenzweig EB, et al. Implications of the FDA warning against the use of sildenafil for the treatment of pediatric pulmonary hypertension. *Am J Respir Crit Care Med.* 2012 Dec 6. [Epub ahead of print].

Baseline characteristics and follow-up in patients with normal haemodynamics versus borderline mean pulmonary arterial pressure in systemic sclerosis: results from the PHAROS registry

Bae S, Saggar R, Bolster MB, et al (Univ of California, Los Angeles; St Joseph Hosp and Med Ctr, Phoenix, AZ; Med Univ of South Carolina, Charleston; et al)
Ann Rheum Dis 71:1335-1342, 2012

Background.—Patients with normal (mean pulmonary arterial pressure (mPAP) ≤ 20 mm Hg) and borderline mean pulmonary pressures (21−24 mm Hg) are "at risk" of developing pulmonary hypertension (PH). The objectives of this analysis were to examine the baseline characteristics in systemic sclerosis (SSc) with normal and borderline mPAP and to explore long-term outcomes in SSc patients with borderline mPAP versus normal haemodynamics.

Methods.—PHAROS is a multicentre prospective longitudinal cohort of patients with SSc "at risk" or recently diagnosed with resting PH on right heart catheterisation (RHC). Baseline clinical characteristics, pulmonary function tests, high-resolution CT, 2-dimensional echocardiogram and RHC results were analysed in normal and borderline mPAP groups.

Results.—206 patients underwent RHC (results showed 35 normal, 28 borderline mPAP, 143 resting PH). There were no differences in the baseline demographics. Patients in the borderline mPAP group were more likely to have restrictive lung disease (67% vs 30%), fibrosis on high-resolution CT and a higher estimated right ventricular systolic pressure on echocardiogram (46.3 vs 36.2 mm Hg; $p < 0.05$) than patients with normal haemodynamics. RHC revealed higher pulmonary vascular resistance and more elevated mPAP on exercise (≥30; 88% vs 56%) in the borderline mPAP group ($p < 0.05$ for both). Patients were followed for a mean of 25.7 months and 24 patients had a repeat RHC during this period. During follow-up, 55% of the borderline mPAP group and 32% of the normal group developed resting PH ($p = NS$).

Conclusions.—Patients with borderline mPAP have a greater prevalence of abnormal lung physiology, pulmonary fibrosis and the presence of exercise mPAP ≥ 30 mm Hg.

▶ The Pharos registry captured 306 patients with systemic sclerosis. Of those included, 206 had invasive hemodynamic assessment performed. These patients were divided into groups based on resting hemodynamic parameters (mean pulmonary arterial pressure ≤20 normal, 21−24 borderline, ≥25 pulmonary hypertension [PH]). Some of the patients with normal or borderline studies underwent exercise challenge.

Patients defined as borderline were more likely to have reduced forced vital capacity as well as increased fibrosis on high-resolution computed tomography. They also demonstrated higher right ventricular systolic pressure on echo (as expected) as well as higher pulmonary vascular resistance and transpulmonary gradient. In addition, they demonstrated a greater incidence of exercise-induced PH. In a prior study[1] that followed 42 systemic sclerosis patients with exercise-induced PH, 19% developed resting PH and 9.5% died of PH-associated complications within 3 years.

Follow-up data were limited, but 4 of the normal patients demonstrated resting PH representing 32% of the restudied population. This compared with 55% of retested patients who presented with borderline PH. None of normal baseline patients with exercise-induced PH retested demonstrated resting PH.

Data obtained in this registry are clearly incomplete, but the takeaway lesson is that patients with systemic sclerosis who demonstrate borderline resting PH have higher incidence of additional lung pathology and are more likely to demonstrate exercise-induced PH (described as mPAP ≥30). These patients deserve close monitoring and follow-up for progression of disease.

C. D. Spradley, MD

Reference

1. Condliffe R, Kiely DG, Peacock AJ, et al. Connective tissue disease-associated pulmonary arterial hypertension in the modern treatment era. *Am J Respir Crit Care Med.* 2009;179:151-157.

An Evaluation of Long-term Survival From Time of Diagnosis in Pulmonary Arterial Hypertension From the REVEAL Registry

Benza RL, Miller DP, Barst RJ, et al (Allegheny General Hosp, Pittsburgh, PA; ICON Late Phase and Outcomes Res, San Francisco, CA; Columbia Univ College of Physicians and Surgeons, NY; et al)
Chest 142:448-456, 2012

Background.—The Registry to Evaluate Early and Long-term Pulmonary Arterial Hypertension Disease Management (REVEAL Registry) was established to characterize the clinical course, treatment, and predictors of outcomes in patients with pulmonary arterial hypertension (PAH) in the United States. To date, estimated survival based on time of patient enrollment has been established and reported. To determine whether the survival of patients with PAH has improved over recent decades, we assessed survival from time of diagnosis for the REVEAL Registry cohort and compared these results to the estimated survival using the National Institutes of Health (NIH) prognostic equation.

Methods.—Newly or previously diagnosed patients (aged ≥3 months at diagnosis) with PAH enrolled from March 2006 to December 2009 at 55 US centers were included in the current analysis.

Results.—A total of 2,635 patients qualified for this analysis. One-, 3-, 5-, and 7-year survival rates from time of diagnostic right-sided heart catheterization were 85%, 68%, 57%, and 49%, respectively. For patients with idiopathic/familial PAH, survival rates were 91% ± 2%, 74% ± 2%, 65% ± 3%, and 59% ± 3% compared with estimated survival rates of 68%, 47%, 36%, and 32%, respectively, using the NIH equation.

Conclusions.—Comprehensive analysis of survival from time of diagnosis in a large cohort of patients with PAH suggests considerable improvements in survival in the past 2 decades since the establishment of the NIH registry, the effects of which most likely reflect a combination of changes in treatments, improved patient support strategies, and possibly a PAH population at variance with other cohorts.

Trial Registry.—ClinicalTrials.gov; No.: NCT00370214; URL: clinicaltrials.gov.

▶ In 1991, the National Institutes of Health (NIH) published their landmark pulmonary hypertension registry describing survival of patients with pulmonary arterial hypertension (PAH) in the time before directed therapy.[1] At the time, survival at diagnosis was less than 3 years. Soon after the publication of the registry, epoprostenol became available for the treatment of PAH. Today, we have 7 agents available in the United States with a multitude of delivery options representing 3 unique classes of drugs. Agents in a fourth class may soon become commercially available with evidence of efficacy in group 4 disease.

In this setting, the long-term survival data from the Registry to Evaluate Early and Long-term Pulmonary Arterial Hypertension Disease Management (REVEAL) are presented. The REVEAL Registry included 2635 patients and showed significant improvement in survival for the group (Fig 2 in the original article) and for subgroups of PAH (Fig 3 in the original article). Fig 5 in the original article compares REVEAL Registry data with the NIH data.

Findings of the REVEAL Registry show long-term benefit that was not seen in the recent French registry.[2] This can be accounted for by an increase in therapeutic options as well as differences in definitions of incident and prevalent patient groups.

It is unscrupulous to apply registry survival statistics to individual patients. Still, in my practice, I frequently use the NIH regression equation to provide natural history survival data to patients who are resistant to the sometimes cumbersome and life-changing therapies. On the basis of the data, a patient who would have a median survival of 2.8 years in 1991 can now expect to live more than 7 years with appropriate therapy. Now I have another tool to show patients the potential benefits of therapy.

C. D. Spradley, MD

References

1. D'Alonzo GE, Barst RJ, Ayres SM, et al. Survival in patients with primary pulmonary hypertension. Results from a national prospective registry. *Ann Intern Med.* 1991;115:343-349.
2. Humbert M, Sitbon O, Chaouat A, et al. Survival in patients with idiopathic, familial, and anorexigen-associated pulmonary arterial hypertension in the modern management era. *Circulation.* 2010;122:156-163.

5 Community-Acquired Pneumonia

Introduction

Epidemiology of community-acquired pneumonia and factors that predict severity of disease/prognosis continued in 2012 to be common themes in the literature on this topic.

From the epidemiology perspective, I have included studies on the expected impact of pneumococcal pneumonia as the population ages, the natural history of community-acquired pneumonia in COPD patients, and the impact of pneumonia on pregnancy. Other studies in this section address influenza-associated pneumonia in the H1N1 influenza pandemic and the prevalence of methicillin-resistant staphylococcus in community-acquired infection. The final article in the epidemiology area reports a rather unusual occurrence. The authors postulated that falling mortality rates from pneumonia might be due to alternative coding by physicians rather than any real changes in mortality. Their suggestion is that physicians have changed how they code pneumonias (to, eg, respiratory failure) to avoid having to report quality (performance) measures. This is only a supposition at present, but if proven, could have a profound impact on the accuracy of pneumonia reporting the country.

The search for accurate biomarker and other predictors of disease severity/outcome and antibiotic management continues. A really nice meta-analysis of data on use of procalcitonin to initiate and manage antibiotic treatment is included as well as a comparison of different natriuretic peptides for predicting pneumonia severity. Other studies report on glucose levels as predictors of mortality in patients admitted with community-acquired pneumonia and factors that can help predict outcomes of parapneumonic effusions. The final article in this group tried to identify patient factors that could predict in-hospital versus post-hospital 30-day death rates within the Medicare population.

A group of miscellaneous studies includes a critical pathway description of community-acquired pneumonia management designed to ensure appropriate, rapid de-escalation of intravenous antibiotic therapy to achieve reduction in length of stay and cost, a metaanalysis of mortality in macrolide-based treatment regimens, and a metaanalysis and systematic analysis of pneumonia in patients using angiotensin converting inhibitors and receptor blockers.

One final study is a negative treatment study. A large sepsis study had suggested that tifacogin, a recombinant tissue factor pathway inhibitor, might be effective in reducing mortality in severe community-acquired pneumonia. This report begged for study reported here using this drug as part of management. It was not a beneficial drug when studied as a primary management strategy.

Janet R. Mauer, MD, MBA

Aging Population and Future Burden of Pneumococcal Pneumonia in the United States

Wroe PC, Finkelstein JA, Ray GT, et al (Harvard Med School and Harvard Pilgrim Health Care Inst, Boston, MA; Children's Hosp Boston, MA; Kaiser Permanente, Oakland, CA; et al)

J Infect Dis 205:1589-1592, 2012

Pneumococcal pneumonia is concentrated among the elderly. Using a decision analytic model, we projected the future incidence of pneumococcal pneumonia and associated healthcare utilization and costs accounting for an aging US population. Between 2004 and 2040, as the population increases by 38% pneumococcal pneumonia hospitalizations will increase by 96% (from 401 000 to 790 000), because population growth is fastest in older age groups experiencing the highest rates of pneumococcal disease. Absent intervention, the total cost of pneumococcal pneumonia will increase by $2.5 billion annually, and the demand for healthcare services

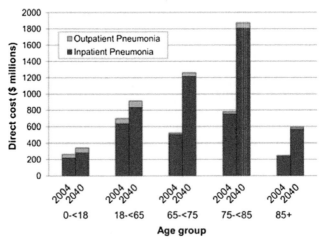

FIGURE 2.—Direct costs by age of outpatient and inpatient pneumococcal pneumonia, 2004 and 2040. All costs are held constant in 2007 dollars. (Reprinted from Wroe PC, Finkelstein JA, Ray GT, et al. Aging population and future burden of pneumococcal pneumonia in the United States. *J Infect Dis.* 2012;205:1589-1592, by permission of Oxford University Press.)

for pneumococcal pneumonia, especially inpatient capacity, will double in coming decades (Fig 2).

▶ This article provides a projection of the anticipated growth in cases of pneumonia over the next 20-plus years. I have included it to increase awareness of 1 of the main diseases that will rise dramatically as the population older than age 65 increases to approximately 20% of the total population by 2040. Unlike many other chronic diseases that will increase significantly, this is an acute process that will have a big impact on rising health care costs. Sixty percent of hospitalizations for pneumococcal community-acquired pneumonia are in patients that are 65 years of age or older. Hospitalizations for all-cause pneumonia are expected to double to 2.6 million per year by 2040 (about 790 000 will be for pneumococcal disease), but because there will be a relatively greater increase in the proportion of the oldest age groups in the general population, the numbers of patients hospitalized will increase proportionately and the numbers hospitalized in the oldest age groups will increase dramatically (Fig 2). This will be reflected in the overall cost of treating pneumonia. A mitigating strategy would be to focus on immunizing a high percentage of the older population against pneumococcal pneumonia and influenza.

J. R. Maurer, MD

Pneumonia and pregnancy outcomes: a nationwide population-based study
Chen Y-H, Keller J, Wang I-T, et al (Taipei Med Univ Hosp, Taiwan)
Am J Obstet Gynecol 207:288.e1-288.e7, 2012

Objective.—Using 2 nationwide population-based datasets, this study aimed to assess the risk of adverse pregnancy outcomes, including low birthweight (LBW), preterm birth, small for gestational age (SGA), cesarean section (CS), lower Apgar score, and preeclampsia/eclampsia, between women with and without pneumonia.

Study Design.—This study included 1462 women who had been hospitalized with pneumonia during pregnancy and used 7310 matched women without pneumonia as a comparison group.

Results.—Compared to women without pneumonia, conditional logistic regression analyses showed that the adjusted odds ratios for LBW, preterm birth, SGA, CS, Apgar scores < 7 at 5 minutes, and preeclampsia/eclampsia in women with pneumonia were 1.73 (95% confidence interval [CI], 1.41−2.12), 1.71 (95% CI, 1.42−2.05), 1.35 (95% CI, 1.17−1.56), 1.77 (95% CI, 1.58−1.98), 3.86 (95% CI, 1.64−9.06), and 3.05 (95% CI, 2.01−4.63), respectively.

Conclusion.—Women with pneumonia during pregnancy had significantly higher risk of LBW, preterm birth, SGA, low Apgar scores infants, CS, and preeclampsia/eclampsia, compared to unaffected women.

▶ Studies focusing on pneumonia in pregnant women have had conflicting results in terms of the impact of pneumonia on fetal outcomes. The reasons for these discrepancies are attributed to several factors. Most of the studies are small, often confined to the experience of 1 hospital. This has resulted in limited sample size and potentially inadequate control of confounding factors. The authors of this study sought to overcome some of these limitations by reporting the results of 2 nationwide, population-based databases and used a clearly defined set of fetal outcome parameters. The databases used were the Taiwan National Health Insurance Research Dataset and the Taiwan national birth certificate registry. The limitations of this study are that it uses retrospective data and may not be generalizable to other populations. However, it does provide very useful data using a large number of patients. The multiple, significant negative impacts of maternal pneumonia on fetal well-being should be carefully considered when pregnant women present with this uncommon, but not rare disease. In the United States, pneumonia complicates between .5 and 1.5 pregnancies per 1000.[1]

J. R. Maurer, MD

Reference

1. Shariatzadeh MR, Marrie TJ. Pneumonia during pregnancy. *Am J Med.* 2006;119: 872-876.

Association of Diagnostic Coding With Trends in Hospitalizations and Mortality of Patients With Pneumonia, 2003-2009
Lindenauer PK, Lagu T, Shieh M-S, et al (Baystate Med Ctr, Springfield, MA)
JAMA 307:1405-1413, 2012

Context.—Recent reports suggest that the mortality rate of patients hospitalized with pneumonia has steadily declined. While this may be the result of advances in clinical care or improvements in quality, it may also represent an artifact of changes in diagnostic coding.

Objective.—To compare estimates of trends in hospitalizations and inpatient mortality among patients with pneumonia using 2 approaches to case definition: one limited to patients with a principal diagnosis of pneumonia, and another that includes patients with a secondary diagnosis of pneumonia if the principal diagnosis is sepsis or respiratory failure.

Design, Setting, and Participants.—Trends study using data from the 2003-2009 releases of the Nationwide Inpatient Sample.

Main Outcome Measures.—Change in the annual hospitalization rate and change in inpatient mortality over time.

Results.—From 2003 to 2009, the annual hospitalization rate for patients with a principal diagnosis of pneumonia declined 27.4%, from 5.5 to 4.0 per 1000, while the age- and sex-adjusted mortality decreased from 5.8% to 4.2% (absolute risk reduction [ARR], 1.6%; 95% CI, 1.4%-1.9%; relative risk reduction [RRR], 28.2%; 95% CI, 25.2%-31.2%). Over the same period, hospitalization rates of patients with a principal diagnosis of sepsis and a secondary diagnosis of pneumonia increased 177.6% from 0.4 to 1.1 per 1000, while inpatient mortality decreased from 25.1% to 22.2%

(ARR, 3.0%; 95% CI, 1.6%-4.4%; RRR, 12%; 95% CI, 7.5%-16.1%); hospitalization rates for patients with a principal diagnosis of respiratory failure and a secondary diagnosis of pneumonia increased 9.3% from 0.44 to 0.48 per 1000 and mortality declined from 25.1% to 19.2% (ARR, 6.0%; 95% CI, 4.6%-7.3%; RRR, 23.7%; 95% CI, 19.7%-27.8%). However, when the 3 groups were combined, the hospitalization rate declined only 12.5%, from 6.3 to 5.6 per 1000, while the age- and sex-adjusted inpatient mortality rate increased from 8.3% to 8.8% (AR increase, 0.5%; 95% CI, 0.1%-0.9%; RR increase, 6.0%; 95% CI, 3.3%-8.8%). Over this same time frame, the age-, sex-, and comorbidity-adjusted mortality rate declined from 8.3% to 7.8% (ARR, 0.5%; 95% CI, 0.2%-0.9%; RRR, 6.3%; 95% CI, 3.8%-8.8%).

Conclusions.—From 2003 to 2009, hospitalization and inpatient mortality rates for patients with a principal diagnosis of pneumonia decreased substantially, whereas hospitalizations with a principal diagnosis of sepsis or respiratory failure accompanied by a secondary diagnosis of pneumonia increased and mortality declined. However, when the 3 pneumonia diagnoses were combined, the decline in the hospitalization rate was attenuated and inpatient mortality was little changed, suggesting an association of these results with temporal trends in diagnostic coding.

▶ The US health care system is undergoing major changes in the way care is delivered. One of the drivers of change is the concept of value, which stresses improvement in the quality of care delivered. A frontline approach to quality assessment is the use of performance measures in which providers are required to report on their adherence to performance measures that are relevant to their practices. One of the areas in which several performance measures have been implemented is community-acquired pneumonia. Since the implementation of community-acquired pneumonia treatment performance measures several years ago, publicly reported mortality rates appear to be decreasing significantly. This has occurred despite the lack of any remarkable breakthroughs in management of pneumonia. Could such a change have occurred by just adhering to evidence-based guidelines and other standard of care measures as required by the performance measures? Possibly. But the authors of this study doubted that and looked at coding of diagnoses to determine if providers were using alternative codes (eg, respiratory failure instead of pneumonia) to circumvent the need to report performance measures. This seemed likely because the rates of hospitalization for pneumonia decreased significantly during this period. In fact, the data in the abstract above suggest that alternate coding likely designed to circumvent the need to report performance measures has been used. Unfortunately, the net result of this can be inaccurate reporting of common diseases, which has many potential ripple effects.

J. R. Maurer, MD

Influenza-Associated Pneumonia Among Hospitalized Patients With 2009 Pandemic Influenza A (H1N1) Virus—United States, 2009

Jain S, for the 2009 Pandemic Influenza A (H1N1) Virus Hospitalizations Investigation Team (Ctrs for Disease Control and Prevention, Atlanta, GA)
Clin Infect Dis 54:1221-1229, 2012

Background.—Pneumonia was a common complication among hospitalized patients with 2009 pandemic influenza A H1N1 [pH1N1] in the United States in 2009.

Methods.—Through 2 national case series conducted during spring and fall of 2009, medical records were reviewed. A pneumonia case was defined as a hospitalized person with laboratory-confirmed pH1N1 virus and a chest radiographic report consistent with pneumonia based on agreement among 3 physicians.

Results.—Of 451 patients with chest radiographs performed, 195 (43%) had pneumonia (spring, 106 of 237 [45%]; fall, 89 of 214 [42%]). Compared with 256 patients without pneumonia, these 195 patients with pneumonia were more likely to be admitted to the intensive care unit (52% vs 16%), have acute respiratory distress syndrome (ARDS; 26% vs 2%), have sepsis (18% vs 3%), and die (17% vs 2%; $P < .0001$). One hundred eighteen (61%) of the patients with pneumonia had $\geq$ 1 underlying condition. Bacterial infections were reported in 13 patients with pneumonia and 2 patients without pneumonia. Patients with pneumonia, when compared with patients without pneumonia, were equally likely to receive influenza antiviral agents (78% vs 79%) but less likely to receive antiviral agents within $\leq$ 2 days of illness onset (28% vs 50%; $P < .0001$).

TABLE 4.—Multivariable Analysis of Select Characteristics Among US Patients Hospitalized With 2009 Pandemic Influenza A (H1N1) With Pneumonia as the Outcome (n = 421)

	Adjusted Odds Ratio (95% Confidence Interval)	P Value
Age, years		
<2	0.4 (.2–.9)	.03
2–17	0.6 (.3–1.1)	.10
18–49	1.0 (.6–1.7)	.90
≥50	Reference	...
Race and ethnicity		
Non-Hispanic black	1.1 (.7–2.0)	.65
Hispanic	1.4 (.8–2.5)	.22
Other	1.7 (.7–4.5)	.26
Unknown	0.9 (.4–1.9)	.76
Non-Hispanic White	Reference	...
Asthma or chronic obstructive pulmonary disease	0.4 (.3–.7)	< .01
Neurological disease	2.2 (1.2–4.4)	.02
Severe illness on presentation[a]	3.3 (2.1–5.2)	< .01
Spring vs fall season	0.8 (.5–1.3)	.38

[a]Defined as shortness of breath or tachypnea, and tachycardia.

Conclusions.—Hospitalized patients with pH1N1 and pneumonia were at risk for severe outcomes including ARDS, sepsis, and death; antiviral treatment was often delayed. In the absence of accurate pneumonia diagnostics, patients hospitalized with suspected influenza and lung infiltrates on chest radiography should receive early and aggressive treatment with antibiotics and influenza antiviral agents (Table 4).

▶ In spring 2009, the Centers for Disease Control and Prevention (CDC) confirmed the first cases of what was to be pandemic H1N1 Influenza A.[1] Since then, H1N1 has continued to be a major Influenza strain throughout the world. In the year after the first cases in the United States were confirmed, an estimated 61 million people became infected, 274 000 were hospitalized, and 12 500 died.[2] One of the major complications leading to death is pneumonia. In this series, many of the patients with pneumonia had relatively delayed institution of antiviral agents (even though the influenza pandemic was well-reported and widely recognized in the country). Physicians may have believed that the pneumonias were primarily caused by bacterial superinfection; however, bacterial infections were documented in only 13 of the cases. Possibly the most important message to take away from this—because pneumonia was associated with a 17% death rate—is to institute antiviral and antibacterial drugs on admission if H1N1 infection is known to be active in the community. Reyes et al,[3] in a study of Spanish patients with H1N1 infection and pneumonia, also recommended combined antiviral and antibacterial treatment in patients presenting with pneumonia because of the difficulty in differentiating between the 2 etiologies rapidly enough to provide life-saving therapy. Coinfection occurred in 33% of this patient population, somewhat higher than in the US report, however, overall death rate was very similar to the US reported death rate. As has been previously reported, in both studies, the patients were younger than patients who typically present with community acquired pneumonia and present with more severe disease, often requiring intensive care management. H1N1 continues to be a major active influenza strain that reemerges each flu season and infects millions more people. In addition to aggressively promoting flu vaccinations, physicians should recognize the different demographic and presentation of influenza pneumonia to ensure early appropriate treatment (Table 4).

J. R. Maurer, MD

References

1. Dawood FS, Jain S, Finelli L, et al; Novel Swine-Origin Influenza A (H1N1) Virus Investigation Team. Emergence of a novel swine-origin influenza A (H1N1) virus in humans. *N Engl J Med.* 2009;360:2605-2615.
2. Shrestha SS, Swerdlow DL, Borse RH, et al. Estimating the burden of 2009 pandemic influenza A (H1N1) in the United States (April 2009-April 2010). *Clin Infect Dis.* 2011;52:S75-S82.
3. Reyes S, Montull B, Martinez R, et al. Risk factors of A/H1N1 etiology in pneumonia and its impact on mortality. *Respir Med.* 2011;105:1404-1411.

The natural history of community-acquired pneumonia in COPD patients: A population database analysis

Müllerova H, Chigbo C, Hagan GW, et al (GlaxoSmithKline Res and Development, Uxbridge, Middlesex, UK; Stockwell Lodge Med Centre, Cheshunt, UK; Respiratory Med Development Centre, GlaxoSmithKline, Stockley Park, UK; et al)
Respir Med 106:1124-1133, 2012

Background.—Patients with Chronic Obstructive Pulmonary Disease (COPD) are at higher risk of developing Community-Acquired Pneumonia (CAP) than patients in the general population. However, no studies have been performed in general practice assessing longitudinal incidence rates for CAP in COPD patients or risk factors for pneumonia onset.

Methods.—A cohort of COPD patients aged $\geq$ 45 years, was identified in the General Research Practice Database (GPRD) between 1996 and 2005, and annual and 10-year incidence rates of CAP evaluated. A nested case-control analysis was performed, comparing descriptors in COPD patients with and without CAP using conditional logistic regression generating odds ratios (OR) and 95% confidence intervals (CI).

Results.—The COPD cohort consisted of 40,414 adults. During the observation period, 3149 patients (8%) experienced CAP, producing an incidence rate of 22.4 (95% CI 21.7—23.2) per 1000 person years. 92% of patients with pneumonia diagnosis had suffered only one episode. Multivariate modelling of pneumonia descriptors in COPD indicate that age over 65 years was significantly associated with increased risk of CAP. Other independent risk factors associated with CAP were co-morbidities including congestive heart failure (OR 1.4, 95% CI 1.2—1.6), and dementia (OR 2.6, 95% CI 1.9—3.). Prior severe COPD exacerbations requiring hospitalization (OR 2.7, 95% CI 2.3—3.2) and severe COPD requiring home oxygen or nebulised therapy (OR 1.4, 95% CI 1.1—1.6) were also significantly associated with risk of CAP.

Conclusion.—COPD patients presenting in general practice with specific co-morbidities, severe COPD, and age > 65 years are at increased risk of CAP (Fig 2).

▶ When chronic obstructive pulmonary disease (COPD) patients get community-acquired pneumonia (CAP), studies suggest they tend to require hospitalization and have more severe courses and worse clinical outcomes than patients who do not have underlying lung disease.[1,2] Many studies have focused on the most severely ill COPD patients with CAP; these studies do not necessarily provide generalizable data to the entire population of COPD patients. Authors of the current study attempted to get a more comprehensive view of CAP in COPD by doing a longitudinal evaluation of a typical UK general practice population of COPD patients. Their goal was to assess incidence, natural history, and risk factors for CAP in a generic COPD population. In this COPD population, patients with mild disease comprised 7.6%, patients with moderate disease 75.7%, and patients with severe disease 17.1%. During the 9-year observation period, 8% of patients

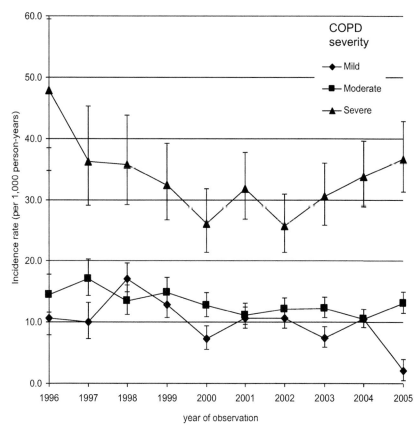

FIGURE 2.—The 1-year incidence rates of community-acquired pneumonia episodes (1996–2005) stratified by COPD severity. Legend: mild patients = not treated during observation period, moderate patients = regular COPD treatment (≥2 prescriptions of the same drug group within six months), severe patients = oxygen or nebulised therapy prescriptions (adapted from Soriano et al.[18]). *Editor's Note*: Please refer to original journal article for full references. (Reprinted from Respiratory Medicine. Müllerova H, Chigbo C, Hagan GW, et al. The natural history of community-acquired pneumonia in COPD patients: a population database analysis. *Respir Med*. 2012;106:1124-1133, Copyright 2012, with permission from Elsevier.)

had an episode of CAP. Of those who had CAP during this period, 60% died (though not necessarily related to the CAP), whereas only 20% of patients without CAP died. This may be because age older than 80 and severity of COPD were both highly associated with development of CAP (Fig 2). Interestingly, both patients with and without CAP had similar inhaled corticosteroid use—arguing against the finding in some reports that inhaled corticosteroids are associated with higher rates of pneumonia—but those with CAP had higher use of long-acting beta agonists. Overall, patients with COPD had about 10 times the rate of pneumonia as the total population of adult patients registered in general practice in the United Kingdom. This study, because it is database-derived, has some limitations. For example, chest radiographs were not available to confirm diagnoses of pneumonia. In addition, the length of CAP episodes was hard to determine and some of the diagnoses on COPD might be erroneous because the collection of COPD indices generally in the United Kingdom came into use during the conduct of the study. Prior to that, medical diagnosis only was used to identify COPD.

The value of these data is in helping identify at-risk patients and managing them more closely with an eye to preventing pneumonia whenever possible.

J. R. Maurer, MD

References

1. Molinos L, Clemente MG, Miranda B, et al. Community-acquired pneumonia in patients with and without chronic obstructive pulmonary disease. *J Infect.* 2009; 58:417-424.
2. Chen Y, Stewart P, Dales R, Johansen H, Bryan S, Taylor G. In a retrospective study of chronic obstructive pulmonary disease inpatients, respiratory comorbidities were significantly associated with prognosis. *J Clin Epidemiol.* 2005;58: 1199-1205.

Direct Comparison of Three Natriuretic Peptides for Prediction of Short- and Long-term Mortality in Patients With Community-Acquired Pneumonia

Nowak A, Breidthardt T, Christ-Crain M, et al (Univ Hosp Basel, Switzerland)
Chest 141:974-982, 2012

Background.—Early and accurate risk stratification for patients with community-acquired pneumonia (CAP) is an unmet clinical need.

Methods.—We enrolled 341 unselected patients presenting to the ED with CAP in whom blinded measurements of N-terminal pro-B-type natriuretic peptide (NT-proBNP), midregional pro-atrial natriuretic peptide (MR-proANP), and B-type natriuretic peptide (BNP) were performed. The potential of these natriuretic peptides to predict short- (30-day) and long-term mortality was compared with the pneumonia severity index (PSI) and CURB-65 (confusion, urea plasma level, respiratory rate, BP, age over 65 years). The median follow-up was 942 days.

Results.—NT-proBNP, MR-proANP, and BNP levels at presentation were higher in short-term (median 4,882 pg/mL vs 1,133 pg/mL; 426 pmol/L vs 178 pmol/L; 436 pg/mL vs 155 pg/mL, all $P < .001$) and long-term nonsurvivors (3,515 pg/mL vs 548 pg/mL; 283 pmol/L vs 136 pmol/L; 318 pg/mL vs 103 pg/mL, all $P < .001$) as compared with survivors. Receiver operating characteristics analysis to quantify the prognostic accuracy showed comparable areas under the curve for the three natriuretic peptides to PSI for short-term (PSI 0.76, 95% CI, 0.71-0.81; NT-proBNP 0.73, 95% CI, 0.67-0.77; MR-proANP 0.72, 95% CI, 0.67-0.77; BNP 0.68, 95% CI, 0.63-0.73) and long-term (PSI 0.72, 95% CI, 0.66-0.77; NT-proBNP 0.75, 95% CI, 0.70-0.80; MR-proANP 0.73, 95% CI, 0.67-0.77, BNP 0.70, 95% CI, 0.65-0.75) mortality. In multivariable Cox-regression analysis, NT-proBNP remained an independent mortality predictor (hazard ratio

1.004, 95% CI, 1.00-1.01, $P = .02$ for short-term; hazard ratio 1.004, 95% CI, 1.00-1.01, $P = .001$ for long-term, increase of 300 pg/mL). A categorical approach combining PSI point values and NT-pro-BNP levels adequately identified patients at low, medium, and high short- and long-term mortality risk.

Conclusions.—Natriuretic peptides are simple and powerful predictors of short- and long-term mortality for patients with CAP. Their prognostic accuracy is comparable to PSI.

▶ Biomarkers are now routinely used in conjunction with several clinical/laboratory indices to help stratify patients with community-acquired pneumonia. Probably the most commonly used and well-validated biomarker is procalcitonin, which is also helpful, when measured sequentially, in determining when it is safe to discontinue antibiotics. Another increasingly studied set of biomarkers are the natriuretic proteins including N-terminal pro-B - type natriuretic peptide (NT-proBNP), B-type natriuretic peptide (BNP), and midregional pro-atrial natriuretic peptide (MR-proANP). BNP has been the most studied of these markers. The natriuretic peptides have the added advantage, relative to other biomarkers, of being able to help separate heart failure from pneumonia in patients in whom the distinction is clinically difficult. NT-proBNP has a potential advantage over BNP, as the levels tend to be related to kidney function and, therefore, might better reflect cardiorenal interactions.[1] MR-proANP has an advantage in that it may be easier to measure accurately in primary care settings, and it has similar accuracy to the BNPs for the identification of heart failure. The study by Nowak et al is a direct comparison of the 3 natriuretic peptides to try to determine if any of them is better at predicting poor outcomes from community-acquired pneumonia. In this study, all the natriuretic peptides were excellent predictors of short- and long-term mortality with accuracy equivalent to a clinical index, the Pneumonia Severity Index (PSI). While NT-proBNP was slightly better at long-term outcome prediction, the ease of measurement of MR-proANP may make it more useful as a front-line test. The usefulness of MR-proANP was supported further in a multicenter validation study that included 1359 patients. In this study, measurements of MR-proANP were divided into quartiles and compared with severity using the PSI.[2] The levels of MR-proANP were highly correlated with severity levels and accurately predicted mortality at 30 and 180 days, complementing the PSI.

J. R. Maurer, MD

References

1. Weber M, Hamm C. Role of B-type natriuretic peptide (BNP) and NT-proBNP in clinical routine. *Heart.* 2006;92:843-849.
2. Vazquez M, Jockers K, Christ-Crain M, Zimmerli W, Müller B, Schuetz P. MR-pro-atrial natriuretic peptide (MR-proANP) predicts short- and long-term outcomes in respiratory tract infections: a prospective validation study. *Int J Cardiol.* 2012;156:16-23.

Serum glucose levels for predicting death in patients admitted to hospital for community acquired pneumonia: prospective cohort study

Lepper PM, on behalf of the German Community Acquired Pneumonia Competence Network (CAPNETZ) (Univ Hosp of Saarland, Homburg, Germany; et al)
BMJ 344:e3397, 2012

Objective.—To examine whether acute dysglycaemia predicts death in people admitted to hospital with community acquired pneumonia.

Design.—Multicentre prospective cohort study.

Setting.—Hospitals and private practices in Germany, Switzerland, and Austria.

Participants.—6891 patients with community acquired pneumonia included in the German community acquired pneumonia competence network (CAPNETZ) study between 2003 and 2009.

Main Outcome Measures.—Univariable and multivariable hazard ratios adjusted for sex, age, current smoking status, severity of community acquired pneumonia using the CRB-65 score (confusion, respiratory rate > 30/min, systolic blood pressure $\leq$ 90 mm Hg or diastolic blood pressure $\leq$ 60 mm Hg, and age $\geq$ 65 years), and various comorbidities for death at 28, 90, and 180 days according to serum glucose levels on admission.

Results.—An increased serum glucose level at admission to hospital in participants with community acquired pneumonia and no pre-existing diabetes was a predictor of death at 28 and 90 days. Compared with participants with normal serum glucose levels on admission, those with mild acute hyperglycaemia (serum glucose concentration 6-10.99 mmol/L) had a significantly increased risk of death at 90 days (1.56, 95% confidence interval 1.22 to 2.01; $P < 0.001$), and this risk increased to 2.37 (1.62 to 3.46; $P < 0.001$) when serum glucose concentrations were $\geq$ 14 mmol/L. In sensitivity analyses the predictive value of serum glucose levels on admission for death was confirmed at 28 days and 90 days. Patients with pre-existing diabetes had a significantly increased overall mortality compared with those without diabetes (crude hazard ratio 2.47, 95% confidence interval 2.05 to 2.98; $P < 0.001$). This outcome was not significantly affected by serum glucose levels on admission ($P = 0.18$ for interaction).

Conclusions.—Serum glucose levels on admission to hospital can predict death in patients with community acquired pneumonia without pre-existing diabetes. Acute hyperglycaemia may therefore identify patients in need of intensified care to reduce the risk of death from community acquired pneumonia.

▶ This prospective study was designed to test the hypothesis that glucose serum levels on admission, in the setting of preexisting diabetes, could predict mortality of patients presenting with community-acquired pneumonia. The background for the study, which includes recent, primarily retrospective, studies of patients with preexisting diabetes, has shown mixed results, with some, but not others, showing poorer outcomes.[1,2] Diabetic patients often have multiple comorbidities, such as cardiovascular and peripheral vascular disease, that contribute to mortality in the setting of pneumonia. In addition, patients with diabetes have impaired immunity, and up to one-fourth of patients presenting with community-acquired pneumonia have diabetes.[3] However, it has not been shown that aggressive control of blood sugars in these patients improves the outcomes.[4] One of the strengths of the study is that it was conducted through the German Community-Acquired Pneumonia Competence (CAPNETZ) Network Registry. This study network/registry differs from others in that it has a larger proportion of outpatients with mild pneumonia and patients younger than 60 years than most pneumonia study cohorts. Thus, the percentage of patients with severe enough pneumonia to require admission would be lower than in most cohorts. This study included 6891 patients from 12 centers in Germany that met those requirements; 16.2% had preexisting diabetes. While the study confirms the increased risk of death in diabetic patients overall, the most interesting finding is that nondiabetics (or at least people not known to have diabetes) presenting with hyperglycemia also had an increased risk of death. Further evaluation of the abnormal glucose levels in nondiabetic patients—possibly an excessive stress response or indicator of systemic inflammation—may be helpful in tailoring treatment for these patients.

J. R. Maurer, MD

References

1. Kornum JB, Thomsen RW, Riis A, Lervang HH, Schønheyder HC, Sørensen HT. Type 2 diabetes and pneumonia outcomes: a population-based cohort study. *Diabetes Care.* 2007;30:2251-2257.
2. McAlister FA, Majumdar SR, Blitz S, Rowe BH, Romney J, Marrie TJ. The relation between hyperglycemia and outcomes in 2,471 patients admitted to the hospital with community-acquired pneumonia. *Diabetes Care.* 2005;28:810-815.
3. Abourizk NN, Vora CK, Verma PK. Inpatient diabetology. The new frontier. *J Gen Intern Med.* 2004;19:466-471.
4. Kansagara D, Fu R, Freeman M, Wolf F, Helfand M. Intensive insulin therapy in hospitalized patients: a systematic review. *Ann Intern Med.* 2011;154:268-282.

Procalcitonin to Guide Initiation and Duration of Antibiotic Treatment in Acute Respiratory Infections: An Individual Patient Data Meta-Analysis
Schuetz P, Briel M, Christ-Crain M, et al (Beth Israel Deaconess Med Ctr, Boston, MA; Univ Hosp Basel, Switzerland; et al)
Clin Infect Dis 55:651-662, 2012

Background.—Procalcitonin algorithms may reduce antibiotic use for acute respiratory tract infections (ARIs). We undertook an individual patient data meta-analysis to assess safety of this approach in different ARI diagnoses and different clinical settings.

Methods.—We identified clinical trials in which patients with ARI were assigned to receive antibiotics based on a procalcitonin algorithm or usual care by searching the Cochrane Register, MEDLINE, and EMBASE. Individual patient data from 4221 adults with ARIs in 14 trials were verified and reanalyzed to assess risk of mortality and treatment failure—overall and within different clinical settings and types of ARIs.

Results.—Overall, there were 118 deaths in 2085 patients (5.7) assigned to procalcitonin groups compared with 134 deaths in 2126 control patients (6.3; adjusted odds ratio, 0.94; 95 confidence interval CI, .71—1.23)]. Treatment failure occurred in 398 procalcitonin group patients (19.1) and in 466 control patients (21.9; adjusted odds ratio, 0.82; 95 CI, .71—.97). Procalcitonin guidance was not associated with increased mortality or treatment failure in any clinical setting or ARI diagnosis. Total antibiotic exposure per patient was significantly reduced overall (median [interquartile range], from 8 [5—12] to 4 [0—8] days; adjusted difference in days, −3.47 [95 CI, −3.78 to −3.17]) and across all clinical settings and ARI diagnoses.

Conclusions.—Use of procalcitonin to guide initiation and duration of antibiotic treatment in patients with ARIs was effective in reducing antibiotic exposure across settings without an increase in the risk of mortality or treatment failure. Further high-quality trials are needed in critical-care patients.

▶ The identification of increased levels of procalcitonin and the course of those elevated levels over time has been used as a potent biomarker not only for identification of bacterial pneumonias, as compared with other inflammatory processes or viral pneumonia, but also to predict when adequate treatment has been provided and, in some cases, to provide outcome information. This body of data has led to the development of algorithms and protocols governing multiple aspects of community-acquired pneumonia management ranging from whether initiation of antibiotic therapy is appropriate to appropriate timing for discontinuation of antibiotics. The purpose of the metaanalysis reported here was to assess the safety and efficacy of using procalcitonin protocols as decision aids in individual patients. To do this, the authors used trials in which patients managed with procalcitonin protocols were compared to patients managed with standard care. A significant value in doing this type of metaanalysis is to get a better estimate of the use of procalcitonin protocol use on mortality from pneumonia because most reported individual studies have not been powered to be able to show statistically significant differences in mortality. The authors confirmed that patients managed with procalcitonin algorithms had less exposure to antibiotics primarily from less initiation at presentation and, to a lesser degree, fewer days on antibiotic treatment. Furthermore, the patients on procalcitonin protocols did not have a higher rate of treatment failure. However, not enough data are available yet to draw conclusions about mortality rates in 1 subgroup of patients, the critically ill patients.

In another large study focusing on procalcitonin-guided antibiotic use for pneumonia in "real-life" settings, Albrich et al collected data from 1759 patients included in a large detailed database from a prospective observational, international, multicenter, quality-control survey (ProREAL). The patients presented to both inpatient and outpatient settings and their treatment was guided by a procalcitonin decision support protocol that was posted on a website. Physicians and support staff were encouraged to use the website to guide management; however, the remainder of the work-up was not prescribed. Ultimately more than 86% of the patients had confirmed pneumonia. Adherence to the protocol varied by diagnosis, but more dramatically by country: in Switzerland, there was 75.8% compliance, in France 73.5%, and in the United States 33.5%. Overall, the compliance rate was 68.2%. The main finding in these "real-life" treatment settings was that outcomes were not worse at 30 days and protocol-guided patients had less antibiotic exposure.[1]

Both the meta-analysis describe here and this large retrospective database study support the routine use of procalcitonin protocols/algorithms as decision support tools for the initial and ongoing management of bacterial pneumonia. This confirms what has become a fairly routine approach worldwide, but apparently with widely varying adherence.

J. R. Maurer, MD

Reference

1. Albrich WC, Dusemund F, Bucher B, et al; ProREAL Study Team. Effectiveness and safety of procalcitonin-guided antibiotic therapy in lower respiratory tract infections in "real life": an international, multicenter poststudy survey (ProREAL). *Arch Intern Med.* 2012;172:715-722.

Predictive factors, microbiology and outcome of patients with parapneumonic effusion

Falguera M, Carratalà J, Bielsa S, et al (Universitat de Lleida, Spain; Universitat de Barcelona, Spain)
Eur Respir J 38:1173-1179, 2011

We aimed to determine the incidence, clinical consequences and microbiological findings related to the presence of pleural effusion in community-acquired pneumonia, and to identify predictive factors for empyema/complicated parapneumonic effusion.

We analysed 4,715 consecutive patients with community-acquired pneumonia from two acute care hospitals. Patients were classified into three groups: no pleural effusion, uncomplicated parapneumonic effusion and empyema/complicated parapneumonic effusion.

A total of 882 (19%) patients had radiological evidence of pleural fluid, of whom 261 (30%) met criteria for empyema/complicated parapneumonic effusion. The most important event related to the presence of uncomplicated parapneumonic effusion was a longer hospital stay. Relevant clinical and microbiological consequences were associated with empyema/complicated parapneumonic effusion. Five independent baseline characteristics could predict the development of empyema/complicated parapneumonic effusion: age <60 yrs ($p = 0.012$), alcoholism ($p = 0.002$), pleuritic pain ($p = 0.002$), tachycardia >100 beats·min^{-1} ($p = 0.006$) and leukocytosis >15,000 mm^{-3} ($p < 0.001$). A higher incidence of anaerobes and Gram-positive cocci was found in this subgroup of patients.

We conclude that only the development of empyema/complicated parapneumonic effusion carried relevant consequences; this condition should be suspected in the presence of some baseline characteristics and managed by using antimicrobials active against Gram-positive cocci and anaerobes.

▶ This is a large study that better characterizes parapneumonic effusions and identifies those patients with community-acquired pneumonia who are likely to develop parapneumonic effusion. And, of those who develop an effusion, it identifies those who are likely to develop a complicated effusion or empyema. Large studies of the outcomes of parapneumonic effusions are surprisingly uncommon. This is a Spanish study conducted over a 13-year period and including more than 4700 patients. This large cohort allowed the authors to identify 5 patient characteristics that were risk factors for complicated effusions/empyemas. Of patients with an effusion who had all 5 risk factors, 15 of 19 (79%) had complicated effusions; of those with 4 risk factors, the proportion with complicated effusion decreased to 55%; and of those with 3 or fewer risk factors, it is less than 50%. These effusions were also more often associated with specific types of organisms. Using information from both patient characteristics and infecting organisms to complement each other may allow early intervention in complicated effusions and improved outcomes.

J. R. Maurer, MD

Prevalence of Methicillin-Resistant *Staphylococcus aureus* as an Etiology of Community-Acquired Pneumonia
Moran GJ, for the EMERGEncy ID NET Study Group (David Geffen School of Medicine at the Univ of California at Los Angeles (UCLA), Sylmar; et al)
Clin Infect Dis 54.1126-1133, 2012

Background.—Methicillin-resistant *Staphylococcus aureus* (MRSA) is a common cause of skin infections. Recent case series describe severe community-acquired pneumonia (CAP) caused by MRSA, but the prevalence and risk factors are unknown.

Methods.—We prospectively enrolled adults hospitalized with CAP from 12 university-affiliated emergency departments during the winter–spring of 2006 and 2007. Clinical information and culture results were collected, and factors associated with MRSA were assessed.

Results.—Of 627 patients, 595 (95%) had respiratory (50%) and/or blood cultures (92%) performed. A pathogen was identified in 102 (17%); MRSA was identified in 14 (2.4%; range by site, 0%–5%) patients and in 5% of patients admitted to the intensive care unit. Two (14%) MRSA pneumonia patients died. All 9 MRSA isolates tested were pulsed-field type USA300. Features significantly associated with isolation of MRSA (as compared with any other or no pathogen) included patient history of MRSA; nursing home admission in the previous year; close contact in the previous month with someone with a skin infection; multiple infiltrates or cavities on chest radiograph; and comatose state, intubation, receipt of pressors, or death in the emergency department.

Conclusions.—Methicillin-resistant *Staphylococcus aureus* remains an uncommon cause of CAP. Detection of MRSA was associated with more severe clinical presentation.

▶ Methicillin-resistant *Staphylococcus aureus* (MRSA) infections of the skin and soft tissues have become common in the United States. MRSA is, in fact, now often identified as the causal organism in community-acquired infections of these tissues. Increasingly, case reports and case series are also documenting MRSA as an organism in community acquired pneumonia. The current article adds to the available literature in this area because it is a prospective, multicenter observational prevalence study of patients admitted to the hospital during 2 consecutive influenza seasons. Thus for the first time we have an idea of percent of community-acquired pneumonia resulting from MRSA based on population-based data. And although it was low (ranging from 0 to 5% at the different centers), the presentation tended to be severe: 14% of MRSA patients died. Of interest is the finding that the strain of MRSA in all 9 patients tested was pulsed-field type USA300. In a related publication by Lessa et al,[1] the authors looked more closely at the strain types of MRSA in a series of pneumonia and bloodstream infections. Initially, USA300 was most commonly seen in community-acquired skin and soft-tissue infections, but as noted in the study by Moran et al, it has been seen increasingly in pneumonia patients. Hospital-acquired infections have been historically more commonly associated with USA100. It has been unclear if the MRSA strain predicts outcome, however. Lessa et al determined the strains of MRSA from 2 groups of patients—1 with catheter-associated bloodstream infections and 1 with community-acquired pneumonia. The authors were unable to show that MRSA strain USA300 was associated with worse outcomes than strain USA100; in fact, in patients with pneumonia, MRSA USA100 was associated with worse outcomes. MRSA is an uncommon, but growing cause of community-acquired pneumonia and should be considered in any patient presenting with a severe presentation.

J. R. Maurer, MD

Reference

1. Lessa FC, Mu Y, Ray SM, et al; Active Bacterial Core surveillance (ABCs); MRSA Investigators of the Emerging Infections Program. Impact of USA300 methicillin-resistant *Staphylococcus aureus* on clinical outcomes of patients with pneumonia or central line-associated bloodstream infections. *Clin Infect Dis.* 2012;55: 232-241.

Predictors of In-Hospital vs Postdischarge Mortality in Pneumonia

Metersky ML, Waterer G, Nsa W, et al (Univ of Connecticut School of Medicine, Farmington; Univ of Western Australia, Perth; Oklahoma Foundation for Med Quality, Oklahoma City)

Chest 142:476-481, 2012

Background.—Many patients who die within 30 days of admission to the hospital for pneumonia die after discharge. Recently, 30-day mortality for patients with pneumonia became a publicly reported performance measure, meaning that hospitals are, in part, being measured based on how the patient fares after discharge from the hospital. This study was undertaken to determine which factors predict in-hospital vs postdischarge mortality in patients with pneumonia.

Methods.—This was a retrospective analysis of a database of 21,223 patients on Medicare aged 65 years and older admitted to the hospital between 2000 and 2001. Multivariate logistic regression analyses were performed to determine the association between 26 patient characteristics and the timing of death (in-hospital vs postdischarge) among those patients who died within 30 days of hospital admission.

Results.—Among the 21,223 patients, 2,561 (12.1%) died within 30 days of admission: 1,343 (52.4%) during the hospital stay, and 1,218 (47.6%) after discharge. Multivariate logistic regression demonstrated that seven factors were significantly associated with death prior to discharge: systolic BP < 90 mm Hg, respiration rate > 30/min, bacteremia, arterial pH < 7.35, BUN level > 11 mmol/L, arterial Po_2 < 60 mm Hg or arterial oxygen saturation < 90%, and need for mechanical ventilation. Some underlying comorbidities were associated with a nonstatistically significant trend toward death after discharge.

Conclusions.—Of elderly patients dying within 30 days of admission to the hospital, approximately one-half die after discharge from the hospital. Comorbidities, in general, were equally associated with death in the hospital and death after discharge.

▶ Surgical outcomes have long been reported in terms of 30-day mortality rates or complication rates. As medical management becomes more closely monitored through performance measures, a 30-day timeframe is frequently being adopted by Centers for Medicare and Medicaid Services (CMS) as well as third-party payers to assess quality of care. Physicians have not traditionally practiced in terms of 30-day outcomes, so they have little experience in managing acute event—like community-acquired pneumonia (CAP) requiring admission that has an average 5-day stay—with an eye on the posthospital mortality at 30 days. The first step in understanding any necessary changes in practice that are required to improve outcomes is to determine what patient or pneumonia characteristics impact postadmission mortality rates. Once this is better understood, appropriate interventions can potentially be designed to improve outcomes. In this study, about half the patients dying within 30 days died after discharge from the hospital. Interestingly, some previous studies[1-3] have suggested that patient status (ie, comorbidities, functional status) were more predictive of post-hospital discharge than the pneumonia severity; however, this study suggests that comorbidities were similarly present in in-hospital and posthospital deaths and that mortality was most closely correlated with the severity of the pneumonia. The authors did use the large retrospective CMS database that, while large, has the limitation of retrospective and somewhat incomplete data. Clearly, more research is required to better define the areas that are most closely associated with mortality and warrant more intense management.

J. R. Maurer, MD

References

1. Mortensen EM, Coley CM, Singer DE, et al. Causes of death for patients with community-acquired pneumonia: results from the Pneumonia Patient Outcomes Research Team cohort study. *Arch Intern Med.* 2002;162;1059-1064.
2. Marrie TJ, Wu L. Factors influencing in-hospital mortality in community-acquired pneumonia: a prospective study of patients not initially admitted to the ICU. *Chest.* 2005;127:1260-1270.
3. Capelastegui A, España PP, Quintana JM, et al. Development of a prognostic index for 90-day mortality in patients discharged after admission to hospital for community-acquired pneumonia. *Thorax.* 2009;64:496-501.

Macrolide-Based Regimens and Mortality in Hospitalized Patients With Community-Acquired Pneumonia: A Systematic Review and Meta-analysis

Asadi L, Sligl WI, Eurich DT, et al (Univ of Alberta, Edmonton, Canada; et al)
Clin Infect Dis 55:371-380, 2012

Background.—Macrolides are used to treat pneumonia despite increasing antimicrobial resistance. However, the immunomodulatory properties of macrolides may have a favorable effect on pneumonia outcomes. Therefore, we systematically reviewed all studies of macrolide use and mortality among patients hospitalized with community-acquired pneumonia (CAP).

Methods.—All randomized control trials (RCTs) and observational studies comparing macrolides to other treatment regimens in adults hospitalized with CAP were identified through electronic databases and gray literature searches. Primary analysis examined any macrolide use and mortality; secondary analysis compared Infectious Diseases Society of America/American Thoracic Society guideline-concordant macrolide/beta-lactam combinations vs respiratory fluoroquinolones. Random effects models were used to generate pooled risk ratios (RRs) and evaluate heterogeneity (I^2).

Results.—We included 23 studies and 137 574 patients. Overall, macrolide use was associated with a statistically significant mortality reduction compared with nonmacrolide use (3.7% [1738 of 47 071] vs 6.5% [5861 of 90 503]; RR, 0.78; 95% confidence interval [CI], .64−.95; $P = .01$; $I^2 = 85\%$). There was no survival advantage and heterogeneity was reduced when analyses were restricted to RCTs (4.6% [22 of 479] vs 4.1% [25 of 613]; RR, 1.13; 95% CI, .65−1.98; $P = .66$; $I^2 = 0\%$) or to patients treated

Study or Subgroup	Macrolide/Beta-lactam Events	Total	Fluoroquinolone Events	Total	Weight	Risk Ratio M-H, Random, 95% CI	Risk Ratio M-H, Random, 95% CI
Arnold 2009 [17]	44	456	20	354	10.0%	1.71 (1.03–2.84)	
Asadi 2012 [2]	22	265	209	2241	11.6%	0.89 (.58–1.36)	
Blasi 2008 [18]	47	559	33	363	11.5%	0.92 (.60–1.41)	
Dambrava 2008 [22]	7	370	2	83	2.2%	0.79 (.17–3.71)	
Frei 2003 [23]	17	872	17	649	7.7%	0.74 (.38–1.45)	
Frei 2006 [24]	3	255	4	102	2.4%	0.30 (.07–1.32)	
Lin 2007 [25]	0	24	1	26	0.6%	0.36 (.02–8.43)	
Lodise 2007 [26]	14	240	19	227	7.7%	0.70 (.36–1.36)	
Marass 2007 [27]	17	96	17	254	8.2%	2.65 (1.41–4.97)	
Menendez 2005 [30]	22	534	9	214	6.6%	0.98 (.46–2.09)	
Menendez 2012 [38]	43	1096	45	1792	11.7%	1.56 (1.04–2.36)	
Portier 2005 [32]	7	175	6	174	4.1%	1.16 (.40–3.38)	
Querol-Ribelles 2005 [33]	25	209	15	250	8.4%	1.99 (1.08–3.68)	
Reyes-Calzada 2007 [34]	21	244	0	11	0.8%	2.11 (.14–32.73)	
Welte 2005 [36]	5	77	6	200	3.7%	2.16 (.68–6.89)	
Zervos 2004 [37]	3	102	5	110	2.7%	0.65 (.16–2.64)	
Total (95% CI)		5574		7050	100.0%	1.17 (.91–1.50)	
Total events	297		408				

Heterogeneity: $\tau^2 = 0.09$; $\chi^2 = 26.43$, df = 15 ($P = .03$); $I^2 = 43\%$
Test for overall effect: $Z = 1.23$ ($P = .22$)

0.01 0.1 1 10 100
Macrolide/Beta-lactam   Fluoroquinolone

FIGURE 3.—Guideline-concordant macrolide/beta-lactam therapy versus respiratory fluoroquinolone monotherapy and mortality (n = 16). *Abbreviations*: CI, confidence interval; M-H, Mantel-Haenszel. (Reprinted from Asadi L, Sligl WI, Eurich DT, et al Macrolide-based regimens and mortality in hospitalized patients with community-acquired pneumonia: a systematic review and meta-analysis. *Clin Infect Dis*. 2012;55:371-380, by permission of the Infectious Diseases Society of America.)

with guideline-concordant antibiotics (macrolide/beta-lactam, 5.3% [297 of 5574] vs respiratory fluoroquinolones, 5.8% [408 of 7050]; RR, 1.17; 95% CI, .91–1.50; $P = .22$; $I^2 = 43\%$).

Conclusions.—In hospitalized patients with CAP, macrolide-based regimens were associated with a significant 22% reduction in mortality compared with nonmacrolides; however, this benefit did not extend to patients studied in RCTs or patients that received guideline-concordant antibiotics. Our findings suggest guideline concordance is more important than choice of antibiotic when treating CAP (Fig 3).

▶ Several studies have suggested that adding a macrolide antibiotic in the treatment regimen of a hospitalized patient with community-acquired pneumonia (CAP) is independently associated with a lower mortality rate. The purpose of this metaanalysis was to assess the available literature on macrolide-based regimens to either confirm or refute this possibility. The theoretical reason for a better outcome for macrolides is that in addition to the antibiotic effect, their immunomodulary and antiinflammatory properties add an extra benefit. This type of benefit is recognized in chronic inflammatory airway diseases, but not proven in acute inflammatory processes. The authors conclude that there is a lower mortality in patients using macrolide regimens. However, this conclusion should be interpreted with care—even though 135 000 patients are included in the study—because there are several issues with the metaanalysis. First, there was significant heterogeneity in the antibiotic regimens to which the macrolide-containing regimens were compared. In fact, in subgroup analysis of 16 studies in which guideline concordant macrolide-containing regimens were compared with fluoroquinolone-containing regimens, mortality rates were similar (Fig 3). Additionally, the studies included in the review were very heterogeneous. Observational studies and randomized controlled trials were included; sources of the population data included large administrative databases and clinically rich databases. The authors suggest that the finding of reduced mortality may be due to confounding because younger, less ill patients are more likely to receive macrolides; however, they were unable to assess this because of the heterogeneity of the data. Probably the most important finding of this study is that in guideline-concordant treatment, mortality is not significantly different. Following the guidelines for appropriate clinical situations, regardless of the treatment regimen, should improve outcomes.

J. R. Maurer, MD

Recombinant Tissue Factor Pathway Inhibitor in Severe Community-acquired Pneumonia: A Randomized Trial
Wunderink RG, on behalf of the CAPTIVATE Trial Group (Northwestern Univ Feinberg School of Medicine, Chicago, IL; et al)
Am J Respir Crit Care Med 183:1561-1568, 2011

Rationale.—Severe community-acquired pneumonia (sCAP) is a leading cause of death worldwide. Adjunctive therapies for sCAP are needed to further improve outcome. A systemic inhibitor of coagulation, tifacogin (recombinant human tissue factor pathway inhibitor) seemed to provide mortality benefit in the sCAP subgroup of a previous sepsis trial.

Objectives.—Evaluate the impact of adjunctive tifacogin on mortality in patients with sCAP.

Methods.—A multicenter, randomized, placebo-controlled, double-blind, three-arm study was conducted from July 2005 to June 2008 at 188 centers in North and South America, Europe, South Africa, Asia, Australia, and New Zealand. Adults with sCAP were randomized to receive a continuous intravenous infusion of tifacogin 0.025 mg/kg/h, tifacogin 0.075 mg/kg/h, or matching placebo over 96 hours.

Measurements and Main Results.—Severity-adjusted 28-day all-cause mortality. Of 2,138 randomized patients, 946, 238, and 918 received tifacogin 0.025 mg/kg/h, tifacogin 0.075 mg/kg/h, and placebo, respectively. Tifacogin 0.075 mg/kg/h was discontinued after the first interim analysis according to prespecified futility criterion. The 28-day all-cause mortality rates were similar between the 0.025 mg/kg/h (18%) and placebo groups (17.9%) ($P = 0.56$). Greater reduction in prothrombin fragment 1 + 2 and thrombin antithrombin complexes levels relative to baseline throughout the first 96 hours was found with tifacogin 0.025 mg/kg/h than with placebo. The incidence of adverse events and serious adverse events were comparable between the tifacogin 0.025 mg/kg/h and placebo groups.

Conclusions.—Tifacogin showed no mortality benefit in patients with sCAP despite evidence of biologic activity.

▶ Recombinant tissue factor pathway inhibitor has been demonstrated to reduce lung injury, inflammation, and mortality in animal models. It does this presumably by restoring regulation of tissue factor pathways. Severe community acquired pneumonia is often associated with septic parameters: hypotension, hypercoagulability, and disruption of the microcirculation. This leads to end organ damage. Tissue factor—expressed on alveolar epithelial cells, endothelial cells, and inflammatory cells—can be excessive and can initiate the coagulation and inflammatory cascades that result in organ dysfunction. A subgroup analysis of the Optimized Phase 3 Tifacogin in Multicenter International Sepsis Phase III trial[1] using tifacogin in severe sepsis suggested that there might be improved survival in that group of patients with severe community-acquired pneumonia. Thus, this prospective trial was initiated that included only patients with severe community-acquired pneumonia. Unfortunately, no benefit was shown. Severe community acquired pneumonia and sepsis are very complicated diseases; finding adjunctive treatments that will improve outcomes have proved extremely elusive. The search continues.

J. R. Maurer, MD

Reference

1. Abraham E, Reinhart K, Opal S, et al. Efficacy and safety of tifacogin (recombinant tissue factor pathway inhibitor) in severe sepsis: a randomized controlled trial. *JAMA*. 2003;290:238-247.

Risk of pneumonia associated with use of angiotensin converting enzyme inhibitors and angiotensin receptor blockers: systematic review and meta-analysis
Caldeira D, Alarcão J, Vaz-Carneiro A, et al (Univ of Lisbon, Portugal)
BMJ 345:e4260, 2012

Objective.—To systematically review longitudinal studies evaluating use of angiotensin converting enzyme (ACE) inhibitors or angiotensin receptor blockers (ARBs) and risk of pneumonia.

Design.—Systematic review and meta-analysis.

Data Sources.—Medline through PubMed, Web of Science with conference proceedings (inception to June 2011), and US Food and Drug Administration website (June 2011). Systematic reviews and references of retrieved articles were also searched.

Study Selection.—Two reviewers independently selected randomised controlled trials and cohort and case-control studies evaluating the use of ACE inhibitors or ARBs and risk of pneumonia and retrieved characteristics of the studies and data estimates.

Data Synthesis.—The primary outcome was incidence of pneumonia and the secondary outcome was pneumonia related mortality. Subgroup analyses were carried according to baseline morbidities (stroke, heart failure, and chronic kidney disease) and patients' characteristics (Asian and non-Asian). Pooled estimates of odds ratios and 95% confidence intervals were derived by random effects meta-analysis. Adjusted frequentist indirect comparisons between ACE inhibitors and ARBs were estimated and combined with direct evidence whenever available. Heterogeneity was assessed using the I^2 test.

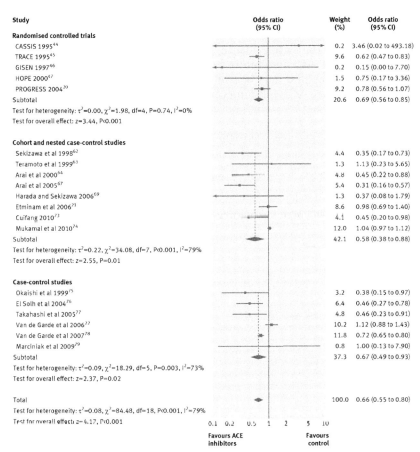

FIGURE 2.—Risk of pneumonia with use of angiotensin converting enzyme (ACE) inhibitors compared with control treatment. (Reprinted from Caldeira D, Alarcão J, Vaz-Carneiro A, et al. Risk of pneumonia associated with use of angiotensin converting enzyme inhibitors and angiotensin receptor blockers: systematic review and meta-analysis. *BMJ.* 2012;345:e4260, with permission from the BMJ Publishing Group Ltd.)

Results.—37 eligible studies were included. ACE inhibitors were associated with a significantly reduced risk of pneumonia compared with control treatment (19 studies: odds ratio 0.66, 95% confidence interval 0.55 to 0.80; $I^2 = 79\%$) and ARBs (combined direct and indirect odds ratio estimate 0.69, 0.56 to 0.85). In patients with stroke, the risk of pneumonia was also lower in those treated with ACE inhibitors compared with control treatment (odds ratio 0.46, 0.34 to 0.62) and ARBs (0.42, 0.22 to 0.80). ACE inhibitors were associated with a significantly reduced risk of pneumonia among Asian patients (0.43, 0.34 to 0.54) compared with non-Asian patients (0.82, 0.67 to 1.00; $P < 0.001$). Compared with control treatments, both ACE inhibitors (seven studies: odds ratio 0.73, 0.58 to 0.92; $I^2 = 51\%$) and ARBs (one randomised controlled trial: 0.63, 0.40 to 1.00) were associated with a decrease in pneumonia related mortality, without differences between interventions.

Conclusions.—The best evidence available points towards a putative protective role of ACE inhibitors but not ARBs in risk of pneumonia. Patient populations that may benefit most are those with previous stroke and Asian patients. ACE inhibitors were also associated with a decrease in pneumonia related mortality, but the data lacked strength (Fig 2).

▶ There has been a keen interest in nonantibiotic drugs and their potential impact on increasing or decreasing the risk of pneumonia. This interest has come largely from secondary observations in studies of these drugs that were conducted to determine the drug's effectiveness for its marketed therapeutic goal or to compare it with a similar drug marketed for the same therapeutic goal. This is true of the studies analyzed here. In this systematic review and metaanalysis, the authors selected all experimental and observational studies they could find evaluating angiotensin-converting enzyme inhibitors (ACEi) and angiotensin-converting enzyme receptor blockers (ARBs), which were generally studied for their effectiveness as antihypertensives, role in prevention of cardiac events or cerebrovascular events, therapeutic impact on diabetic renal disease, or their usefulness in managing congestive heart failure. The authors identified 37 usable studies from a search result of 807 studies. The studies generally either compared ACEi and ARBs with each other or to controls. In only 2 of the studies was pneumonia specifically identified as an outcome measure and in those that reported pneumonia, it was not always reported the same way (eg, in some cases only fatal disease, in some only severe disease, in some just whether or not it occurred). The types of studies evaluated were predominantly randomized controlled studies (n = 18), but also included 11 cohort studies, 2 nested case-control studies, and 6 case control studies. To the authors' credit, they used a standard quality tool for observational studies to identify those at risk of bias and they observed that the finding of pneumonia risk reduction was consistent across the different methodology study types (Fig 2). Nevertheless, there are some limitations in using a variety of different types of studies, and this might create some bias in the results. Another potential source of bias is that patients from different care settings were included in the studies as well as patients with different baseline comorbidities. The compelling findings—that patients on ACEis, but not ARBs have significant reduced risk of pneumonia—begs for a large prospective randomized trial for confirmation. The potential value of ACEi in reducing risk of pneumonia is of particular interest because many of the patients requiring these drugs are either elderly or have certain comorbid diseases such as diabetes mellitus or heart failure that are associated with both high pneumonia risk and death from pneumonia. More research is also needed to better define why ACEis, but generally not ARBs, appear to be associated with this risk reduction and if it relates to the different influences on bradykinin levels of these drugs.

J. R. Maurer, MD

Effect of a 3-Step Critical Pathway to Reduce Duration of Intravenous Antibiotic Therapy and Length of Stay in Community-Acquired Pneumonia: A Randomized Controlled Trial

Carratalà J, Garcia-Vidal C, Ortega L, et al (Univ of Barcelona, Spain; SCIAS-Hosp de Barcelona, Spain; et al)
Arch Intern Med 172:922-928, 2012

Background.—The length of hospital stay (LOS) for community-acquired pneumonia (CAP) varies considerably, even though this factor has a major impact on the cost of care. We aimed to determine whether the use of a 3-step critical pathway is safe and effective in reducing duration of intravenous antibiotic therapy and length of stay in hospitalized patients with CAP.

Methods.—We randomly assigned 401 adults who required hospitalization for CAP to follow a 3-step critical pathway including early mobilization and use of objective criteria for switching to oral antibiotic therapy and for deciding on hospital discharge or usual care. The primary end point was LOS. Secondary end points were the duration of intravenous antibiotic therapy, adverse drug reactions, need for readmission, overall case-fatality rate, and patients' satisfaction.

Results.—Median LOS was 3.9 days in the 3-step group and 6.0 days in the usual care group (difference, −2.1 days; 95% CI, −2.7 to −1.7; *P* < .001). Median duration of intravenous antibiotic therapy was 2.0 days in the 3-step group and 4.0 days in the usual care group (difference, −2.0 days; 95% CI, −2.0 to −1.0; *P* < .001). More patients assigned to usual care experienced adverse drug reactions (4.5% vs 15.9% [difference, −11.4 percentage points; 95% CI, −17.2 to −5.6 percentage points; *P* < .001]). No significant differences were observed regarding subsequent readmissions, case fatality rate, and patients' satisfaction with care.

Conclusions.—The use of a 3-step critical pathway was safe and effective in reducing the duration of intravenous antibiotic therapy and LOS for CAP and did not adversely affect patient outcomes. Such a strategy will help optimize the process of care of hospitalized patients with CAP, and hospital costs would be reduced.

Trial Registration.—isrctn.org Identifier: ISRCTN17875607.

▶ Community-acquired pneumonia (CAP) is very common, accounting for more than 1.3 million hospitalizations per year in the United States. It is the eighth most common cause of death and is a particularly common killer in the elderly.[1] The Centers for Medicare and Medicaid Services has recognized the high cost of this illness and focused on it in developing some of its first clinical quality improvement measures. Those initial measures focused on rapid administration of antibiotics and proper selection of antibiotics and preventative care (vaccinations).[2] However, the largest cost component of pneumonia management—in the United States, estimated at more than $40 billion per year—is the cost of hospitalization for those more severely ill patients who require intravenous drugs. Carratalà et al have attempted to address this cost by carefully structuring the management of the hospitalized patient to ensure that appropriate progression in the management course occurs. The 3 steps in the critical pathway included 1) early mobilization defined as movement to an upright position for at least 20 minutes in the first 24 hours with ongoing progressive mobilization; 2) change from intravenous to oral antibiotics when vital signs stabilized and included patient becoming afebrile; and 3) once on oral antibiotics, discharge as soon as the oxygenation was adequate on room air and the mental status had reached baseline. In a randomized trial, adherence to this critical pathway approach reduced length of stay by a third with similar outcomes. In a different approach to better management of antibiotic therapy in hospitalized CAP patients, Avdic et al performed a prospective trial with an antibiotic stewardship intervention aimed at decreasing antibiotic therapy, increasing the use of microbiology results to streamline therapy, and decreasing duplicate therapy within 24 hours. The authors were able to provide education and feedback to the ordering physicians to significantly reduce the days of antibiotic use and appropriately narrow antibiotic choices.[3]

These studies demonstrate that multiple areas remain to improve the management of CAP. Quality of care measures are moving beyond initial antibiotic care to antibiotic stewardship and reductions in cost of care while improving outcomes.

J. R. Maurer, MD

References

1. Buie VC, Owings MF, DeFrances CJ, Golosinskiy A. National hospital discharge survey. 2006 summary. National Center for Health Statistics. *Vital Health Stat.* 2010;13:37.
2. Bratzler DW, Nsa W, Houck PM. Performance measures for pneumonia: are they valuable, and are process measures adequate? *Curr Opin Infect Dis.* 2007;20: 182-189.
3. Avdic E, Cushinotto LA, Hughes AH, et al. Impact of an antimicrobial stewardship intervention on shortening the duration of therapy for community-acquired pneumonia. *Clin Infect Dis.* 2012;54:1581-1587.

6　Lung Transplantation

Introduction

This year's chapter on Lung Transplantation starts with some exciting and innovative developments in donor and pre-transplant candidate management. The use of non heart beating donors is becoming increasingly common in transplant centers around the world. Little data is yet available on survivals following the use of this type of donor. However, the Australian centers have formed a collaborative—a great idea—so they can present their data on survivals collectively. More long-term outcome information should be coming soon. Another approach to increasing donors, championed by the Toronto Lung Transplant Group, is to retrieve donor lungs that might not appear acceptable for transplant, then manage them "ex vivo" for several hours to determine whether they will be adequate for transplantation. Though time and resource consumptive, this could greatly increase the donor pool. In the "pre-transplant" area, I have also included articles that comment on the impact of donor smoking on recipient outcome. From the candidate perspective, I have included an important observational paper documenting the importance of hypoalbuminemia as a prognostic factor. But the really big news for transplant candidates is the use of new, smaller and more easily deployed ECMO devices to oxygenate very ill pre-transplant patients to bridge them to transplant. The present lung allocation system encourages this approach because it allows sickest first allotment of organs. This approach also is extremely resource intensive and time will tell how widely it will be used.

Post-transplant immunosuppression has gradually been switched from cyclosporine to tacrolimus in most centers, because it is more tolerable medication and because it has been presumed to be associated with lower rates of bronchiolitis obliterans syndrome. Actual documentation of lower rates of rejection has been hard to come by with well-designed clinical trials, but I have included a randomized, prospective study that is the best supportive evidence so far. Sirolimus, on the other hand, has not proved to be as effective as has been hoped when it was first introduced with the documentation of renal toxicity and interstitial lung problems over 10 or so years of use. Documented recently has been an association with cavitary lung disease noted in the article by Banerjee et al. Of particular interest is the report of a survey of transplant centers that asked about the assessment and management of lung rejection. This survey noted wide variability in the way that different centers manage these issues—not a surprising finding, but one that makes it difficult to make progress in resolving the ongoing negative impact of this problem.

Several articles on new or new aspects of long-term post-transplant survival are included. Some document potential complications, but one that shows the impact of structured exercise training after transplant I found particularly interesting. It suggests that post-transplant exercise training improves long-term function. Such programs are not commonly employed even though it has been well documented that post-transplants only recover 40 to 60 percent of normal exercise capacity. To be able to improve post-transplant quality of life in such an easy manner is a great opportunity for programs and their patients.

Janet R. Mauer, MD, MBA

Clinical *Ex Vivo* Lung Perfusion—Pushing the Limits
Aigner C, Slama A, Hötzenecker K, et al (Med Univ of Vienna, Austria)
Am J Transplant 12:1839-1847, 2012

Ex vivo lung perfusion (EVLP) provides the ability to evaluate donor lungs before transplantation. Yet, limited prospective clinical data exist with regard to its potential to recondition unacceptable donor lungs. This paper summarizes the results of a prospective study of lung transplantation using only initially unacceptable donor lungs, which were improved by EVLP for 2—4 h. From March 2010—June 2011, 13 lungs were evaluated *ex vivo*. Median donor PaO_2 at FiO_2 1.0/PEEP5 was 216 mmHg (range 133—271). Four lungs, all with trauma history, showed no improvement and were discarded. Nine lungs improved to a ΔPO_2 higher than 350 mmHg. Median PvO_2 at final assessment in these lungs was 466 mmHg (range 434—525). These lungs were transplanted with a median total ischemic time of 577 min (range 486—678). None of the patients developed primary graft dysfunction grades 2 or 3 within 72 h after transplantation. One patient with secondary pulmonary hypertension was left on a planned prolonged extracorporeal membrane oxygenation postoperatively. Median intubation time was 2 days. Thirty-day mortality was 0%. During the observation period, 119 patients received standard lung transplantation with comparable perioperative outcome. EVLP has a significant potential to improve the quality of otherwise unacceptable donor lungs.

▶ Multiple approaches have been used in the past decade to increase the donor pool. The first approach was to make donor organ criteria less strict. After multiple institutions reported acceptable outcomes with less than pristine donor organs, a number of transplant centers initiated retrieval of organs from donors after the donors had experienced clinical death. These approaches have been very effective as evidenced by a near doubling of the lung transplants performed over the past 10 years.[1] This study reports on a third—and the most recent—approach to increasing the donor pool. Using this technique, called ex vivo lung perfusion, the lung transplant team retrieves donor organs that would not be acceptable for transplant even under relaxed criteria. Initially lungs are flushed with a standard preservation solution, cooled, and taken to the transplant center where they are warmed up to a normothermic temperature, ventilated, and perfused at a rate that is a set percentage of typical cardiac output. The perfusion solution contains red cells so that oxygenation and oxygen consumption can be measured across the pulmonary vasculature. If, after 2 to 4 hours of perfusion adequate oxygenation is observed and other functional parameters are stable, the lungs are considered suitable for transplant. This technique, originally reported by the Toronto group,[2] is being adopted by an increasing number of centers. It is resource and time intensive, but appears to have acceptable early outcomes. Its impact in increasing the donor pool, while promising, is still uncertain.

J. R. Maurer, MD

References

1. Stehlik J, Edwards LB, Kucheryavaya AY, et al; International Society of Heart and Lung Transplantation. The Registry of the International Society for Heart and Lung Transplantation: 29th Official Adult Heart Transplant Report—2012. *J Heart Lung Transplant*. 2012;31(10):1052-1064.
2. Cypel M, Yeung JC, Hirayama S, et al. Technique for prolonged normothermic ex vivo lung perfusion. *J Heart Lung Transplant*. 2008;27:1319-1325.

Excellent Clinical Outcomes From a National Donation-After-Determination-of-Cardiac-Death Lung Transplant Collaborative
Levvey BJ, Harkess M, Hopkins P, et al (Alfred Hosp and Monash Univ, Melbourne, Australia; St Vincent's Hosp, Darlinghurst, Sydney, Australia; The Prince Charles Hosp, Chermside, Brisbane, Australia; et al)
Am J Transplant 12:2406-2413, 2012

Donation-after-Determination-of-Cardiac-Death (DDCD) donor lungs can potentially increase the pool of lungs available for Lung Transplantation (LTx). This paper presents the 5-year results for Maastricht category III DDCD LTx undertaken by the multicenter Australian National DDCD LTx Collaborative. The Collaborative was developed to facilitate interaction with the Australian Organ Donation Authority, standardization of definitions, guidelines, education and audit processes. Between 2006 and 2011 there were 174 actual DDCD category III donors (with an additional 37 potentially suitable donors who did not arrest in the mandated 90 min postwithdrawal window), of whom 71 donated lungs for 70 bilateral LTx and two single LTx. In 2010 this equated to an "extra" 28% of donors utilized for LTx. Withdrawal to pulmonary arterial flush was a mean of 35.2 ± 4.0 min (range 18—89). At 24 h, the incidence of grade 3 primary graft dysfunction was 8.5% [median PaO_2/FiO_2 ratio 315 (range 50—507)]. Overall the incidence of grade 3 chronic rejections was 5%. One- and 5-year actuarial survival was 97% and 90%, versus 90% and 61%, respectively, for 503 contemporaneous brain-dead donor lung transplants. Category III DDCD LTx therefore provides a significant, practical, additional quality source of transplantable lungs.

▶ One of the approaches to increasing the donor pool to better match supply to demand of donor lung grafts has been to use organs retrieved after clinical death. The difficulty in doing this is to be able to preserve the lung function so that the reasonable outcomes are achieved. There are several categories of non—heart-beating donors, first classified in a 1995 article by Kootstra et al from Maastricht[1] and still widely used. Categories I and II are called "uncontrolled" and refer to patients brought to the emergency department deceased or who arrest and undergo unsuccessful resuscitation. These are less desirable donors and have not been widely used because of concerns about organ quality. Categories III and IV are called "controlled" because these donor organs are retrieved from patients who have nonsurvivable cerebral injuries and are fully maintained on life support or have experienced brain stem death (typical cadaveric donor criteria) and are allowed to cardiac arrest before organs are retrieved. The removal of life support can be timed so that organ retrieval teams are available within a few minutes of the actual cardiac arrest. Category III includes a large number of potential donors, but also an ethically difficult group because, although these patients could not survive off of life support, at the same time they are not technically brain stem dead. Over the past 15 years, with the institution of appropriate safeguards and protocols to ensure clinical death before organ retrieval, there has been increasing acceptance of the use of Category III donors. The study by Levvey et al presents the Australian experience using Category III non—heart-beating donors. The most important aspect of this report, I think, is that it illustrates how a concerted effort can result in a national, rational approach to a potentially controversial approach to increasing the donor pool. The Australian lung transplant centers were able to create a National Donation-after-Determination-of-Cardiac-Death (DDCD) Lung Transplant Collaborative with relatively consistent management of the donors among all institutions and, as a result, are able here to report 1 of the largest experiences to date with excellent outcomes. Large single-center experiences in the United States and elsewhere using DDCD donors are also beginning to be reported.[2] However, the creation of national or international protocols and management as has been done in Australia is a model approach and should be adopted by other countries to both standardize management and retrieval of and increase the number of and enable standardized reporting of the outcomes of non—heart-beating donor organs.

J. R. Maurer, MD

References

1. Kootstra G, Daemen JH, Oomen AP. Categories of non-heart-beating donors. *Transplant Proc.* 1995;27:2893-2894.
2. Mason DP, Brown CR, Murthy SC, et al. Growing single-center experience with lung transplantation using donation after cardiac death. *Ann Thorac Surg.* 2012;94:406-412.

Outcome of critically ill lung transplant candidates on invasive respiratory support

Gottlieb J, Warnecke G, Hadem J, et al (Hannover Med School, Germany)
Intensive Care Med 38:968-975, 2012

Purpose.—Lung transplantation (LTx) of patients on mechanical ventilation (MV) or extracorporeal support (ECS) is controversial because of impaired survival. Prognostic factors to predict survival should be identified.

Methods.—A retrospective analysis was performed in a single centre of all ventilated LTx-candidates awarded an Eurotransplant (ET) high-urgency (HU) status between November 2004 and July 2009. Clinical data were collected on the first day of HU-status from intubated patients with an approved HU status. Single parameters as well as the lung allocation score (LAS), the Sequential Organ Failure Assessment score (SOFA) and the Simplified Acute Physiology Score (SAPS 2) were calculated. The association of these variables with survival was evaluated.

Results.—A total of 100 intubated patients (median age 38 years, 56% female) fulfilled the inclusion criteria, of whom 60 also required ECS. The main indications were cystic fibrosis (25%) and idiopathic pulmonary fibrosis (24%). Median time with HU status was 12 days [interquartile range (IQR) 6−21 days]. Sixty patients were transplanted, five were weaned from mechanical ventilation and 38 died while on the wait list. One-year-survival rates were 57, 36 and 5% for transplanted patients, all candidates and non-transplanted candidates, respectively ($p < 0.001$). A SAPS score > 24 (median 30, IQR 27−35), a procalcitonin level of > 0.5 µg/l (median 0.4, IQR 0.1−1.4 µg/l) and any escalation of bridging strategy were independently associated with mortality ($p = 0.021$, = 0.003, and < 0.001, respectively). The LAS (median 88, IQR 8−90) did not predict survival ($p = 0.92$).

Conclusions.—High-urgency LTx improves survival in critically ill intubated candidates. Higher SAPS scores, escalating therapy and an abnormal procalcitonin level were associated with a poor outcome.

▶ The 2012 transplant literature was replete with publications about the use of extraordinary measures to bridge critically ill patients to transplant. Although a small number of successful lung transplant patients maintained preoperatively on mechanical ventilation and fewer maintained on short periods of extracorporeal membrane oxygenation (ECMO) have appeared as case reports or very small series previously, use of these approaches has burgeoned recently. The adoption of these preoperative maintenance approaches is multinational as illustrated by the article abstracted and by Javidfar et al.[1] Two changes have fueled the increased use of ECMO. The first was a change in the approach to the allocation of available donor organs to recipient candidates from a system of giving the organs to patients who had waited the longest to a system that allocates organs to sickest candidates first. This meant that more critically ill patients may receive transplants because they are at the top of the waitlist. The second change has been major technological advances in the application of ECMO. These have included the development of venovenous systems that can allow a patient to be somewhat mobile, pumpless arteriovenous systems to remove carbon dioxide, and streamlined arteriovenous systems that are the best at correcting hypoxemia. Using modern ECMO, oxygenation often can be adequately maintained by modern ECMO (either venovenous or arteriovenous) without intubating the patient. This means the patient may be able to be awake, eat, and otherwise interface with caregivers. Some institutions have reported modified rehabilitation approaches including walking and other exercises. Overall the survival numbers using ECMO have been variable, though better than in the initial case reports using these modalities. Gottlieb et al report data on the largest group of patients from a single European institution. Of the 57 patients transplanted, 32 survived 1 year—a 56% survival. Javidfar et al report an American experience of 10 patients bridged to transplant, all of whom were alive at the time the study was published.[1] These approaches to bridging patients to transplant are seductive and undoubtedly will proliferate. What I don't see discussed or mentioned much in these reports is the resource cost of these approaches. This is concerning and needs to be factored into this invasive preoperative management, especially at a time when medical costs are spiraling out of control. Perhaps it would be best initially to limit the use of these approaches to well-designed studies in specific institutions until the cost-benefit of such approaches can be better understood.

J. R. Maurer, MD

Reference

1. Javidfar J, Brodie D, Iribarne A, et al. Extracorporeal membrane oxygenation as a bridge to lung transplantation and recovery. *J Thorac Cardiovasc Surg.* 2012;144: 716-721.

Effect of donor smoking on survival after lung transplantation: a cohort study of a prospective registry
Bonser RS, on behalf of members of the Cardiothoracic Advisory Group to NHS Blood and Transplant and the Association of Lung Transplant Physicians (UK)
(Univ Hosp Birmingham NHS Foundation Trust, UK; et al)
Lancet 380:747-755, 2012

Background.—The risk that a positive smoking history in lung donors could adversely affect survival of transplant recipients causes concern. Conversely, reduction of the donor pool by exclusion of donors with positive smoking histories could compromise survival of patients waiting to receive a transplant. We examined the consequences of donor smoking on post-transplantation survival, and the potential effect of not transplanting lungs from such donors.

Methods.—We analysed the effect of donor smoking on 3 year survival after first adult lung transplantation from brain-dead donors done between July 1, 1999, and Dec 31, 2010, by Cox regression modelling of data from the UK Transplant Registry. We estimated the effect of acceptance of lungs from donors with positive smoking histories on survival and compared it

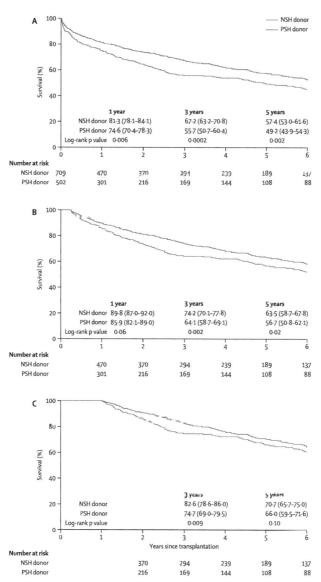

FIGURE 2.—Kaplan—Meier unadjusted survival of patients based on donor smoking status (A) and for patients alive 90 days (B) and 1 year (C) after transplantation. NSH = negative smoking history. PSH = positive smoking history. (Reprinted from The Lancet, Bonser RS, on behalf of members of the Cardiothoracic Advisory Group to NHS Blood and Transplant and the Association of Lung Transplant Physicians (UK). Effect of donor smoking on survival after lung transplantation: a cohort study of a prospective registry. *Lancet.* 2012;380:747-755. Copyright 2012 with permission from Elsevier.)

with the effect of remaining on the waiting list for a potential transplant from a donor with a negative smoking history donor, by analysing all waiting-list registrations during the same period with a risk-adjusted sequentially stratified Cox regression model.

Findings.—Of 1295 lung transplantations, 510 (39%) used lungs from donors with positive smoking histories. Recipients of such lungs had worse 3 year survival after transplantation than did those who received lungs from donors with negative smoking histories (unadjusted hazard ratio [HR] 1·46, 95% CI 1·20—1·78; adjusted HR 1·36, 1·11—1·67). Independent factors affecting survival were recipient's age, donor—recipient cytomegalovirus matching, donor—recipient height difference, donor's sex, and total ischaemic time. Of 2181 patients registered on the waiting list, 802 (37%) died or were removed from the list without receiving a transplant. Patients receiving lungs from donors with positive smoking histories had a lower unadjusted hazard of death after registration than did those who remained on the waiting list (0·79, 95% CI 0·70—0·91). Patients with septic or fibrotic lung disease registered in 1999—2003 had risk-adjusted hazards of 0·60 (95% CI 0·42—0·87) and 0·39 (0·28—0·55), respectively.

Interpretation.—In the UK, an organ selection policy that uses lungs from donors with positive smoking histories improves overall survival of patients registered for lung transplantation, and should be continued. Although lungs from such donors are associated with worse outcomes, the individual probability of survival is greater if they are accepted than if they are declined and the patient chooses to wait for a potential transplant from a donor with a negative smoking history. This situation should be fully explained to and discussed with patients who are accepted for lung transplantation (Fig 2).

▶ In the late 20th century when lung transplant was just coming into its own, transplant centers generally used very strict criteria in accepting donor organs. These included such things as lack of any infiltrate, no significant airway colonization, minimal levels of arterial partial pressure of oxygen when ventilated with 100% oxygen, and no history of smoking by the donor. These criteria effectively restricted the donor lung retrieval rate to less than 20% of available donors. About 15 years ago, a successful effort was made to expand the donor pool considerably. To do this, restrictions such as smoking history was relaxed. The Bonser et al study is 1 of the first to evaluate whether donor smoking has an impact on survival of the recipient in large prospective cohorts. The article compares survival in 2 groups of recipients, 1 group received nonsmoking donors and 1 received smoking donors. These are large multicenter cohorts (more than 500 each) from a prospective registry and a significant portion were followed for at least 3 years. On the limitation side, it was not possible to know the amount of smoking in the donors (estimates were used), so relative cumulative effects of smoking could not be discerned. Nevertheless, when other patient-related factors were taken into account smoking history in the donor definitely resulted in lower recipient survival (Fig 2), especially in the early posttransplant period—as previously reported in smaller cohorts.[1] The authors argue, however, that more years of life are gained by using these donors than are lost by early deaths after transplant. That is undoubtedly true. However, it seems that an approach that would avoid current smokers and those with high pack-year histories might be prudent.

J. R. Maurer, MD

Reference

1. Oto T, Griffiths AP, Levvey B, et al. A donor history of smoking affects early but not late outcome in lung transplantation. *Transplantation*. 2004;78:599-606.

Hypoalbuminemia and Early Mortality After Lung Transplantation: A Cohort Study
Baldwin MR, Arcasoy SM, Shah A, et al (Columbia Univ, NY; et al)
Am J Transplant 12.1250-1267, 2012

Hypoalbuminemia predicts disability and mortality in patients with various illnesses and in the elderly. The association between serum albumin concentration at the time of listing for lung transplantation and the rate of death after lung transplantation is unknown. We examined 6808 adults who underwent lung transplantation in the United States between 2000 and 2008. We used Cox proportional hazard models and generalized additive models to examine multivariable-adjusted associations between serum albumin and the rate of death after transplantation. The median follow-up time was 2.7 years. Those with severe (0.5—2.9 g/dL) and mild hypoalbuminemia (3.0—3.6 g/dL) had posttransplant adjusted mortality rate ratios of 1.35 (95% CI: 1.12—1.62) and 1.15 (95% CI: 1.04—1.27), respectively. For each 0.5 g/dL decrease in serum albumin concentration the 1-year and overall mortality rate ratios were 1.48 (95% CI: 1.21—1.81) and 1.26 (95% CI: 1.11—1.43), respectively. The association between hypoalbuminemia and posttransplant mortality was strongest in recipients with cystic fibrosis and interstitial lung disease. Hypoalbuminemia is an independent risk factor for death after lung transplantation. The authors find that pretransplant hypoalbuminemia is independently associated with early mortality after lung transplantation.

▶ Nutrition is often an issue for patients with progressive lung disease who are potential candidates for lung transplantation. This study, using a national database of lung transplant patients in whom surgery was performed between 2000 and 2008 is the first large-scale attempt to correlate poor nutrition—and possibly higher rates of systemic inflammation with which hypoalbuminemia is also associated—with outcomes. It shows clearly that hypoalbuminemic patients are at higher risk of death in the early posttransplant period. This should not be surprising because similar lower survivals have been shown in nourished apparently healthy elderly patients and in other pulmonary diseases.[1,2] But albumin levels are rarely followed in patients awaiting transplant. How can this study help us? It should prompt further investigation into whether increased systemic inflammation or other unidentified organ dysfunction is a major factor in these patients because these may not be remediable issues and may portend poor prognosis, which is important in patient counseling. For those whose hypoalbuminemia is primarily nutritional, paying attention to improving pretransplant nutrition may prove life-saving.

J. R. Maurer, MD

References

1. Zisman DA, Kawut SM, Lederer DJ, et al. Serum albumin concentration and waiting list mortality in idiopathic interstitial pneumonia. *Chest.* 2009;135:929-935.
2. Reuben DB, Cheh AL, Harris TB, et al. Peripheral blood markers of inflammation predict mortality and functional decline in high functioning community-dwelling older persons. *J Am Geriatr Soc.* 2002;50:638-644.

Tacrolimus and cyclosporine have differential effects on the risk of development of bronchiolitis obliterans syndrome: Results of a prospective, randomized international trial in lung transplantation

Treede H, for the European and Australian Investigators in Lung Transplantation (Univ Heart Ctr Hamburg, Germany; et al)
J Heart Lung Transplant 31:797-804, 2012

Background.—Chronic lung allograft dysfunction, which manifests as bronchiolitis obliterans syndrome (BOS), is recognized as the primary cause of morbidity and mortality after lung transplantation. In this study we assessed the efficacy and safety of two de novo immunosuppression protocols to prevent BOS.

Methods.—Our study approach was a multicenter, prospective, randomized (1:1) open-label superiority investigation of de novo tacrolimus vs cyclosporine, with both study arms given mycophenolate mofetil and prednisolone after lung transplantation. Cytolytic induction therapy was not employed. Patients were stratified at entry for cystic fibrosis. Primary outcome was incidence of BOS 3 years after transplant (intention-to-treat analysis). Secondary outcomes were survival and incidence of acute rejection, infection and other adverse events.

Results.—Group demographic data were well matched: 110 of 124 tacrolimus vs 74 of 125 cyclosporine patients were treated per protocol ($p < 0.01$ by chi-square test). Cumulative incidence of BOS Grade ≥ 1 at 3 years was 11.6% (tacrolimus) vs 21.3% (cyclosporine) (cumulative incidence curves, $p = 0.037$ by Gray's test, pooled over strata). Univariate proportional subdistribution hazards regression confirmed cyclosporine as a risk for BOS (HR 1.97, 95% CI 1.04 to 3.77, $p = 0.039$). Three-year cumulative incidence of acute rejection was 67.4% (tacrolimus) vs 74.9% (cyclosporine) ($p = 0.118$ by Gray's test). One- and 3-year survival rates were 84.6% and 78.7% (tacrolimus) vs 88.6% and 82.8% (cyclosporine) ($p = 0.382$ by log-rank test). Cumulative infection rates were similar ($p = 0.91$), but there was a trend toward new-onset renal failure with tacrolimus ($p = 0.09$).

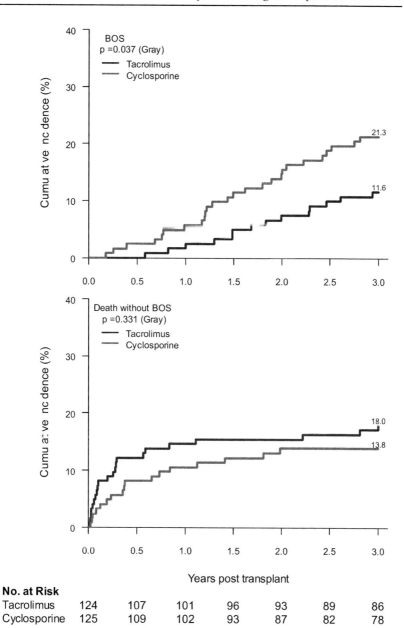

No. at Risk							
Tacrolimus	124	107	101	96	93	89	86
Cyclosporine	125	109	102	93	87	82	78

FIGURE 3.—Cumulative incidence of BOS ($p = 0.037$ by Gray's test) and death without BOS ($p = 0.331$ by Gray's test) for the tacrolimus and cyclosporine groups. (Reprinted from The Journal of Heart and Lung Transplantation, Treede H, for the European and Australian Investigators in Lung Transplantation. Tacrolimus and cyclosporine have differential effects on the risk of development of bronchiolitis obliterans syndrome: results of a prospective, randomized international trial in lung transplantation. *J Heart Lung Transplant*. 2012;31:797-804. Copyright 2012, with permission from the International Society for Heart Transplantation.

Conclusions.—Compared with cyclosporine, de novo tacrolimus use was found to be associated with a significantly reduced risk for BOS Grade ≥ 1 at 3 years despite a similar rate of acute rejection. However, no survival advantage was detected (Fig 3).

▶ Prospective, randomized trials comparing different approaches to treatment remain uncommon in lung transplantation. Trials that are multicenter and multicontinental are even rarer. This one is particularly important because it compares the 2 available calcineurin inhibitors—a necessary type of immunosuppression for lung transplant recipients—with a primary outcome of bronchiolitis obliterans syndrome (BOS) and several secondary outcomes including survival. The study was carried out over 3 years so that adequate time would elapse to get a good sense of the rates of BOS in each group. This is an important study because both of these drugs have significant toxicities, although they are somewhat different from each other. Because of a growing perception—though not proof—of tacrolimus' superiority in reducing acute and chronic rejection and an improved patients' acceptance rate, it has gradually replaced cyclosporine as the primary calcineurin inhibitor used in lung transplant recipients. This anecdotal transition to tacrolimus has begged for some "comparative effectiveness research" to either support or refute the perception. This is the first robustly designed trial with a sufficient duration to address the question. The results supported previous, smaller studies in that tacrolimus-treated participants experienced a lower rate of BOS than cyclosporine (Fig 3). There was no survival advantage, but that may be because the trial did not last long enough to detect a survival difference.

Most complications were similar in the 2 regimens, except notably the development of renal disease that was more common in tacrolimus patients. The investigators are to be congratulated on performing this difficult but much-needed study and are encouraged to use their consortium to continue comparing different management approaches aimed at improving the treatment of lung transplant recipients.

J. R. Maurer, MD

Cavitatory lung disease in thoracic transplant recipients receiving sirolimus
Banerjee SK, Santhanakrishnan K, Tsui S, et al (Papworth Hosp NHS Trust, Cambridge, UK)
J Heart Lung Transplant 31:548-551, 2012

Sirolimus is a potent immunosuppressant agent that has utility in solid-organ transplantation (SOT), particularly for its renal-sparing effects. However, lung toxicity can be a significant issue and a variety of different lung injury patterns have been described. We report an unrecognized association of sirolimus with lung cavitation in patients who have undergone cardiothoracic transplantation. Between 1996 and 2010, lung and heart transplant patients received sirolimus-based immunosuppression as a second-line agent after initial therapy with calcineurin inhibitors. All cases of sirolimus-induced lung cavities were recorded and a retrospective review of the case notes of these patients was undertaken. A total of 9 patients were identified. Clinical symptoms, time to first cavity and mean levels were variable. Some patients showed complete resolution, whereas others had persistent cavitatory lung lesions. Patients who developed persistent lung cavities had a worse outcome than those who did not have cavitation.

▶ Sirolimus (rapamycin) was Food and Drug Administration—approved in the United States in September 1999 and was eagerly awaited by transplant physicians because it was reputed to cause less renal toxicity than the calcineurin inhibitors (cyclosporine and tacrolimus), which are necessary immunosuppressants for most types of solid organ transplant. Although it is associated with less renal disease, it does have renal toxicity and required relabeling in 2008 to reflect this. In addition—and of particular import for lung transplant physicians—it and other molecular target of rapamycin (mTOR) inhibitors also have pulmonary toxicity that appears more commonly in patients with underlying lung disease. The primary manifestation of this toxicity is interstitial pneumonitis that has limited its use as a calcineurin inhibitor-sparing agent in the lung transplant population. The article by Banerjee et al is included here because it is to my knowledge the first published of another type of pulmonary toxicity, cavitary disease, which was accompanied by significant morbidity and mortality. It is not clear why this might occur; however, the ability to interfere with a cell reproduction at the G1 phase significantly impairs protein synthesis and may interfere with fibroblast proliferation and lung healing. Impaired healing has been observed in multiple other contexts such as the healing of bronchial anastomoses,[1] so it is generally avoided as an early posttransplant immunosuppressive. Whatever the mechanism, this is yet another reason to carefully weigh the risks and benefits before using an mTOR inhibitor.

J. R. Maurer, MD

Reference

1. King-Biggs MB, Dunitz JM, Park SJ, Kay Savik S, Mertz MI. Airway anastomotic dehiscence associated with use of sirolimus immediately after lung transplantation. *Transplantation.* 2003;75:1437-1443

SaLUTaRy: Survey of lung transplant rejection
Gordon IO, Bhorade S, Vigneswaran WT, et al (Univ of Chicago, IL)
J Heart Lung Transplant 31:972-979, 2012

Background.—The International Society for Heart and Lung Transplantation (ISHLT) guidelines on the interpretation of lung rejection in pulmonary allograft biopsy specimens were revised most recently in 2007. The goal of our study was to determine how these revisions, along with nuances in the interpretation and application of the guidelines, affect patient care.

Methods.—A Web-based survey was e-mailed to pathologists and pulmonologists identified as being part of the lung transplant team at institutions in the United States with active lung transplant programs as determined from the Organ Procurement and Transplantation Network Web site (http://optn.transplant.hrsa.gov/members/directory.asp).

Results.—Grades B1 and B2 in asymptomatic patients would fall into the same treatment group under the 2007 classification, which combines B1 and B2 into B1R. Also, some pulmonologists would not interpret a pathologic diagnosis of lymphocytic bronchiolitis as grade B rejection, resulting in under-treatment of these patients. Regarding bronchiolitis obliterans, most pulmonologists would treat the patient differently if there were an active mononuclear inflammatory infiltrate, and most pathologists would comment on the presence of such an infiltrate, contrary to the 2007 guidelines, which discourage reporting this infiltrate. We also found discrepancies among pathologists in their interpretation of airway lymphocytic infiltrates, whether eosinophils can be present in bronchial-associated lymphoid tissue, and whether airway inflammation represents rejection or bacterial infection.

Conclusions.—The issue of grading and treating airway inflammation in pulmonary allograft biopsy specimens continues to be problematic, despite revised ISHLT guidelines. Clarification of guidelines for pathologists and pulmonologists using evidence-based criteria could lead to improved communication and patient care.

▶ Evidence-based guidelines are generally much easier to write than they are to implement.[1] One might think this holds true for common diseases such as chronic obstructive pulmonary disorder and asthma because thousands of physicians or several specialties care for them. Conversely, one might think that implementation of carefully crafted guidelines designed to optimize diagnosis and management of a serious complication of lung transplantation would be readily and eagerly embraced by the small group of very specialized physicians that manage these patients. Surprise! This enlightening survey by a Chicago-based transplant group illustrates that it is just as difficult to implement best-evidence guidelines in lung transplantation as it is in the more common and highly prevalent diseases. Unfortunately, the failure or inability to implement such guidelines may impact outcomes of patients or increase costs of care. Maybe even more importantly, it makes it difficult to assess—and potentially improve—current treatment because of the heterogeneity of approaches among institutions. Hopefully, this will be a bit of a "wake up call" to lung transplant physicians and encourage more consistent approaches to evaluation and management.

J. R. Maurer, MD

Reference

1. Grimshaw JM, Thomas RE, MacLennan G, et al. Effectiveness and efficiency of guideline dissemination and implementation strategies. *Health Technol Assess.* 2004;8:iii-iv, 1−72.

A Targeted Peritransplant Antifungal Strategy for the Prevention of Invasive Fungal Disease After Lung Transplantation: A Sequential Cohort Analysis

Koo S, Kubiak DW, Issa NC, et al (Brigham and Women's Hosp, Boston, MA)
Transplantation 94:281-286, 2012

Background.—Lung transplant recipients are at high risk of invasive fungal disease (IFD), particularly invasive aspergillosis and candidiasis. The antifungal strategy that optimally balances effective reduction of IFD with a minimum of toxicity remains undefined; universal triazole prophylaxis is common at lung transplantation (LT) centers, despite the well-known toxicities and costs of this approach.

Methods.—We implemented an antifungal strategy in March 2007 targeted at LT recipients at highest risk for IFD based on our institutional epidemiology. All patients received inhaled amphotericin B during their initial LT hospitalization, bilateral lung transplant recipients received 7 to 10 days of micafungin, and only patients with growth of yeast or mold in their day-of-transplant cultures received further oral antifungal therapy tailored to their fungal isolate.

Results.—IFD events were assessed in sequential cohorts composed of 82 lung transplant recipients before and 83 patients after the implementation of this targeted antifungal strategy. We observed a sharp decline in IFD; in the second cohort, 87%, 91%, and 96% of patients were free of IFD, invasive candidiasis, and invasive aspergillosis at 1 year. Only 19% of patients in the second cohort received systemic antifungal therapy beyond the initial LT hospitalization, and no patients experienced antifungal drug-related toxicity or IFD-associated mortality.

Conclusions.—The targeted antifungal strategy studied seems to be a reasonable approach to reducing post-LT IFD events while limiting treatment-related toxicities and costs.

▶ Invasive fungal disease, particularly with *Aspergillus* sp, has been a significant problem for posttransplant lung recipients. This has resulted in an intensive strategy in many centers to continue antifungal prophylaxis for a long period following transplant. Several strategies have been used, but triazole prophylaxis is predominant because it is oral and easily administered. Initially, itraconazole was the preferred agent; however, when voriconazole was approved in 2002, it quickly replaced other drugs as the prophylactic of choice. Its appeal is both its high level of activity against most common invasive fungal species as well as high bioavailability. It did not take long, however, for reports of the darker side of voriconazole to appear.[1] Its biggest drawback is hepatotoxicity in half or more of lung transplant recipients, especially if started early after transplant.[2] But reports of other problems are also beginning to appear. High cumulative exposures of voriconazole also seem to be associated with increased risk of non-melanoma skin cancers,[3,4] even greater than the known risk with just immunosuppressive medication. In view of these issues, some centers as noted in the present article have abandoned a "shotgun" approach to antifungal prophylaxis.

In this case, only high-risk patients, particularly those still growing fungi after initial prophylaxis, were continued on posthospitalization drug. The strategy was successful in reducing medication complications and without an increase in morbidity or mortality. Undoubtedly it was significantly cost-saving as well. This targeted approach has many potential advantages including its patient-centeredness and should be implemented whenever appropriate in any number of situations where a "shotgun" approach is now used.

J. R. Maurer, MD

References

1. Husain S, Paterson DL, Studer S, et al. Voriconazole prophylaxis in lung transplant recipients. *Am J Transplant*. 2006;6:3008-3016.
2. Luong ML, Hosseini-Moghaddam SM, Singer LG, et al. Risk factors for voriconazole hepatotoxicity at 12 weeks in lung transplant recipients. *Am J Transplant*. 2012;12:1929-1935.
3. Zwald FO, Spratt M, Lemos BD, et al. Duration of voriconazole exposure: an independent risk factor for skin cancer after lung transplantation. *Dermatol Surg*. 2012;38:1369-1374.
4. Singer JP, Boker A, Metchnikoff C, et al. High cumulative dose exposure to voriconazole is associated with cutaneous squamous cell carcinoma in lung transplant recipients. *J Heart Lung Transplant*. 2012;31:694-699.

Exercise Training After Lung Transplantation Improves Participation in Daily Activity: A Randomized Controlled Trial
Langer D, Burtin C, Schepers L, et al (KULeuven, Tervuursevest, Heverlee, Belgium; et al)
Am J Transplant 12:1584-1592, 2012

The effects of exercise training after lung transplantation have not been studied in a randomized controlled trial so far. We investigated whether 3 months of supervised training, initiated immediately after hospital discharge, improve functional recovery and cardiovascular morbidity of patients up to 1 year after lung transplantation. Patients older than 40 years, who experienced an uncomplicated postoperative period, were eligible for this single blind, parallel group study. Sealed envelopes were used to randomly allocate patients to 3 months of exercise training (n = 21) or a control intervention (n = 19). Minutes of daily walking time (primary outcome), physical fitness, quality of life and cardiovascular morbidity were compared between groups adjusting for baseline assessments in a mixed models analysis. After 1 year daily walking time in the treated patients (n = 18) was 85 ± 27 min and in the control group (n = 16) 54 ± 30 min (adjusted difference 26 min [95% CI 8−45 min, $p = 0.006$]). Quadriceps force ($p = 0.001$), 6-minute walking distance ($p = 0.002$) and self-reported physical functioning ($p = 0.039$) were significantly higher in the intervention group. Average 24 h ambulatory blood pressures were significantly lower in the treated patients ($p \leq 0.01$). Based on these results patients should be strongly encouraged to participate in an exercise training intervention after lung transplantation.

▶ Ongoing preoperative pulmonary rehabilitation is a standard component of virtually every lung transplant program. Postoperative pulmonary rehabilitation, on the other hand, is rarely prescribed. This is interesting because at best, even with intensive preoperative rehabilitation, patients undergoing transplant are very deconditioned. Several studies have documented that the activity level of patients undergoing transplant remains impaired after transplant[1-3] and others have shown that posttransplant exercise capacity is typically no more than 40% to 60% of predicted normal values.[4] Proposed etiology for this impaired functional capacity have ranged from impaired muscle function because of prolonged periods of sedentary life styles to mitochondrial or other metabolic changes induced by the calcineurin inhibitor immunosuppression. Perhaps because of these postulated reasons for impaired function and the presumption that they are not reparable by exercise, few data have been reported on the impact of postoperative pulmonary rehabilitation. The investigation by Langer et al is a very welcome contribution because it is a randomized trial that demonstrates that a significant improvement in function can be achieved in a standard postoperative exercise program. The improvement continued throughout the 1-year follow-up. Interestingly, the only significant differences in health-related quality of life were in physical functioning and role limitations between the groups. Despite this, the improved functional capacity undoubtedly resulted in greater participation in family and other activities that would integrate them more fully back into the family unit. These results make a strong case for postoperative pulmonary rehabilitation in lung transplant recipients despite the known muscle changes that are considered irreparable.

J. R. Maurer, MD

References

1. Lands LC, Smountas AA, Mesiano G, et al. Maximal exercise capacity and peripheral skeletal muscle function following lung transplantation. *J Heart Lung Transplant.* 1999;18:113-120.
2. Maury G, Langer D, Verleden G, et al. Skeletal muscle force and functional exercise tolerance before and after lung transplantation: a cohort study. *Am J Transplant.* 2008;8:1275-1281.
3. Leung TC, Ballman KV, Allison TG, et al. Clinical predictors of exercise capacity 1 year after cardiac transplantation. *J Heart Lung Transplant.* 2003;22:16-27.
4. Mathur S, Reid WD, Levy RD. Exercise limitation in recipients of lung transplants. *Phys Ther.* 2004;84:1178-1187.

Changes in Neurocognitive Functioning Following Lung Transplantation

Hoffman BM, Blumenthal JA, Carney RC, et al (Duke Univ Med Ctr, Durham, NC; Washington Univ, St Louis, MO)
Am J Transplant 12:2519-2525, 2012

Although neurocognitive impairment is relatively common among patients with advanced lung disease, little is known regarding changes in neurocognition following lung transplantation. We therefore administered 10 tests of neurocognitive functioning before and 6 months following lung transplantation and sought to identify predictors of change. Among the 49 study participants, native diseases included chronic obstructive pulmonary disease (n = 22), cystic fibrosis (n = 12), nonfibrotic diseases (n = 11) and other (n = 4). Although composite measures of executive function and verbal memory scores were generally within normal limits both before and after lung transplantation, verbal memory performance was slightly better posttransplant compared to baseline ($p < 0.0001$). Executive function scores improved in younger patients but worsened in older patients ($p = 0.03$). A minority subset of patients (29%) exhibited significant cognitive decline (i.e. >1 standard deviations on at least 20% of tests) from baseline to posttransplant. Patients who declined were older ($p < 0.004$) and tended to be less educated ($p = 0.07$). Lung transplantation, like cardiac revascularization procedures, appears to be associated with cognitive decline in a subset of older patients, which could impact daily functioning posttransplant.

▶ This is an important study because the investigators assessed the cognitive function in a cohort of lung transplant candidates and then assessed it again 6 months after they received their grafts so that individual pre- and postfunction could be compared. The most important finding of the study was that 29% of patients had a significant decline in cognitive function 6 months after surgery. This type of change can have a major impact on one's quality of life and that of one's family as well as the ability to manage the considerable self-care required while on immunosuppressive drugs. Although the current study identified only older age as a risk factor, further investigations that identify specific risk factor—in addition to age—for this type of change in potential transplant candidates should be undertaken so that candidates can be better informed about the risk. This is particularly important because the number of older patients receiving lung transplants has steadily increased over the past decade and continues to do so. Known impacts on cognitive function have been attributed to some posttransplant immunosuppressive agents, notably steroids and calcineurin inhibitors. If these and/or other risks can be identified, opportunities exist to minimize the impacts in the posttransplant patient.

J. R. Maurer, MD

Risk of Post-Lung Transplant Renal Dysfunction in Adults With Cystic Fibrosis

Quon BS, Mayer-Hamblett N, Aitken ML, et al (Univ of Washington, Seattle; Seattle Children's Hosp, WA)
Chest 142:185-191, 2012

Background.—Cystic fibrosis (CF) is one of the leading indications for lung transplantation. The incidence and pre-lung transplant risk factors for posttransplant renal dysfunction in the CF population remain undefined.

Methods.—We conducted a cohort study using adults ($\geq$ 18 years old) in the CF Foundation Patient Registry from 2000 to 2008 to determine the incidence of post-lung transplant renal dysfunction, defined by an estimated glomerular filtration rate of < 60 mL/min/1.73 m^2. Multivariable Cox proportional hazards modelling was used to identify independent pretransplant risk factors for post-lung transplant renal dysfunction.

Results.—The study cohort included 993 adult lung transplant recipients with CF, with a median follow-up of 2 years. During the study period, 311 individuals developed renal dysfunction, with a 2-year risk of 35% (95% CI, 32%-39%). Risk of posttransplant renal dysfunction increased substantially with increasing age (25 to < 35 years vs 18 to < 25 years: hazard ratio [HR], 1.60; 95% CI, 1.15-2.23; vs $\geq$ 35 years: HR, 2.45; 95% CI, 1.73-3.47) and female sex (HR, 1.56; 95% CI, 1.22-1.99). CF-related diabetes requiring insulin therapy (HR, 1.30; 95% CI, 1.02-1.67) and pretransplant renal function impairment (estimated glomerular filtration rate, 60-90 mL/min/m^2 vs > 90 mL/min/m^2: HR, 1.58; 95% CI, 1.19-2.12) also increased the risk of posttransplant renal dysfunction.

Conclusions.—Renal dysfunction is common following lung transplant in the adult CF population. Increased age, female sex, CF-related diabetes requiring insulin, and pretransplant renal impairment are significant risk factors.

▶ Though the biggest threats to overall survival of lung transplant patients are bronchiolitis obliterans syndrome (BOS) and various infections, there are many other complications—most related to immunosuppressive medication—that diminish the quality of life of transplant recipients. Among the most pervasive is renal disease. Patients placed on calcineurin inhibitors (either cyclosporine or tacrolimus) have a rather dramatic fall in glomerular filtration rate within a few weeks posttransplant, which tends to be progressive, and, over the course of a few years, results in end-stage renal disease. Most at risk are those patients who are older and who have acute renal dysfunction in the peritransplant period.[1] The International Lung Transplant Registry has reported that approximately 3% to 5% of long-term survivors eventually require dialysis or renal transplant; however, because this is a voluntary registry, it is likely that the longitudinal data underreports the actual scope of renal disease.[2] This study of cystic fibrosis transplant recipients, the first comprehensive study of posttransplant renal disease in a specific population, uses a much better data source, the US Cystic Fibrosis Foundation Patient Registry. The data suggest that renal disease is a much larger problem than previously documented. The registry documents that approximately one third of cystic fibrosis lung recipients followed for only a median of 2 years developed significant renal dysfunction, and of those developing renal dysfunction, 11.9%—or 3.7% of the entire posttransplant population—progressed to end-stage disease over a relatively short time frame. These findings suggest that the problem of renal disease and the attendant hypertension and other systemic morbidities that accompany renal disease are more common than previously appreciated and should be aggressively managed from early posttransplant. That management approach needs to include manipulation of immunosuppressive regimens, strict control of blood pressures, and avoidance of potentially nephrotoxic antibiotics or other drugs.

J. R. Maurer, MD

References

1. Barraclough K, Menahem SA, Dailey M, Thomson NM. Predictors of decline in renal function after lung transplantation. *J Heart Lung Transplant.* 2006;25: 1431-1435.
2. Stehlik J, Edwards LB, Kucheryavaya AY, et al; International Society of Heart and Lung Transplantation. The Registry of the International Society for Heart and Lung Transplantation: 29th Official Adult Heart Transplant Report—2012. *J Heart Lung Transplant.* 2012;31(10):1052-1064.

Survival and Extrapulmonary Course of Connective Tissue Disease After Lung Transplantation

Takagishi T, Ostrowski R, Alex C, et al (Loyola Univ Med Ctr, Louisville, KY)
J Clin Rheumatol 18:283-289, 2012

Background.—Connective tissue disease (CTD)—related lung dysfunction is a common cause of morbidity and mortality; however, few lung transplantations (LTs) are performed in this population secondary to uncertainty regarding the posttransplant survival, outcome, and management.

Objectives.—The objectives were to evaluate the survival and the pulmonary and extrapulmonary courses of CTD after LT.

Methods.—Survival outcomes of patients documented within the Organ Procurement and Transplantation Network who had undergone a LT for CTD were compared with thosewho underwent LT for chronic obstructive pulmonary disease (COPD) and idiopathic pulmonary fibrosis (IPF). In addition, the pulmonary and extrapulmonary courses of the CTD were evaluated after LT.

Results.—From 1991 to 2009, there were 284 documented LT in patients with CTD. Post-LT cumulative survival of patients with CTD was less than that for COPD through 5 years, with a difference that peaked at 1 year (72.7% vs. 83.1%, $P < 0.001$). When patients with CTD were compared with those with IPF, a difference was only noted at 1 year (72.7% vs. 77.7%, $P = 0.049$). There were no documented post-LT pulmonary recurrences of the CTD, and extrapulmonary flares of the CTD were rare

(1 possible flare per 20.3 patient-years and 1 probable flare per 81.0 patient-years).

Conclusions.—Cumulative survival of patients with CTD who underwent LT is similar to those with IPF and slightly less than those with COPD, with an increased risk of mortality that was most prominent at 6 months after transplant followed by subsequent narrowing of the survival differences over time. Lung transplantationmay be aviable therapeutic option for patients with end-stage lung dysfunction resulting from a CTD.

▶ End-stage pulmonary disease as a manifestation of systemic connective tissue disease (CTD) is an uncommon indication for lung transplantation—less than 1% of reported transplants during the period covered by this report.[1] Part of the reason for this small representation in the transplant population is the rarity of the CTDs, but another reason is one that the authors suggest: the reluctance of transplant centers to accept these patients because of fear of progression of their extrapulmonary disease and possible recurrence of pulmonary disease. Previous reports of outcomes in CTD have focused on scleroderma patients who appear to have a similar outcome to non-CTD patients; however, these reports have included only small numbers of patients.[2,3] This study includes all the patients with any type of CTD—scleroderma, Sjogren, rheumatoid arthritis, dermatomyositis, mixed connective tissue, systemic lupus erythematosus—that underwent lung transplant over an 18-year period and is the most comprehensive report of these patients to date. It also includes patients who had both interstitial lung pathology and pulmonary hypertension. A goal of the investigators was to determine if the systemic diseases progressed after transplant. They had specific information about the underlying course of disease in 22 patients, 4 of whom had possible postoperative disease flares consisting of polyarthritis. None of the 22 patients had documented recurrent lung disease. In the broader group of CTD lung recipients, survival (a possible surrogate for recurrent disease) was very similar to that of idiopathic pulmonary fibrosis lung transplant recipients. This report should be reassuring to those transplant centers who have consciously or unconsciously avoided transplanting this type of patient.

J. R. Maurer, MD

References

1. Stehlik J, Edwards LB, Kucheryavaya AY, et al; International Society of Heart and Lung Transplantation. The Registry of the International Society for Heart and Lung Transplantation: 29th Official Adult Heart Transplant Report—2012. *J Heart Lung Transplant.* 2012;31(10):1052-1064.
2. Kubo M, Vensak J, Dauber J, Keenan R, Griffith B, McCurry K. Lung transplantation in patients with scleroderma. *J Heart Lung Transplant.* 2001;20:174-175.
3. Saggar R, Khanna D, Furst DE, et al. Systemic sclerosis and bilateral lung transplantation: a single centre experience. *Eur Respir J.* 2010;36:893-900.

7 Sleep Disorders

Introduction

Another year has passed, and I was once again tasked with selecting the top articles in sleep medicine from the last year. While the majority of the selections in the YEAR BOOK relate to obstructive sleep apnea, its relationship with comorbid disease exclusive of cardiovascular disease was highlighted. I encourage you to read the article by Nieto and colleagues, who established a step-wise association between cancer-related death and sleep-disordered breathing. Longer periods of hypoxia may perhaps evoke angiogenesis in certain types of cancer. There is already an increasing interest in circadian rhythms and cancer chronotherapeutics. Nieto and colleagues have added another interesting link to this area of research. I look forward to seeing additional studies that will examine the impact of CPAP on cancer-related mortality. Review the article entitled "Sleep Disturbances among Soldiers with Combat-Related Traumatic Brain Injury." This study certainly draws attention to the prevalence of OSA, insomnia, and concomitant use of narcotics and benzodiazepines amongst our military.

Also amongst this YEAR BOOK's top articles are studies that relate to both the young and the old(er). The largest study to date on obstructive sleep apnea links adverse outcomes amongst pregnant women with obstructive sleep apnea. I hope this article promotes a more aggressive approach to screening pregnant women for sleep-disordered breathing. Be sure to share "Clinical Practice Guideline: Diagnosis and management of childhood obstructive sleep apnea syndrome" with pediatricians and family medicine practitioners in your area. The article on insomnia and atherosclerosis risk in the elderly is very interesting. While much of the medical research and literature has focused on atherosclerosis and obstructive sleep apnea, we are just beginning to understand effects of insomnia, sleep loss, and deprivation on cardiovascular disease and mortality. Larger population-based studies are shedding light on this much needed area of research.

I have included a significant proportion of articles on obstructive sleep apnea. "Exercise is associated with a reduced incidence of sleep disordered breathing" is hypothesis generating. Meanwhile, hypoglossal nerve stimulation is something we will see more of in the future. This will give our patients a greater number of options to manage obstructive sleep apnea. The article written by Barbé and the Spanish Sleep and Breathing Network should be read by all and deserves special attention. While at a glance, it may seem that CPAP does not mitigate the development of new onset hypertension, I think with a closer look at the article, you will see that it does.

I hope you find the additional selections in this YEAR BOOK thought-provoking. I encourage you to share your thoughts with me and your colleagues.

Shirley F. Jones, MD, FCCP, DABSM

Central Sleep Apnea and Heart Failure

The Treatment of Central Sleep Apnea Syndromes in Adults: Practice Parameters with an Evidence-Based Literature Review and Meta-Analyses
Aurora RN, Chowdhuri S, Ramar K, et al (Johns Hopkins Univ, Baltimore, MD; John D. Dingell VA Med Ctr and Wayne State Univ, Detroit, MI; Mayo Clinic, Rochester, MN; et al)
Sleep 35:17-40, 2012

The International Classification of Sleep Disorders, Second Edition (ICSD-2) distinguishes 5 subtypes of central sleep apnea syndromes (CSAS) in adults. Review of the literature suggests that there are two basic mechanisms that trigger central respiratory events: (1) post-hyperventilation central apnea, which may be triggered by a variety of clinical conditions, and (2) central apnea secondary to hypoventilation, which has been described with opioid use. The preponderance of evidence on the treatment of CSAS supports the use of continuous positive airway pressure (CPAP). Much of the evidence comes from investigations on CSAS related to congestive heart failure (CHF), but other subtypes of CSAS appear to respond to CPAP as well. Limited evidence is available to support alternative therapies in CSAS subtypes. The recommendations for treatment of CSAS are summarized as follows:

- CPAP therapy targeted to normalize the apnea-hypopnea index (AHI) is indicated for the initial treatment of CSAS related to CHF. (STANDARD)
- Nocturnal oxygen therapy is indicated for the treatment of CSAS related to CHF. (STANDARD)
- Adaptive Servo-Ventilation (ASV) targeted to normalize the apnea-hypopnea index (AHI) is indicated for the treatment of CSAS related to CHF. (STANDARD)
- BPAP therapy *in a spontaneous timed (ST)* mode targeted to normalize the apnea-hypopnea index (AHI) may be considered for the treatment of CSAS related to CHF only if there is no response to adequate trials of CPAP, ASV, and oxygen therapies. (OPTION)
- The following therapies have limited supporting evidence but may be considered for the treatment of CSAS related to CHF after optimization of standard medical therapy, if PAP therapy is not tolerated, and if accompanied by close clinical follow-up: acetazolamide and theophylline. (OPTION)

- Positive airway pressure therapy may be considered for the treatment of primary CSAS. (OPTION)
- Acetazolamide has limited supporting evidence but may be considered for the treatment of primary CSAS. (OPTION)
- The use of zolpidem and triazolam may be considered for the treatment of primary CSAS only if the patient does not have underlying risk factors for respiratory depression. (OPTION)
- The following possible treatment options for CSAS related to end-stage renal disease may be considered: CPAP, supplemental oxygen, bicarbonate buffer use during dialysis, and nocturnal dialysis. (OPTION)

▶ This is an excellent article that summarizes the available evidence on management of central sleep apnea. It is well written and brings together a wealth of the published studies about the management of central sleep apnea into a single document. The authors are careful to make distinctions between the different types of central sleep apnea syndromes listed by the International Classification of Sleep Disorders. Because the greatest body of literature is on management of central sleep apnea caused by Cheyne Stokes breathing pattern, the authors evaluate different positive airway pressure devices separate from medical therapy. Outcomes important to congestive heart failure such as left ventricular ejection fraction, heart transplant free survival, and apnea-hypopnea index are focused in this article. Information on cost of therapy is supplied so the reader may glean the financial implications of each line of therapy. Finally, there is a portion of the article about future directions, specifically, studies that are currently underway. I look forward to the SERVE-HF study, which will examine hard outcomes of Adaptive Servo Ventilation on Survival and Hospital Admission in heart failure.

S. F. Jones, MD, FCCP, DABSM

Consequences of Sleep-Disordered Breathing

Obstructive Sleep Apnea Affects Hospital Outcomes of Patients with non-ST-Elevation Acute Coronary Syndromes
Correia LCL, Souza AC, Garcia G, et al (Med School of Bahia, Salvador, Brazil; San Rafael Hosp, Monte Tabor, Salvador/Bahia, Brazil; et al)
Sleep 35:1241-1245, 2012

Study Objective.—We aimed to test the hypothesis that clinically suspected obstructive sleep apnea (OSA) independently predicts worse in-hospital outcome in patients with non-ST elevation acute coronary syndromes.

Design.—At admission, individuals were evaluated for clinical probability of OSA by the Berlin Questionnaire. Primary cardiovascular endpoint was defined as the composite of death, nonfatal myocardial infarction, or refractory angina during hospitalization.

Setting.—Coronary care unit.

Patients.—There were 168 consecutive patients admitted with unstable angina or non-ST elevation acute myocardial infarction.

Measurements and Results.—During a median hospitalization of 8 days, the incidence of cardiovascular events was 13% (12 deaths, 4 nonfatal myocardial infarctions, and 6 refractory anginas.) Incidence of the primary endpoint was 18% in individuals with high probability of OSA, compared with no events in individuals with low probability ($P = 0.002$). After logistic regression adjustment for the Global Registry of Acute Coronary Events (GRACE) risk score, anatomic severity of coronary disease, and hospital treatment, probability of OSA remained an independent predictor of events (odds ratio [OR] = 3.4; 95% confidence interval [CI] = 1.3–9.0; $P = 0.015$). Prognostic discrimination of the GRACE score, measured by a C-statistic of 0.72 (95% CI = 0.59–0.85), was significantly improved to 0.82 (95% CI = 0.73–0.92) after inclusion of OSA probability in the predictive model ($P = 0.03$).

Conclusion.—Considering the independent prognostic and incremental value of suspected OSA, this condition may represent an aggravating factor for patients with non-ST elevation acute coronary syndrome.

▶ The collapse of the upper airway in obstructive sleep apnea (OSA) leads to decrease in oxygen and a surge of sympathetic activity following arousals. This process may be particularly harmful in the patient with acute coronary syndrome. By using the Berlin questionnaire, authors were able to quickly separate those subjects who were likely to have OSA and were able to observe a significant difference in the incidence of major cardiovascular events during hospitalization: death, nonfatal acute myocardial infarction, or refractory unstable angina between groups (Fig 1 in the original article). This study did run into a confounding effect in that patients who had no cardiovascular events had more 3 vessel involvement and higher Global Registry of Acute Coronary Events (GRACE) scores and required surgical revascularization; however, in the logistic regression after controlling for these confounders, OSA was still noted to be an independent risk factor for a major cardiovascular event during hospitalization; this risk was 3.4 times higher. The major limitation of this study is that those patients were never confirmed to have OSA by polysomnography. Although the Berlin questionnaire is a useful tool for screening purposes, its use has the best evidence in the outpatient primary care clinics, not in the hospital, and it has not been validated in this population. Nevertheless, the theory behind the findings does generate additional thoughts that vulnerability to plaque instability and endothelial dysfunction could potentially be modified or mitigated with treatment. This article should provoke additional studies in this area.

S. F. Jones, MD, FCCP, DABSM

Obstructive sleep apnea and the risk of adverse pregnancy outcomes

Chen Y-H, Kang J-H, Lin C-C, et al (Taipei Med Univ, Taiwan; Taipei Med Univ Hosp, Taiwan)
Am J Obstet Gynecol 206:136.e1-136.e5, 2012

Objective.—We examined the risk of adverse pregnancy outcomes, including low birthweight (LBW), preterm birth, small for gestational age (SGA), cesarean section (CS), low Apgar score (at 5 minutes after delivery), and preeclampsia in pregnant women with and without obstructive sleep apnea (OSA).

Study Design.—Our subjects included 791 women with OSA and 3955 randomly selected women without OSA. We performed conditional logistic regression analyses to examine the risks of adverse pregnancy outcomes between women with and without OSA.

Results.—Compared with women without OSA, adjusted odds ratios for LBW, preterm birth, SGA infants, CS, and preeclampsia in women with OSA were 1.76 (95% confidence interval [CI], 1.28−2.40), 2.31 (95% CI, 1.77−3.01), 1.34 (95% CI, 1.09−1.66), 1.74 (95% CI, 1.48−2.04), and 1.60 (95% CI, 2.16−11.26), respectively.

Conclusion.—Pregnant women with OSA are at increased risk for having LBW, preterm, and SGA infants, CS, and preeclampsia, compared with pregnant women without OSA.

▶ Understanding maternal and neonatal complications associated with obstructive sleep apnea (OSA) is a very important field, and this study represents the largest to date. Using 2 large population datasets from Taiwan, Chen and colleagues compared risk for adverse outcomes in 791 women with OSA and compared them with a control group of 3955 women without OSA. Risk for low birth weight, preterm birth, small for gestational age infants, cesarean section, and preeclampsia were all higher in women with OSA. This study lends greater evidence for screening efforts for OSA in this population. Although this study was performed in a Taiwanese population and limits generalizing its results to other ethnicities, the study is still quite meaningful, particularly because of its large study sample. A smaller study conducted by Louis et al was conducted in 57 pregnant women with OSA in the United States with results similar to those noted by Chen.[1]

S. F. Jones, MD, FCCP, DABSM

Reference

1. Louis JM, Auckley D, Sokol RJ, Mercer BM. Maternal and neonatal morbidities associated with obstructive sleep apnea complicating pregnancy. *Am J Obstet Gynecol.* 2010;202:261.e1-261.e5.

A 3-year longitudinal study of sleep disordered breathing in the elderly

Sforza E, Gauthier M, Crawford-Achour E, et al (PRES Université de Lyon, Saint-Etienne, France)
Eur Respir J 40:665-672, 2012

Limited and controversial data exist on the natural evolution of sleep disordered breathing (SDB) in untreated individuals. This study examines the evolution of SDB over a 3-yr period in a community-based sample of elderly subjects.

From the initial cohort of 854 healthy subjects aged mean $\pm$ SD 68.4 $\pm$ 0.8 yrs, 519 untreated subjects accepted clinical and instrumental follow-up 3.6 $\pm$ 1.6 yrs later. SDB was defined as a respiratory disturbance index (RDI) >15 events·h^{-1}.

At baseline, 202 (39%) subjects had an RDI $\leq$ 15 events·h^{-1} and 317 (61%) had an RDI > 15 events·h^{-1}. 3 yrs later, 280 (54%) subjects were non-SDB and 239 (46%) had SDB. Between evaluations, the RDI decreased from 22.3 $\pm$ 16.2 to 16.4 $\pm$ 13.0 events·h^{-1}, with a greater decrease in the number of cases with an RDI > 30 events·h^{-1} that in those with RDI $\geq$ 30 events·h^{-1}. In the non-SDB group, 81% had a stable RDI and 19% increased their RDI by a mean of 13.7 events·h^{-1}. In the SDB group, the RDI decreased to values $\leq$ 15 events·h^{-1} in 36.6% of cases, 63.4% still having SDB. The RDI changes did not depend on weight changes.

In healthy elderly subjects, the prevalence and severity of SDB did not show a tendency toward natural worsening, some cases having improvement or a remission independent of weight changes. These findings also suggest that in the elderly, natural SDB progression is still hypothetical.

▶ We still have a lot to learn about the natural progression of sleep-disordered breathing and what drives it. Sforza and colleagues expand our knowledge with this study of 519 untreated subjects 65 years of age over a period of 3 years. A total of 61% of subjects had sleep-disordered breathing diagnosed (respiratory disturbance index of > 15 events per hour). Despite lack of treatment, there were decreases in blood pressure and respiratory disturbance index without any change in the degree of sleepiness at 3-year follow-up. A total of 36% of subjects who had respiratory disturbance index (RDI) greater than 15 at baseline now had RDI $\leq$15 events per hour. The change in the RDI was not due to changes in weight. Although this may indicate that age alone is not a significant modifier of sleep-disordered breathing, the details deserve a better look. Much like other longitudinal studies of sleep-disordered breathing in the elderly,[1] the changes in the respiratory disturbance index are small over time. In this particular study by Sforza and colleagues, the changes in body mass index were very small (on average < 0.5 kg/m^2). The study was conducted in France in otherwise healthy older patients. The results of this study may not be applicable in the US population where we see increasing rates of obesity. Furthermore, the change in the RDI alone may not reflect harder clinical outcomes such as cardiovascular disease and stroke and their impacts.

S. F. Jones, MD, FCCP, DABSM

Reference

1. Silva GE, An MW, Goodwin JL, et al. Longitudinal evaluation of sleep-disordered breathing and sleep symptoms with change in quality of life: the Sleep Heart Health Study (SHHS). *Sleep.* 2009;32:1049-1057.

Cardiovascular Mortality in Obstructive Sleep Apnea in the Elderly: Role of Long-Term Continuous Positive Airway Pressure Treatment: A Prospective Observational Study

Martínez-García M-A, Campos-Rodríguez F, Catalán-Serra P, et al (La Fe Univ and Polytechnic Hosp, Valencia, Spain; Valme Univ Hosp, Seville, Spain; Requena General Hosp, Valencia, Spain)
Am J Respir Crit Care Med 186:909-916, 2012

Rationale.—Obstructive sleep apnea (OSA) is a risk factor for cardiovascular death in middle-aged subjects, but it is not known whether it is also a risk factor in the elderly.

Objectives.—To investigate whether OSA is a risk factor for cardiovascular death and to assess whether continuous positive airway pressure (CPAP) treatment is associated with a change in risk in the elderly.

Methods.—Prospective, observational study of a consecutive cohort of elderly patients (≥65 yr) studied for suspicion of OSA between 1998 and 2007. Patients with an apnea—hypopnea index (AHI) less than 15 were the control group. OSA was defined as mild to moderate (AHI, 15—29) or severe (AHI, ≥30). Patients with OSA were classified as CPAP-treated (adherence ≥4 h/d) or untreated (adherence < 4 h/d or not prescribed). Participants were monitored until December 2009. The end point was cardiovascular death. A multivariate Cox survival analysis was used to determine the independent impact of OSA and CPAP treatment on cardiovascular mortality.

Measurements and Main Results.—A total of 939 elderly were studied (median follow-up, 69 mo). Compared with the control group, the fully adjusted hazard ratios for cardiovascular mortality were 2.25 (confidence interval [CI], 1.41 to 3.61) for the untreated severe OSA group, 0.93 (CI, 0.46 to 1.89) for the CPAP-treated group, and 1.38 (CI, 0.73 to 2.64) for the untreated mild to moderate OSA group.

Conclusions.—Severe OSA not treated with CPAP is associated with cardiovascular death in the elderly, and adequate CPAP treatment may reduce this risk.

▶ How is this different than other studies and what we already know? While we know that obstructive sleep apnea (OSA) is associated with increased cardiovascular events, this association has primarily been seen in middle aged men.[1] The association between OSA and cardiovascular mortality in elderly people is not known. However, in practice, many of us extrapolate that data to the elderly without any real evidence.

Martínez-García and colleagues are the first to show that severe untreated obstructive sleep apnea is associated with increased cardiovascular mortality in patients 65 years and older, specifically from stroke and congestive heart failure. This risk is approximately 4-fold versus patients without OSA. Interestingly, increased cardiovascular mortality from ischemic heart disease was not significant. The study cannot determine the cause of this, but other studies have noticed this finding as well.[2] This study also shows that use of continuous positive airway pressure was associated with a reduced risk of cardiovascular mortality. The reduced risk of mortality was similar to that in subjects without OSA and those with moderate disease.

The authors should be commended for several things in this study: the mean follow-up of 69 months and completed follow-up in 99.5% of subjects and large sample size, just to name a few.

S. F. Jones, MD, FCCP, DABSM

References

1. Marin JM, Carrizo SJ, Vicente E, Agusti AG. Long-term cardiovascular outcomes in men with obstructive sleep apnoea-hypopnoea with or without treatment with continuous positive airway pressure: an observational study. *Lancet.* 2005;365: 1046-1053.
2. Lavie P, Lavie L. Unexpected survival advantage in elderly people with moderate sleep apnoea. *J Sleep Res.* 2009;18:397-403.

Sleep-disordered Breathing and Cancer Mortality: Results from the Wisconsin Sleep Cohort Study
Nieto FJ, Peppard PE, Young T, et al (Univ of Wisconsin—Madison)
Am J Respir Crit Care Med 186:190-194, 2012

Rationale.—Sleep-disordered breathing (SDB) has been associated with total and cardiovascular mortality, but an association with cancer mortality has not been studied. Results from *in vitro* and animal studies suggest that intermittent hypoxia promotes cancer tumor growth.

Objectives.—The goal of the present study was to examine whether SDB is associated with cancer mortality in a community-based sample.

Methods.—We used 22-year mortality follow-up data from the Wisconsin Sleep Cohort sample (n = 1,522). SDB was assessed at baseline with full polysomnography. SDB was categorized using the apnea-hypopnea index (AHI) and the hypoxemia index (percent sleep time below 90% oxyhemoglobin saturation). The hazards of cancer mortality across levels of SDB severity were compared using crude and multivariate analyses.

Measurements and Main Results.—Adjusting for age, sex, body mass index, and smoking, SDB was associated with total and cancer mortality in a dose—response fashion. Compared with normal subjects, the adjusted relative hazards of cancer mortality were 1.1 (95% confidence interval [CI], 0.5—2.7) for mild SDB (AHI, 5—14.9), 2.0 (95% CI, 0.7—5.5) for moderate SDB (AHI, 15—29.9), and 4.8 (95% CI, 1.7—13.2) for severe

TABLE 2.—Adjusted Relative Hazards of Total and Cancer Mortality According to Sleep-Disordered Breathing Categories

SDB (AHI Range)	All-Cause Mortality	Cancer Mortality
Absent (<5)	1.0	1.0
Mild SDB (5—14.9)	1.8 (1.1—2.8)	1.1 (0.5—2.7)
Moderate SDB (15—29.9)	1.1 (0.5—2.5)	2.0 (0.7—5.5)
Severe SDB (≥30)*	3.4 (1.7—6.7)	4.8 (1.7—13.2)
P for trend	0.0014	0.0052

Definition of abbreviations: AHI = apnea-hypopnea index; BMI = body mass index; CI = confidence interval; CPAP = continuous positive airway pressure; SDB ¼ sleep-disordered breathing.
Data are presented as adjusted relative hazard (95% CI). Adjusted for age (time scale), sex, BMI, BMI², and smoking.
*Includes participants who were subject to CPAP treatment during the polysomnography study (n = 9).

TABLE 3.—Adjusted Relative Hazards of Cancer Mortality According to Hypoxemia Index

Hypoxemia Index*	Relative Hazards of Cancer Mortality (95% CI)
Percentile < 73 (<0.8% of the time)	1.0
Percentile 73—89 (0.8—3.6% of the time)	1.6 (0.6—4.4)
Percentile 90—97 (3.6—11.2% of the time)	2.9 (0.9—9.8)
Percentile > 97 (.11.2% of the time)	8.6 (2.6—28.7)
P for trend	0.0008

Definition of abbreviations: AHI = apnea-hypopnea index; BMI = body mass index; CI = confidence interval.
Adjusted for age (time scale), sex, BMI, BMI², and smoking. Hypoxemia index = percent sleep time below 90% oxyhemoglobin saturation; analyses based on a subset of 1,306 participants on whom O_2 saturation data were available.
*Cut-offs defined according to the same percentile distribution as that resulting from the standard AHI cut-offs used in this study (AHI = 5, 15, and 30).

SDB (AHI ≥ 30) (*P*-trend = 0.0052). For categories of increasing severity of the hypoxemia index, the corresponding relative hazards were 1.6 (95% CI, 0.6—4.4), 2.9 (95% CI, 0.9—9.8), and 8.6 (95% CI, 2.6—28.7).

Conclusions.—Our study suggests that baseline SDB is associated with increased cancer mortality in a community-based sample. Future studies that replicate our findings and look at the association between sleep apnea and survival after cancer diagnosis are needed (Tables 2 and 3).

▶ This article is the first to demonstrate an association between sleep-disordered breathing and cancer-related death. In Tables 2 and 3, the severity of sleep-disordered breathing and the percent of time with hypoxia show a stepwise increase in cancer mortality. Fig 1 in the original article depicts that severe sleep-disordered breathing had the lowest survival rates. The etiology of this is not known, but the authors suggest that hypoxia-mediated tumor growth may play a role. The limitations of this study include the small number of cancer-related deaths in this population (n = 50). Further studies need to be performed to confirm these results and, if possible, the effect of continuous positive airway pressure on cancer death.

S. F. Jones, MD, FCCP, DABSM

CPAP Treatment and Benefits

Association Between Treated and Untreated Obstructive Sleep Apnea and Risk of Hypertension

Marin JM, Agusti A, Villar I, et al (Hosp Universitario Miguel Servet, Zaragoza, Spain; Thorax Inst, Barcelona, Spain; Aragon Inst of Health Sciences, Zaragoza, Spain; et al)

JAMA 307:2169-2176, 2012

Context.—Systemic hypertension is prevalent among patients with obstructive sleep apnea (OSA). Short-term studies indicate that continuous positive airway pressure (CPAP) therapy reduces blood pressure in patients with hypertension and OSA.

Objective.—To determine whether CPAP therapy is associated with a lower risk of incident hypertension.

Design, Setting, and Participants.—A prospective cohort study of 1889 participants without hypertension who were referred to a sleep center in Zaragoza, Spain, for nocturnal polysomnography between January 1, 1994, and December 31, 2000. Incident hypertension was documented at annual follow-up visits up to January 1, 2011. Multivariable models adjusted for confounding factors, including change in body mass index from baseline to censored time, were used to calculate hazard ratios (HRs) of incident hypertension in participants without OSA (controls), with untreated OSA, and in those treated with CPAP therapy according to national guidelines.

Main Outcome Measure.—Incidence of new-onset hypertension.

Results.—During 21 003 person-years of follow-up (median, 12.2 years), 705 cases (37.3%) of incident hypertension were observed. The crude incidence of hypertension per 100 person-years was 2.19 (95% CI, 1.71-2.67) in controls, 3.34 (95% CI, 2.85-3.82) in patients with OSA ineligible for CPAP therapy, 5.84 (95% CI, 4.82-6.86) in patients with OSA who declined CPAP therapy, 5.12 (95% CI, 3.76-6.47) in patients with OSA nonadherent to CPAP therapy, and 3.06 (95% CI, 2.70-3.41) in patients with OSA and treated with CPAP therapy. Compared with controls, the adjusted HRs for incident hypertension were greater among patients with OSA ineligible for CPAP therapy (1.33; 95% CI, 1.01-1.75), among those who declined CPAP therapy (1.96; 95% CI, 1.44-2.66), and among those nonadherent to CPAP therapy (1.78; 95% CI, 1.23-2.58), whereas the HR was lower in patients with OSA who were treated with CPAP therapy (0.71; 95% CI, 0.53-0.94).

Conclusion.—Compared with participants without OSA, the presence of OSA was associated with increased adjusted risk of incident hypertension; however, treatment with CPAP therapy was associated with a lower risk of hypertension.

▶ This article by Marin and colleagues lend supportive evidence that patients with obstructive sleep apnea (OSA) are at risk for the development of new-onset hypertension. In addition, this study shows that use of continuous positive airway pressure (CPAP), particularly in those with severe OSA, seems to mitigate the development of new-onset hypertension. This study advances the literature to the question of "Is there a causal link between OSA and incident hypertension?" The long-term follow-up of study subjects (median 12.2 years) and the measurement and inclusion of significant covariates in the analysis (change in body mass index, cigarette smoking, and alcohol consumption) strengthen this study's findings. It is interesting that even after controlling for body mass index, the risk of incident hypertension was lower in subjects treated with CPAP compared with the other groups, a suggestion that CPAP therapy may be protective against the development of new-onset hypertension.

While the observational nature of the study may lead some to criticize the findings, I believe that such a study design is very acceptable and appropriate. Specifically, research subjects were not randomly assigned to the arms of the study; instead, groups were separated based on the treatment received or not received (either by patient choice or national guidelines). This may have introduced bias in that patients who choose CPAP are those who are more likely to choose healthy behaviors. However, the authors reported similar adherence rates to cholesterol medications among subjects in all groups, which refutes that the significant differences noted in the subjects who were treated with CPAP are due to healthy behaviors. A take-home point is that clinicians should screen obese and overweight patients for OSA and that institution of therapy reduces risk of incident hypertension regardless of weight increase.

S. F. Jones, MD, FCCP, DABSM

Obstructive Sleep Apnea: Effects of Continuous Positive Airway Pressure on Cardiac Remodeling as Assessed by Cardiac Biomarkers, Echocardiography and Cardiac MRI
Colish J, Walker JR, Elmayergi N, et al (St Boniface General Hosp, Winnipeg, Manitoba, Canada; Univ of Manitoba, Winnipeg, Canada)
Chest 141:674-681, 2012

Background.—Obstructive sleep apnea (OSA) is associated with an increased risk of cardiovascular morbidity and mortality. Although previous echocardiographic studies have demonstrated shortterm improvement in cardiovascular remodeling in patients with OSA receiving continuous positive airway pressure (CPAP) therapy, a long-term study incorporating cardiac biomarkers, echocardiography, and cardiac MRI (CMR) has not been performed to date.

Methods.—A prospective study of 47 patients with OSA was performed between 2007 and 2010. Cardiac biomarkers, including C-reactive protein (CRP), N-terminal pro-B-type natriuretic peptide (NT-proBNP), and troponin T (TnT), were measured at baseline and serially over 1 year. All patients underwent baseline and serial transthoracic echocardiography (TTE) and CMR to assess cardiac remodeling.

Results.—Following 12 months of CPAP therapy, levels of CRP, NT-proBNP, and TnT did not change significantly from normal baseline values. As early as 3 months after initiation of CPAP, TTE revealed an improvement in right ventricular end-diastolic diameter, left atrial volume index, right atrial volume index, and degree of pulmonary hypertension, which continued to improve over 1 year of follow-up. Finally, left ventricular mass, as determined by CMR, decreased from 159 ± 12 g/m^2 to 141 ± 8 g/m^2 as early as 6 months into CPAP therapy and continued to improve until completion of the study at 1 year.

Conclusion.—Both systolic and diastolic abnormalities in patients with OSA can be reversed as early as 3 months into CPAP therapy, with progressive improvement in cardiovascular remodeling over 1 year as assessed by both TTE and CMR.

▶ Obstructive sleep apnea (OSA) is an independent risk factor for pulmonary hypertension.[1] The findings of significant reductions in right atrial and right ventricular measures based on echo in as little as 3 months after continuous positive airway pressure (CPAP) use is significant with further improvements up to a year (Fig 1 in the original article). Similar reductions in right atrial and right ventricular measures using cardiac magnetic resonance imaging (MRI) in this study support the evidence that CPAP can reverse cardiac abnormalities. The use of cardiac MRI is a strength in this study because often echocardiography is difficult to perform and interpret in obese individuals. The longer follow-up in this study (1 year) is also a strength. The authors chose to study patients with no evidence of cardiac disease or hypertension, so it is not surprising to me that there were no observed differences in cardiac biomarkers. However, the significant changes noted on echocardiography and cardiac MRI in subjects *without* clinical evidence of cardiac disease questions if similar results will be found in those *with* cardiac disease. Further research is needed. There are some limitations to this study, such as lack of a control group (untreated OSA), but inclusion of sham CPAP in a population with severe OSA (such as this study) would be unethical.

S. F. Jones, MD, FCCP, DABSM

Reference

1. Alchanatis M, Tourkohoriti G, Kakouros S, Kosmas E, Podaras S, Jordanoglou JB. Daytime pulmonary hypertension in patients with obstructive sleep apnea: the effect of continuous positive airway pressure on pulmonary hemodynamics. *Respiration.* 2001;68:566-572.

Control of OSA During Automatic Positive Airway Pressure Titration in a Clinical Case Series: Predictors and Accuracy of Device Download Data
Huang H-CC, Hillman DR, McArdle N (The Canberra Hosp, Woden, ACT, Australia; Sir Charles Gairdner Hosp, Nedlands WA, Australia)
Sleep 35:1277-1283, 2012

Study Objectives.—To investigate the factors associated with physiologic control of obstructive sleep apnea (OSA) during automatic positive airway pressure (APAP) titration in a clinical series. To also assess the usefulness of apnea-hypopnea index (AHI) data downloaded from the APAP device (Dev AHI).

Design.—Retrospective review of a consecutive series of patients with OSA who underwent APAP titration (Autoset Spirit, ResMed, Bella Vista, New South Wales, Australia) with simultaneous polysomnographic (PSG) monitoring in the sleep laboratory.

Setting.—Tertiary sleep clinic.

Participants.—There were 190 consecutive patients with OSA referred for APAP titration.

Measurements and Results.—There were 58% of patients who achieved optimal or good control of OSA (titration PSG AHI < 10, or at least 50% reduction in AHI if diagnostic AHI < 15/hr) during APAP titration. The independent predictors of titration PSG AHI were a history of cardiac disease and elevated central apnea and arousal indices during the diagnostic study. Although the median and interquartile range (IQR) AHI from the device (7.0, 3.9-11.6 events/hr) was only slightly less than the PSG AHI (7.8, 3.9-14.4 events/hr, $P = 0.04$) during titration, case-by-case agreement between the two measures was poor (chi-square < 0.001).

Conclusion.—In a clinical sample control of OSA during APAP titration is often poor, and close clinical follow-up is particularly needed in patients with a history of cardiac disease or with high arousal or central apnea indices on the diagnostic study. Device AHI does not reliably assess control during APAP titration, and PSG assessment may be required if clinical response to treatment is poor. The findings relate to the ResMed AutoSet device and may not apply to other devices.

▶ Using autotitrating positive airway pressure (APAP) downloads to determine clinical response to treatment is common in clinical practice. However, this approach is contingent on how well the device is able to accurately assess the residual apnea hypopnea index and the measures of central apneas. Unfortunately, with the variety of APAP devices available today, the numbers on the download depend on the proprietary algorithm of the manufacturer. Without knowledge of how the device measures hypopneas and apneas, we cannot make fair comparisons.

The basis of the APAP device is to deliver the minimum effective pressure needed in response to dynamic changes in upper airway resistance or flow. The findings that higher device apnea-hypopnea indexes are seen in certain populations (cardiac disease, poor sleep efficiency, higher arousals and awakenings during the diagnostic polysomnographic monitoring) suggest that a blanketed approach to using APAP is not ideal. Appropriate selection of patients and close clinical follow-up is necessary. Failure to respond to therapy should signal to the provider that a continuous positive airway pressure titration in the laboratory is needed.

S. F. Jones, MD, FCCP, DABSM

Effect of Continuous Positive Airway Pressure on the Incidence of Hypertension and Cardiovascular Events in Nonsleepy Patients With Obstructive Sleep Apnea: A Randomized Controlled Trial

Barbé F, for the Spanish Sleep and Breathing Network (IRB Lleida, Spain; et al)
JAMA 307:2161-2168, 2012

Context.—Continuous positive airway pressure (CPAP) is the first-line treatment for patients with symptomatic obstructive sleep apnea (OSA). However, its indication for all patients with sleep-disordered breathing, regardless of daytime symptoms, is unclear.

Objective.—To evaluate the effect of CPAP treatment on the incidence of hypertension or cardiovascular events in a cohort of nonsleepy patients with OSA.

Design, Setting, and Patients.—Multicenter, parallel-group, randomized controlled trial in 14 teaching hospitals in Spain. Between May 2004 and May 2006, 725 consecutive patients were enrolled who had an apnea-hypopnea index of $20 \, h^{-1}$ or greater and an Epworth Sleepiness Scale score of 10 or less (scores range from 0-24, with values < 10 suggesting no daytime sleepiness). Exclusion criteria were previous cardiovascular event, physical or psychological incapacity, chronic disease, or drug or alcohol addiction. Follow-up ended in May 2009.

Intervention.—Patients were allocated to receive CPAP treatment or no active intervention. All participants received dietary counseling and sleep hygiene advice.

Main Outcome Measures.—Incidence of either systemic hypertension (taking antihypertensive medication or blood pressure greater than 140/90 mm Hg) or cardiovascular event (nonfatal myocardial infarction, nonfatal stroke, transient ischemic attack, hospitalization for unstable angina or arrhythmia, heart failure, or cardiovascular death).

Results.—Seven hundred twenty-three patients underwent follow-up for a median of 4 (interquartile range, 2.7-4.4) years (1 patient from each group did not receive allocated treatment); 357 in the CPAP group and 366 in the control group were included in the analysis. In the CPAP group there were 68 patients with new hypertension and 28 cardiovascular events (17 unstable angina or arrhythmia, 3 nonfatal stroke, 3 heart failure, 2 nonfatal myocardial infarction, 2 transient ischemic attack, 1 cardiovascular death). In the control group there were 79 patients with new hypertension and 31 cardiovascular events (11 unstable angina or arrhythmia, 8 nonfatal myocardial infarction, 5 transient ischemic attack, 5 heart failure, 2 nonfatal stroke). The hypertension or cardiovascular event incidence density rate was 9.20 per 100 person-years (95% CI, 7.36-11.04) in the CPAP group and 11.02 per 100 person-years (95% CI, 8.96-13.08) in the control group. The incidence density ratio was 0.83 (95% CI, 0.63-1.1; $P = .20$).

Conclusions.—In patients with OSA without daytime sleepiness, the prescription of CPAP compared with usual care did not result in a statistically significant reduction in the incidence of hypertension or cardiovascular events. However, the study may have had limited power to detect a significant difference.

Trial Registration.—clinicaltrials.gov Identifier: NCT00127348.

▶ In my practice, I find it challenging to address the benefits of continuous positive airway pressure (CPAP) in my patients who are not sleepy. During follow-up, patients often report no perceived benefit from using the device—there is no improvement in how they feel when waking up, no difference in drowsiness during the day, etc. But one must remember these people were not drowsy to start. So how does one tout the benefits of CPAP in nonsleepy individuals when the benefits are not subject to feelings or symptoms? I prefer to explain the benefits of CPAP from the standpoint of lower cardiovascular morbidity and mortality, as this effect has been observed previously.[1] In this article, Barbé and colleagues aimed to evaluate the effect of CPAP treatment on the incidence of hypertension or cardiovascular events in a cohort of nonsleepy patients with obstructive sleep apnea (OSA). Although overall the effect of CPAP on the development of incident hypertension was insignificant, I think we should be careful not to offer such a blanketed statement to our patients. Median follow-up was 4 years (range 2.7-4.4 years), which is still short. Furthermore, half of the patients enrolled had hypertension at the time of enrollment and hence could only fulfill the primary outcome of measurement by development of cardiovascular event within the short study duration. The authors suggest that the study may have suffered from limited power to detect significant differences between groups, a statement with which I agree. The power analysis was based on a cohort of sleepy patients. Furthermore, the post hoc analysis did show significant improvement in the incidence of hypertension or cardiovascular event in subjects who used CPAP for more than 4 hours per night. This finding is in line with other studies. In summary, though at first glance it appears that CPAP may not benefit nonsleepy patients with OSA, the fine details do support its use.

S. F. Jones, MD, FCCP, DABSM

Reference

1. Marin JM, Carrizo SJ, Vicente E, Agusti AG. Long-term cardiovascular outcomes in men with obstructive sleep apnoea-hypopnoea with or without treatment with continuous positive airway pressure: an observational study. *Lancet.* 2005;365: 1046-1053.

Continuous Positive Airway Pressure Treatment of Sleepy Patients with Milder Obstructive Sleep Apnea: Results of the CPAP Apnea Trial North American Program (CATNAP) Randomized Clinical Trial

Weaver TE, Mancini C, Maislin G, et al (Univ of Illinois at Chicago College of Nursing; Univ of Pennsylvania School of Nursing, Philadelphia; Univ of Pennsylvania School of Medicine, Philadelphia; et al)
Am J Respir Crit Care Med 186:677-683, 2012

Rationale.—Twenty-eight percent of people with mild to moderate obstructive sleep apnea experience daytime sleepiness, which interferes with daily functioning. It remains unclear whether treatment with continuous positive airway pressure improves daytime function in these patients.

Objectives.—To evaluate the efficacy of continuous positive airway pressure treatment to improve functional status in sleepy patients with mild and moderate obstructive sleep apnea.

Methods.—Patients with self-reported daytime sleepiness (Epworth Sleepiness Scale score > 10) and an apnea-hypopnea index with 3% desaturation and from 5 to 30 events per hour were randomized to 8 weeks of active or sham continuous positive airway pressure treatment. After the 8-week intervention, participants in the sham arm received 8 weeks of active continuous positive airway pressure treatment.

Measurements and Main Results.—The Total score on the Functional Outcomes of Sleep Questionnaire was the primary outcome measure. The adjusted mean change in the Total score after the first 8-week intervention was 0.89 for the active group (n = 113) and −0.06 for the placebo group (n = 110) (P = 0.006). The group difference in mean change corresponded to an effect size of 0.41 (95% confidence interval, 0.14-0.67). The mean (SD) improvement in Functional Outcomes of Sleep Questionnaire Total score from the beginning to the end of the crossover phase (n = 91) was 1.73 ± 2.50 ($t[90] = 6.59$; P < 0.00001) with an effect size of 0.69.

Conclusions.—Continuous positive airway pressure treatment improves the functional outcome of sleepy patients with mild and moderate obstructive sleep apnea.

▶ The practice parameters of the American Academy of Sleep Medicine support a standard recommendation for use of continuous positive airway pressure (CPAP) in patients with moderate to severe obstructive sleep apnea (OSA) resulting from a multitude of supportive data from randomized controlled trials.[1] However, the level of recommendation for use of CPAP to treat mild OSA is optional because of conflicting evidence from previous studies. The authors aimed to evaluate the effect of CPAP on functional study in patients with mild OSA but with self-reported sleepiness based on the Epworth Sleepiness Scale score. Subjects were randomized to therapeutic or sham CPAP for 8 weeks. Those who received sham CPAP then used therapeutic CPAP for another 8 weeks. The strength of this article lies in the use of sham CPAP. Previous studies that examine the effect of CPAP in mild OSA patients with sleepiness used oral placebo tablets, quite different from CPAP, and hence introduced potential bias to their results.[2] To eliminate this potential source of bias, a study would have to include a sham CPAP intervention, a not-so-easy task because of the known effectiveness of CPAP in treating patients with severe sleep apnea and its effect on reducing cardiovascular events. Fortunately, this population has milder degrees of OSA and are otherwise healthy individuals with stable medical problems, so the ethical problem was avoided. The findings from this article support use of CPAP to statistically reduce sleepiness and improve productivity, vigilance, and activity. However, CPAP induced only a mean change in Epworth was of −2.6. The mean Epworth at baseline in CPAP group was 15.21, which indicates that patients were still sleepy despite therapeutic CPAP. Why is this the case? Participant's use of CPAP was just 4 hours. It is not clear from the study why device adherence was less than expected, but this is most likely the reason for persistent sleepiness in this study. Nevertheless, based on this study, patients with mild OSA and subjective sleepiness should be offered CPAP as its use does improve functional outcomes.

S. F. Jones, MD, FCCP, DABSM

References

1. Kushida CA, Littner MR, Hirshkowitz M, et al. Practice parameters for the use of continuous and bilevel positive airway pressure devices to treat adult patients with sleep-related breathing disorders. *Sleep.* 2006;29:375-380.
2. Engleman HM, Kingshott RN, Wraith PK, Mackay TW, Deary IJ, Douglas NJ. Randomized placebo-controlled crossover trial of continuous positive airway pressure for mild sleep Apnea/Hypopnea syndrome. *Am J Respir Crit Care Med.* 1999; 159:461-467.

Non-CPAP Treatment of Sleep-Disordered Breathing

Exercise Is Associated with a Reduced Incidence of Sleep-disordered Breathing

Awad KM, Malhotra A, Barnet JH, et al (Brigham and Women's Hosp, Boston, MA; Univ of Wisconsin School of Medicine and Public Health—Madison)
Am J Med 125:485-490, 2012

Background.—The effect of exercise on sleep-disordered breathing is unknown. While diet and weight loss have been shown to reduce the severity of sleep-disordered breathing, it is unclear whether exercise has an independent effect.

Methods.—A population-based longitudinal epidemiologic study of adults measured the association between exercise and incidence and severity of sleep-disordered breathing. Hours of weekly exercise were assessed by 2 mailed surveys (1988 and 2000). Sleep-disordered breathing was assessed by 18-channel in-laboratory polysomnography at baseline and at follow-up.

Results.—Associations were modeled using linear and logistic regression, adjusting for body mass index, age, sex, and other covariates. Hours of exercise were associated with reduced incidence of mild (odds ratio 0.76, $P = .011$) and moderate (odds ratio 0.67, $P = .002$) sleep-disordered breathing. A decrease in exercise duration also was associated with worsening sleep-disordered breathing, as measured by the apnea-hypopnea index ($\beta = 2.368$, $P = .048$). Adjustment for body mass index attenuated these effects.

Conclusions.—Exercise is associated with a reduced incidence of mild and moderate sleep-disordered breathing, and decreasing exercise is associated with worsening of sleep-disordered breathing. The effect of exercise on sleep-disordered breathing appears to be largely, but perhaps not entirely, mediated by changes in body habitus.

▶ Recommendations for food modification and exercise are standard recommendations to our patients with obstructive sleep apnea forming the pillars of a weight loss program. Although weight loss does reduce the severity of sleep-disordered breathing and in many cases can be curative, the authors in this study aimed to determine if there is an independent effect of exercise on sleep-disordered breathing. Using data from the Wisconsin Sleep Cohort, a longitudinal study of a middle-aged population, Awad and colleagues report that exercising anywhere from 1 to 4 hours per week reduced the incidence of new-onset mild or moderate sleep-disordered breathing over a follow-up period of 8 years. Despite the fact that the population studied gained weight (on average the group went from overweight to obese), the risk of incident OSA in exercisers did not completely equate to those who did not exercise at all with an odds ratio of 0.65 and 0.74 for mild to moderate obstructive sleep apnea, respectively, in those subjects who exercised ≥4 hours per week. Although the *P* values are technically insignificant, there is some evidence that exercise has a protective effect independent of body mass index. The authors describe the possible ways: (1) through increase in upper airway muscle tone, (2) changes in distribution of body fat, and/or (3) alteration in control of breathing and arousal threshold. Exploration is needed to discover the mechanisms behind these findings.

S. F. Jones, MD, FCCP, DABSM

Long-term follow-up of patients operated with Uvulopalatopharyngoplasty from 1985 to 1991

Värendh M, Berg S, Andersson M (Lund Univ, Sweden)
Respir Med 106:1788-1793, 2012

Objectives.—Short-term outcome and side effects after Uvulopalatopharyngoplasty (UPPP) are well recognized. However, there is a lack of knowledge of the long-term outcome and side effects after this surgery. This study was completed to investigate the outcome and side effects 20 years after UPPP for snoring and obstructive sleep apnoea.

Methods.—Medical records of patients who underwent UPPP surgery for sleep apnoea and snoring between 1985 and 1991 were investigated retrospectively. A specific questionnaire focusing on the present health profile, side effects of previous UPPP surgery and present sleeping patterns of patients was mailed out.

Results.—UPPP patients, 186 (including 11 females) were identified. Of these, 35 (19%) had passed away and 7 (4%) were not located. 129 patients (mean: age 68 years, range 43—83) of the possible 144 patients answered the questionnaire (response rate 90%). At follow-up, 41 patients (32%) used continuous positive airway pressure (CPAP). 66 of the patients (52%) were satisfied with the result of the operation, but 61 (47%) were not satisfied. 49 patients (38%) reported persistent side effects (problems with nasal regurgitation 18 (14%), swallowing 26 (20%), changed voice 15 (12%), and pain in the oral cavity 15 (12%).

Conclusion.—Almost 50% of patients operated with UPPP were not satisfied with the result of the operation after about 20 years, and one third used CPAP at follow-up. A large proportion of patients still experienced side effects, which, after this time, are likely to be permanent.

▶ I like the simplicity behind this study, which is to investigate the current status of patients who received Uvulopalatopharyngoplasty between 1985 and 1991. The authors are commended for a survey response rate of 90%, which is hard to accomplish. Thirty-two percent of those studied were using continuous positive airway pressure (CPAP). However, the number with sleep apnea is more as an additional 13% of non-CPAP users actually reported having obstructive sleep apnea. Hence, a total of 55 of 129 subjects (34%) continue to have obstructive sleep apnea despite surgery. It is not surprising that surgical satisfaction and choice were closely related to use of CPAP (CPAP users were not satisfied). Nearly 40% of subjects still experience side effects, which indicate that these are permanent. It is possible that the number of subjects who undergo this procedure today may experience fewer side effects, particularly as Uvulopalatopharyngoplasty has been modified because of associated velopharyngeal insufficiency. Because of the nonselective nature of those subjects who received Uvulopalatopharyngoplasty during this period, the results were less than optimal for many. As a result, one-third of patients reported using CPAP. With 50% of patients not satisfied with the result of Uvulopalatopharyngoplasty in this study, there is an unmet need to compare effectiveness of different surgical techniques and standardize the definition of success in the area of surgical therapies for obstructive sleep apnea.

S. F. Jones, MD, FCCP, DABSM

Acute Upper Airway Responses to Hypoglossal Nerve Stimulation during Sleep in Obstructive Sleep Apnea

Schwartz AR, Barnes M, Hillman D, et al (Johns Hopkins School of Medicine, Baltimore, MD; Austin Hosp, Melbourne, Australia; Sir Charles Gairdner Hosp, Perth, Australia; et al)

Am J Respir Crit Care Med 185:420-426, 2012

Rationale.—Hypoglossal nerve stimulation (HGNS) recruits lingual muscles, reduces pharyngeal collapsibility, and treats sleep apnea.

Objectives.—We hypothesized that graded increases in HGNS relieve pharyngeal obstruction progressively during sleep.

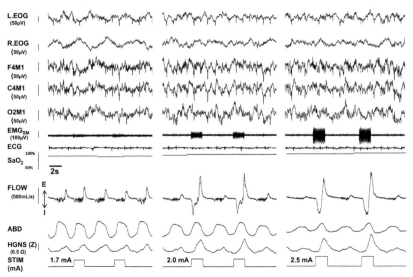

FIGURE 1.—Representative polysomnographic recording examples of hypoglossal nerve stimulation (HGNS) response at low (1.7 mA, *left panel*), moderate (2 mA, *middle panel*), and high (2.5 mA, *right panel*) levels of stimulation in one patient. In each panel, two stimulated breaths are shown (stimulation marker signal at bottom and stimulus artifact in EMG_{SM}), and are bracketed by adjacent unstimulated breaths during stable non-REM sleep. Unstimulated breaths displayed evidence of severe inspiratory airflow limitation as characterized by an early plateau in inspiratory flow at a low level and high frequency mid-inspiratory oscillations in airflow, consistent with snoring. During unstimulated breaths, maximal inspiratory airflow did not change across all stimulation levels, indicating that severe inspiratory flow limitation persisted across stimulation levels. In contrast, a graded response in maximal inspiratory airflow (downward direction) was observed with increasing levels of maximal inspiratory airflow as current was increased. Inspiratory airflow limitation persisted at low (*left panel*) and mid-levels (*middle panel*) of stimulation, but was abolished at the highest stimulation level applied (*right panel*). Note time lags of respiratory impedance signal (HGNS [Z]) and stimulus current marker signal (STIM) of approximately 400 ms and approximately 250 ms, respectively, relative to the airflow and ABD signals caused by signal processing and transmission from the implanted neurostimulation device. ABD = abdominal piezoelectric gauge; EMG_{SM} = submental electromyogram; F4M1, C4M1, and O2M1 = electroencephalogram leads; FLOW = tidal airflow; HGNS (Z) = implanted respiratory impedance sensor; L. EOG = left electrooculogram; R. EOG = right electrooculogram; STIM = stimulation current marker signal. (Reprinted from Schwartz AR, Barnes M, Hillman D, et al. Acute upper airway responses to hypoglossal nerve stimulation during sleep in obstructive sleep apnea. *Am J Respir Crit Care Med.* 2012;185:420-426. Official Journal of the American Thoracic Society. © 2012, American Thoracic Society, http://www.ajrccm.org.).)

Methods.—Responses were examined in 30 patients with sleep apnea who were implanted with an HGNS system. Current (milliampere) was increased stepwise during non-REM sleep. Frequency and pulse width were fixed. At each current level, stimulation was applied on alternating breaths, and responses in maximal inspiratory airflow ($V_{I}max$) and inspiratory airflow limitation (IFL) were assessed. Pharyngeal responses to HGNS were characterized by the current levels at which $V_{I}max$ first increased and peaked (flow capture and peak flow thresholds), and by the $V_{I}max$ increase from flow capture to peak ($\Delta V_{I}max$).

Measurements and Main Results.—HGNS produced linear increases in $V_{I}max$ from unstimulated levels at flow capture to peak flow thresholds (215 ± 21 to 509 ± 37 ml/s; mean $\pm$ SE; $P < 0.001$) with increasing current from 1.05 ± 0.09 to 1.46 ± 0.11 mA.$V_I$max increased in all patients and IFL was abolished in 57% of patients (non-IFL subgroup). In the non-IFL compared with IFL subgroup, the flow response slope was greater (1241 ± 199 vs. 674 ± 166 ml/s/mA; $P < 0.05$) and the stimulation amplitude at peak flow was lower (1.23 ± 0.10 vs. 1.80 ± 0.20 mA; $P < 0.05$) without differences in peak flow.

Conclusions.—HGNS produced marked dose-related increases in airflow without arousing patients from sleep. Increases in airflow were of sufficient magnitude to eliminate IFL in most patients and IFL and non-IFL subgroups achieved normal or near-normal levels of flow, suggesting potential HGNS efficacy across a broad range of sleep apnea severity (Fig 1).

▶ The collapsibility of the upper airways leads to obstructive sleep. Although continuous positive airway pressure (CPAP) is an effective therapy, its adherence is far from perfect. Research into alternative yet effective therapies continues. The authors investigate hypoglossal nerve stimulation, a means that reduces collapsibility and reduces airflow obstruction. The population studied is patients with moderate to severe obstructive sleep apnea. A unilateral hypoglossal nerve stimulator was placed and a measurement of airflow at graded intensities of the stimulation was observed. Fig 1 shows inspiratory airflow flattening and graded improvements in airflow following higher intensities of stimulation without electroencephalogram evidence of arousals. Furthermore, every subject enrolled had evidence of significant improvement with hypoglossal nerve stimulation and more than half had a complete response. This may be a promising line of therapy in the future, but further studies definitely need to be done. The subjects enrolled had primarily hypopneas, not apneas, and it is unclear if rapid eye movement—related or positional-related apnea would respond just as well. Although the protocol allowed for hypoglossal nerve stimulation of alternating breaths, primarily to observe and differentiate responses, it is clear that there is not a persistent and maintained effect on airflow without activation. Nevertheless, I for one look forward to more research in this area. Promising alternatives to CPAP are definitely needed.

S. F. Jones, MD, FCCP, DABSM

Surgical vs Conventional Therapy for Weight Loss Treatment of Obstructive Sleep Apnea: A Randomized Controlled Trial
Dixon JB, Schachter LM, O'Brien PE, et al (Monash Univ, Melbourne, Victoria, Australia; et al)
JAMA 308:1142-1149, 2012

Context.—Obstructive sleep apnea (OSA) is strongly related to obesity. Weight loss is recommended as part of the overall management plan for obese patients diagnosed with OSA.

Objective.—To determine whether surgically induced weight loss is more effective than conventional weight loss therapy in the management of OSA.

Design, Setting, and Patients.—A randomized controlled trial of 60 obese patients (body mass index: >35 and <55) with recently diagnosed (<6 months) OSA and an apnea-hypopnea index (AHI) of 20 events/hour or more. These patients had been prescribed continuous positive airway pressure (CPAP) therapy to manage OSA and were identified via accredited community sleep clinics. The trial was conducted between September 2006 and March 2009 by university- and teaching hospital–based clinical researchers in Melbourne, Australia. Patients with obesity hypoventilation syndrome, previous bariatric surgery, contraindications to bariatric surgery, or significant cardiopulmonary, neurological, vascular, gastrointestinal, or neoplastic disease were excluded.

Interventions.—Patients were randomized to a conventional weight loss program that included regular consultations with a dietitian and physician, and the use of very low-calorie diets as necessary (n = 30) or to bariatric surgery (laparoscopic adjustable gastric banding; n = 30).

Main Outcome Measures.—The primary outcome was baseline to 2-year change in AHI on diagnostic polysomnography scored by staff blinded to randomization. Secondary outcomes were changes in weight, CPAP adherence, and functional status.

Results.—Patients lost a mean of 5.1 kg (95% CI, 0.8 to 9.3 kg) in the conventional weight loss program compared with 27.8 kg (95% CI, 20.9 to 34.7 kg) in the bariatric surgery group ($P < .001$). The AHI decreased by 14.0 events/hour (95% CI, 3.3 to 24.6 events/hour) in the conventional weight loss group and by 25.5 events/hour (95% CI, 14.2 to 36.7 events/hour) in the bariatric surgery group. The between-group difference was −11.5 events/hour (95% CI, −28.3 to 5.3 events/hour; $P = .18$). CPAP adherence did not differ between the groups. The bariatric surgery group had greater improvement in the Short Form 36 physical component summary score (mean, 9.3 [95% CI, 0.5 to 18.0]; $P = .04$).

Conclusion.—Among a group of obese patients with OSA, the use of bariatric surgery compared with conventional weight loss therapy did not result in a statistically greater reduction in AHI despite major differences in weight loss.

Trial Registration.—anzctr.org Identifier: 12605000161628.

▶ Preoperative referral for polysomnography prior to bariatric surgery is a common occurrence at my institution. In some cases, I have seen patients lose a significant amount of weight, but the sustainability of the weight loss is variable as is the effect of weight loss on obstructive sleep apnea (OSA). There is a paucity of literature in the area of postsurgical effects of weight loss on OSA because of the lack of many studies with repeat polysomnography after weight loss. The authors of this study aimed to determine whether laparoscopic adjustable gastric banding (Lap-Band) or conventional weight loss was more effective at improving OSA. The study included 60 subjects and the authors are commended for complete datasets on 87% to 93% of the 2 groups, respectively. The data do show that significantly more weight loss occurs in those randomized to Lap-Band over conventional therapy; however, this does not translate to any significant differences between groups regarding reductions in the apnea-hypopnea index (AHI). Both groups still had severe OSA on average. As a whole, there was a positive relationship between the change in weight and the change in AHI, but when the effect was determined separately, the relationship was significant only in the conventional weight loss group. Figure 2 in the original article from this study depicts weight and AHI at baseline, 12 months, and 2 years. It appears that the greatest reduction in body weight occurs within the first 12 months, as does the reduction in AHI. However, at the end of 2 years, there is individual variability in these measures. Some people regained the weight, whereas others did not. Is it possible that this individual variation in weight gain/change exerts a strong effect on the final results of this study and that a larger sample size is needed? It is possible; however, I think one of the take-home points to this study is that even significant amounts of weight loss are not necessarily curative for OSA and that patients need follow-up. Consider repeating polysomnography before discontinuing treatment for OSA.

S. F. Jones, MD, FCCP, DABSM

Non-Pulmonary Sleep

Association of Insomnia and Short Sleep Duration With Atherosclerosis Risk in the Elderly

Nakazaki C, Noda A, Koike Y, et al (Nagoya Univ Graduate School of Medicine, Japan; Chubu Univ, Kasugai, Japan)
Am J Hypertens 25:1149-1155, 2012

Background.—Short sleep duration is associated with an increased risk of cardiovascular disease and all-cause mortality, although a relationship with atherosclerosis in the elderly remains unclear.

Methods.—Eighty-six volunteers aged ≥65 years (mean, 73.6 ± 4.9 years) were evaluated for insomnia. Total sleep time (TST) and sleep efficiency were measured by actigraphy. Subjective symptoms were assessed with the Pittsburgh Sleep Quality Index (PSQI). Atherosclerosis was evaluated using ultrasonographic measurements of carotid intima—media thickness (IMT).

Results.—IMT was significantly greater and sleep efficiency was significantly lower in subjects with TST ≤ 5 h than those with TST > 7 h (1.3 ± 0.5 vs. 0.9 ± 0.3 mm; $P = 0.009$; 91.0 ± 6.0 vs. 81.6 ± 11.3%, $P = 0.03$, respectively). IMT was also significantly greater in the insomnia group than the noninsomnia group (1.3 ± 0.5 vs. 1.1 ± 0.4 mm; $P = 0.03$). IMT was significantly correlated with systolic blood pressure (SBP), diastolic blood pressure (DBP), and TST (SBP: $r = 0.49$, $P < 0.0001$; DBP: $r = 0.33$, $P = 0.0021$; TST: $r = -0.28$, $P = 0.010$). Multiple regression analysis revealed that SBP, TST, and the PSQI were significant contributing factors for increased IMT (SBP: coefficient $\beta = 0.56$, $P = 0.0001$; TST: coefficient $\beta = -0.32$, $P = 0.005$; PSQI: coefficient $\beta = 0.22$, $P = 0.05$).

Conclusions.—High blood pressure, short sleep duration (≤5 h), poor sleep, and insomnia were associated with atherosclerosis risk leading to cardiovascular disease in the elderly.

▶ For so long we thought that insomnia was an indicator of mental problems and that poor health was due primarily to the effects of mental disease rather than insomnia. Only recently, has an association between insomnia, short sleep duration, and cardiovascular morbidity been established,[1,2] so research examining the relationships between sleep disordered breathing and cardiovascular disease received greater popularity. However, I agree that the effect of insomnia on poor health goes both ways.

This study examines the link between insomnia and short sleep duration and atherosclerosis risk (measured by carotid artery intima-media thickness [IMT]) in a population of persons age 65 and older, predominantly female. There appears to be a graded effect between sleep duration and IMT, and shorter sleep duration is associated with higher degrees of vascular thickness/atherosclerotic risk. Because there were no significant differences in the apnea hypopnea index between groups separated by sleep duration, this would support the theory that insomnia and short sleep duration have an independent effect on atherosclerosis development.

S. F. Jones, MD, FCCP, DABSM

References

1. Ikehara S, Iso H, Date C, et al. Association of sleep duration with mortality from cardiovascular disease and other causes for Japanese men and women: the JACC study. *Sleep.* 2009;32:295-301.
2. Vgontzas AN, Liao D, Pejovic S, et al. Insomnia with short sleep duration and mortality: the Penn State cohort. *Sleep.* 2010;33:1159-1164.

Sleep Disturbances Among Soldiers with Combat-Related Traumatic Brain Injury
Collen J, Orr N, Lettieri CJ, et al (Walter Reed Natl Military Med Ctr, Bethesda, MD)
Chest 142:622-630, 2012

Background.—Sleep complaints are common among patients with traumatic brain injury. Evaluation of this population is confounded by polypharmacy and comorbid disease, with few studies addressing combat-related injuries. The aim of this study was to assess the prevalence of sleep disorders among soldiers who sustained combat-related traumatic brain injury.

Methods.—The study design was a retrospective review of soldiers returning from combat with mild to moderate traumatic brain injury. All underwent comprehensive sleep evaluations. We determined the prevalence of sleep complaints and disorders in this population and assessed demographics, mechanism of injury, medication use, comorbid psychiatric disease, and polysomnographic findings to identify variables that correlated with the development of specific sleep disorders.

Results.—Of 116 consecutive patients, 96.6% were men (mean age, 31.1 ± 9.8 years; mean BMI, 27.8 ± 4.1 kg/m^2), and 29.5% and 70.5% sustained blunt and blast injuries, respectively. Nearly all (97.4%) reported sleep complaints. Hypersomnia and sleep fragmentation were reported in 85.2% and 54.3%, respectively. Obstructive sleep apnea syndrome (OSAS) was found in 34.5%, and 55.2% had insomnia. Patients with blast injuries developed more anxiety (50.6% vs 20.0%, $P = .002$) and insomnia (63% vs 40%, $P = .02$), whereas patients with blunt trauma had significantly more OSAS (54.3% vs 25.9%, $P = .003$). In multivariate analysis, blunt trauma was a significant predictor of OSAS (OR, 3.09; 95% CI, 1.02-9.38; $P = .047$).

Conclusions.—Sleep disruption is common following traumatic brain injury, and the majority of patients develop a chronic sleep disorder. It appears that sleep disturbances may be influenced by the mechanism of injury in those with combat-related traumatic brain injury, with blunt injury potentially predicting the development of OSAS.

▶ This article highlights the high prevalence rates of obstructive sleep apnea (OSA) and insomnia in soldiers with traumatic brain injury returning from Afghanistan and Iraq. The rates of obstructive sleep apnea and insomnia were 34.5% and 55.2%, respectively, which are much higher than those in the general population. The average age of subjects in this study was 31 years; subjects were predominantly male with average body mass index of 27.8. Logistic regression analysis did not find an association between body mass index and OSA; instead, it found an association between blunt injury and OSA. Blast injury was associated with insomnia and anxiety. It is not surprising that a large number of patients was on medications for treatment of posttraumatic stress, depression, and anxiety. Nearly half of soldiers were taking narcotics and a quarter were taking benzodiazepines, both of which can worsen sleep-disordered breathing. The retrospective nature of this study is a limitation along with the possible confounding of the mood disorders and drugs. Nevertheless, this study imparts an awareness of the number of sleep-related problems this population develops and should heighten inquiry when caring for these patients.

S. F. Jones, MD, FCCP, DABSM

Sleep Disruption Due to Hospital Noises: A Prospective Evaluation
Buxton OM, Ellenbogen JM, Wang W, et al (Brigham and Women's Hosp, Boston, MA; Cambridge Health Alliance, MA; Cavanaugh Tocci Associates, Sudbury, MA)
Ann Intern Med 157:170-179, 2012

Background.—Sleep plays a critical role in maintaining health and wellbeing; however, patients who are hospitalized are frequently exposed to noise that can disrupt sleep. Efforts to attenuate hospital noise have been limited by incomplete information on the interaction between sounds and sleep physiology.

Objective.—To determine profiles of acoustic disruption of sleep by examining the cortical (encephalographic) arousal responses during sleep to typical hospital noises by sound level and type and sleep stage.

Design.—3-day polysomnographic study.

Setting.—Sound-attenuated sleep laboratory.

Participants.—Volunteer sample of 12 healthy participants.

Intervention.—Baseline (sham) night followed by 2 intervention nights with controlled presentation of 14 sounds that are common in hospitals (for example, voice, intravenous alarm, phone, ice machine, outside traffic, and helicopter). The sounds were administered at calibrated, increasing decibel levels (40 to 70 dBA [decibels, adjusted for the range of normal hearing]) during specific sleep stages.

Measurements.—Encephalographic arousals, by using established criteria, during rapid eye movement (REM) sleep and non-REM (NREM) sleep stages 2 and 3.

Results.—Sound presentations yielded arousal response curves that varied because of sound level and type and sleep stage. Electronic sounds were more arousing than other sounds, including human voices, and there were large differences in responses by sound type. As expected, sounds in NREM stage 3 were less likely to cause arousals than sounds in NREM stage 2; unexpectedly, the probability of arousal to sounds presented in REM sleep varied less by sound type than when presented in NREM sleep and caused a greater and more sustained elevation of instantaneous heart rate.

Limitations.—The study included only 12 participants. Results for these healthy persons may underestimate the effects of noise on sleep in patients who are hospitalized.

Conclusion.—Sounds during sleep influence both cortical brain activity and cardiovascular function. This study systematically quantifies the disruptive capacity of a range of hospital sounds on sleep, providing evidence that is essential to improving the acoustic environments of new and existing health care facilities to enable the highest quality of care.

▶ I have heard so many patients complain about poor sleep while hospitalized. Unfortunately, many health care providers and hospitals pay very little attention to these complaints. Sleep is necessary for proper immune function,[1] and sleep deprivation is associated with memory impairments.[2] Common noises from intravenous alarms and human voices at various decibels (but within usual thresholds) lead to arousals (Fig 2 in the original article) and sympathetic responses in the cardiovascular system, particularly if arousals occur during rapid eye movement sleep. Although not investigated in this study, the cardiovascular response could theoretically worsen cardiovascular health, particularly in the vulnerable (ie, patients in cardiac intensive care unit). Furthermore, sleep loss may be tied to delirium, a condition that affects nearly 80% of patients receiving mechanical ventilation in the intensive care unit.[3]

The authors noted significant arousals in this study of 12 healthy subjects. Keeping in mind that hospitalized patients are generally older, with acute or chronic and often complex medical issues, we can expect that the degree of sleep fragmentation is much worse. Hard outcomes of mortality need further investigation. Consider incorporating quiet times for patients and keeping disruptions to a minimum.

S. F. Jones, MD, FCCP, DABSM

References

1. Gamaldo CE, Shaikh AK, McArthur JC. The sleep-immunity relationship. *Neurol Clin.* 2012;30:1313-1343.
2. Williams HL, Gieseking CF, Lubin A. Some effects of sleep loss on memory. *Percept Mot Skills.* 1966;23:1287-1293.
3. Ely EW, Inouye SK, Bernard GR, et al. Delirium in mechanically ventilated patients: validity and reliability of the confusion assessment method for the intensive care unit (CAM-ICU). *JAMA.* 2001;286:2703-2710.

Self-Reported Sleep Characteristics and Mortality in Older Adults of Mexican Origin: Results From the Hispanic Established Population for the Epidemiologic Study of the Elderly
Howrey BT, Peek MK, Raji MA, et al (Univ of Texas Med Branch, Galveston)
J Am Geriatr Soc 60:1906-1911, 2012

Objectives.—To determine how poor sleep affects the health of older ethnic minorities.

Design.—Cross-sectional study involving a population-based survey.

Setting.—Hispanic Established Population for the Epidemiologic Study of the Elderly (H-EPESE) survey conducted in the southwestern United States.

Participants.—Two thousand two hundred fifty-six Mexican-American men and women aged 65 and older.

Measurements.—The association between self-reported sleep problems and mortality over a 15-year period in a population based sample of older Mexican Americans was examined. Using five waves of data (1993–2008) from the H-EPESE, Cox proportional hazard models stratified according to sex were used to model the risk of death as a function of chronic sleep problems.

Results.—Having any sleeping problems during the last month was associated with greater risk of mortality (hazard ratio = 1.14, 95% confidence interval = 1.00–1.29) in unadjusted models, although the association was attenuated after accounting for covariates.

Conclusions.—Similar factors explained the association between sleep and mortality in men and women: health behaviors, depressive symptoms, and health conditions. These factors are related to stress, and both may

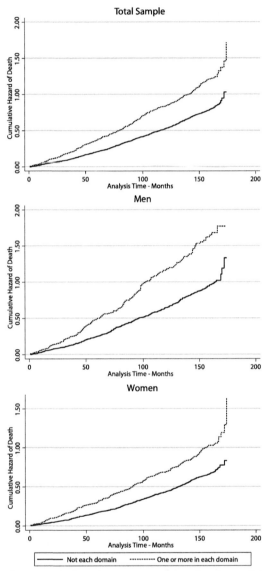

FIGURE.—Cumulative mortality hazard estimates according to sleep characteristics (having ≥1 problems in each sleep domain vs not having a problem in each domain) for the Hispanic Established Population for the Epidemiologic Study of the Elderly: 1993–2007 (N = 2,530). Estimates for the entire sample (top panel), men (middle panel), and women (bottom panel). (Reprinted from Howrey BT, Peek MK, Raji MA, et al. Self-reported sleep characteristics and mortality in older adults of Mexican origin: results from the hispanic established population for the epidemiologic study of the elderly. *J Am Geriatr Soc.* 2012;60:1906-1911, © 2012, American Geriatrics Society and The Authors.)

lead to poor sleep quality. Research is needed to better understand the factors moderating the relationship between sleep, mortality, and sex (Fig).

▶ Few studies have examined sleep in older ethnic populations. This is a cross-sectional study of 2256 Mexican American men and women aged 65 years and older. Nearly 45% of the population was immigrants and the highest level of education completed was fifth grade on average. More women report difficulty falling asleep, waking frequently, difficulty staying asleep, and waking feeling tired compared with men. However, despite better sleep quality, the cumulative mortality hazard estimates are higher in men compared with women after adjustment for medical conditions and health behaviors (Figure). This indicates that there are significant gender differences when it comes to mortality but that sleep quality is linked to comorbid disease and lifestyle choices (smoking). The authors are commended for undertaking a large population based study like this and, particularly, for examining sleep qualities in an understudied population.

S. F. Jones, MD, FCCP, DABSM

Pediatric Sleep-Disordered Breathing

Diagnosis and Management of Childhood Obstructive Sleep Apnea Syndrome
Marcus CL, Brooks LJ, Draper KA, et al (American Academy of Sleep Medicine; American College of Chest Physicians; Merck Company; et al)
Pediatrics 130:576-584, 2012

Objectives.—This revised clinical practice guideline, intended for use by primary care clinicians, provides recommendations for the diagnosis and management of the obstructive sleep apnea syndrome (OSAS) in children and adolescents. This practice guideline focuses on uncomplicated childhood OSAS, that is, OSAS associated with adenotonsillar hypertrophy and/or obesity in an otherwise healthy child who is being treated in the primary care setting.

Methods.—Of 3166 articles from 1999–2010, 350 provided relevant data. Most articles were level II–IV. The resulting evidence report was used to formulate recommendations.

Results and Conclusions.—The following recommendations are made. (1) All children/adolescents should be screened for snoring. (2) Polysomnography should be performed in children/adolescents with snoring and symptoms/signs of OSAS; if polysomnography is not available, then alternative diagnostic tests or referral to a specialist for more extensive evaluation may be considered. (3) Adenotonsillectomy is recommended as the first-line treatment of patients with adenotonsillar hypertrophy. (4) High-risk patients should be monitored as inpatients postoperatively. (5) Patients should be reevaluated postoperatively to determine whether further treatment is required. Objective testing should be performed in patients who are high risk or have persistent symptoms/signs of OSAS after therapy. (6) Continuous positive airway pressure is recommended as treatment if adenotonsillectomy is not performed or if OSAS persists postoperatively. (7) Weight loss is recommended in addition to other therapy in patients who are overweight or obese. (8) Intranasal corticosteroids are an option for children with mild OSAS in whom adenotonsillectomy is contraindicated or for mild postoperative OSAS.

▶ I am happy to see that a new guideline has been published (the last was in 2002). This update is based on a detailed review of 350 articles, though many, many more were screened but not included. This document summarizes the most up-to-date management of pediatric obstructive sleep apnea very well. Although some of these recommendations are well known, such as key action statement 3, which is the recommendation of adenotonsillectomy as the first line of treatment in children with obstructive sleep apnea syndrome (OSAS) and adenotonsillar hypertrophy, this panel also provides a more detailed review of alternative testing for OSAS in children. Based on observational studies, clinicians can use ambulatory polysomnography, nocturnal video recording, or daytime nap polysomnography for testing. This statement received a strength of option instead of strong recommendation or recommendation. Although I agree that some testing is better than no testing, it is important to emphasize that such tests are associated with higher rates of false positives and negatives. Much like use of ambulatory testing in adults suspected to have OSAS, if there is high clinical suspicion, but contradictory ambulatory testing results, one should proceed to the gold standard of in-laboratory full polysomnography. The authors' key action statement 4 regarding monitoring high-risk patients undergoing adenotonsillectomy received a strength of recommendation. Although the rate of complications for adenotonsillectomy are low in general, it is still significant, and careful selection and attention to those patients at highest risk are very important. I would recommend sharing this document with your clinicians caring for children.

S. F. Jones, MD, FCCP, DABSM

8 Critical Care Medicine

Introduction

Welcome to the YEAR BOOK OF PULMONARY DISEASE 2013! As always, science continues to progress in Critical Care and in Pulmonary Medicine. We have some exciting articles within this chapter. The first article is the best one I recall seeing that explains exactly how ECMO (extracorporeal membrane oxygenation) actually works. It's becoming clear that we seem to have plateaued on ventilator strategies for ARDS. Now many centers are turning to ECMO. We have done that here at Scott & White. I believe this is the current state of the art.

As is shown in the second article in this chapter, pharmacotherapy for ARDS is previously heavily researched in mind. However, most likely it is going to be many years before we really have a pharmacologic answer for preventing or derailing the progression of ARDS. Again, I would encourage everyone to read this wonderful article about ECMO, which includes detailed illustrations of the actual cannulations. For example, I did not know that most ECMO for lung support is veno venous.

The third article is a great read. It is from Michael Matthay et al, some of the giants of ARDS research. This article gives the state of the art as to the basic science current knowledge state for the development and progression of ARDS. In addition, there is some very useful information about previous trials for ARDS therapy.

Along the same vein, the fourth article is a groundbreaking one. Everyone must read it! The Berlin definition of ARDS changes our definition of ARDS (I think in good ways). Since ARDS is a syndrome, it is important that we refine and define the syndrome for better understanding and for better research. The survival rate continues to improve. As mentioned above, however, the therapy has plateaued. The current definition of ARDS has not been helpful with defining high-risk patients, nor has it included a component of PEEP. I particularly like the way the authors of the Berlin definition have separated the syndrome into different thirds. They then suggest therapies based on severity third.

The remainder of this chapter continues to have some excellent state-of-the-art articles that I believe everyone will be interested in. There is discussion of frequent complication of airway management across the world, looking at many papers to help categorize better approaches to difficult airways. Ultrasonography continues to be a daily mainstream tool used in the ICU. Again, there is a very nice article enclosed about decision-making for septic patients in ER departments and Critical Care units after use of ultrasound. Oximetery, at least one brand, can now be used for trending hemoglobin concentration. A large study here shows the usefulness of this technology in liver transplants and liver surgery. These are high blood loss operations where tracking hemoglobin from moment to moment would be of tremendous use.

Early mobilization is quickly becoming the standard in Critical Care, or at least it should be. Article 19 shows that we may be able to decrease acquired muscular weakness by rapidly mobilizing our patients.

A new technology continues to improve our care. The 23rd article shows that PCR technology will increase our yield and find some cases of positive organisms that blood cultures may not find. This needs to be done as an adjunct to blood cultures rather than a replacement. VAP continues to drop in incidence as systematic or bundled care is implemented.

I hope you all enjoy reading these articles as much as I have. Every year science continues to provide better information and even some surprises for me. Please read on!

James A. Barker, MD, CPE, FACP, FCCP, FAASM

Acute Respiratory Disorder Syndrome

Venovenous Extracorporeal Membrane Oxygenation in Adults: Practical Aspects of Circuits, Cannulae, and Procedures

Sidebotham D, Allen SJ, McGeorge A, et al (Auckland City Hosp, New Zealand)
J Cardiothorac Vasc Anesth 26:893-909, 2012

Background.—Extracorporeal membrane oxygenation (ECMO) is being used more frequently to manage severe respiratory failure in adults. The two basic forms of ECMO are venoarterial (VA) and venovenous (VV), with VA ECMO supporting lungs and heart and VV ECMO supporting lungs only. VV ECMO is now the preferred mode of extracorporeal support for adults with acute respiratory distress syndrome (ARDS) because it avoids the disadvantages of VA ECMO, specifically, the need for arterial cannulation and upper-body hypoxemia. Instituting ECMO allows ventilator settings to be reduced to "rest" settings, resolving considerable hemodynamic instability associated with ARDS. The technical considerations, physiology, circuit complications, and practical procedures related to the circuit in VV ECMO were documented.

Technical Considerations and Physiology.—In VV ECMO, deoxygenated blood is drained from a cannula usually in the inferior vena cava (IVC), and oxygenated blood is returned through a cannula whose tip is in or close to the right atrium (RA). Because oxygenated blood from the return cannula mixes with deoxygenated blood from the systemic venous return, it

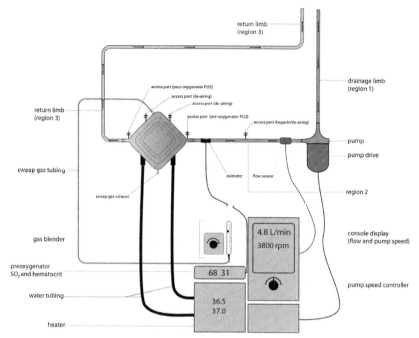

FIGURE 2.—A schematic of the ECMO circuit shown in Figure 1. The only major difference between the circuits shown in Figures 1 and 2 is that the preoxygenator ("venous") oximeter is positioned in the drainage limb (region 1) in the photograph and between the pump and the oxygenator (region 2) in the schematic. Additionally, an air filter is present in the sweep gas tubing in Figure 1 but is not shown in Figure 2. (Reprinted from The Journal of Cardiothoracic and Vascular Anesthesia. Sidebotham D, Allen SJ, McGeorge A, et al. Venovenous extracorporeal membrane oxygenation in adults: practical aspects of circuits, cannulae, and procedures. *J Cardiothorac Vasc Anesth.* 2012;26:893-909, Copyright 2012, with permission from Elsevier.)

is usually impossible to achieve normal arterial oxygen saturation during VV ECMO, so a common target is 86% to 92%. For most adults a circuit flow of 3.0 to 6.0 L/min is needed to achieve oxygen saturation above 86%.

Circuit Concerns.—Basic circuit design involves a centrifugal pump and a polymethylpentene (PMP) oxygenator. The three functional limbs of the circuit are the drainage limb, which extends from the drainage cannula to the pump; the limb between the outflow of the pump and the venous side of the oxygenator; and the return limb, which runs from the arterial side of the oxygenator to the return cannula. Three types of oxygenators use silicone membranes, microporous hollow fiber, and PMP hollow-filter membranes. Each has advantages and disadvantages. The pump can be of the roller or centrifugal type, but centrifugal pumps are the preferred choice for ECMO. Other system components include the pump drive, heater unit, gas blender, console, access ports, inline oxygen saturation monitoring devices, a bridge, and surface coatings.

Cannulas are made of wire-reinforced polyurethane and are accompanied by a guidewire/dilator kit to facilitate percutaneous insertion using the

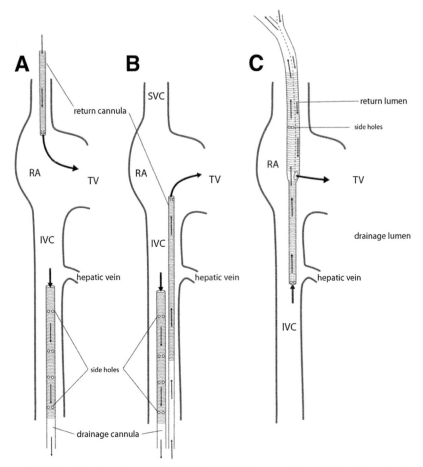

FIGURE 7.—Cannula configurations for VV ECMO. (A) Femoroatrial cannulation: drainage is via a large multiport cannula introduced into a femoral vein and advanced to the mid-IVC; return is via a short cannula introduced into the right internal jugular vein and advanced to the SVC-RA junction. (B) Femorofemoral cannulation: drainage is via a large multiport cannula introduced into a femoral vein and advanced to the mid-IVC; return is via a long cannula introduced into the contralateral femoral vein and advanced to the RA. (C) Double-lumen cannulation: drainage and return are via a double-lumen cannula introduced into the right internal jugular vein. The cannula is advanced until the tip lies in the mid-IVC, just distal to the hepatic vein. Drainage is from the IVC and the SVC, and return is to the RA. See text for details. TV, tricuspid valve. (Reprinted from The Journal of Cardiothoracic and Vascular Anesthesia. Sidebotham D, Allen SJ, McGeorge A, et al. Venovenous extracorporeal membrane oxygenation in adults: practical aspects of circuits, cannulae, and procedures. *J Cardiothorac Vasc Anesth.* 2012;26:893-909, Copyright 2012, with permission from Elsevier.)

Seldinger technique. Configurations are adopted to maximize flow and minimize recirculation. Options include two-cannula, single-cannula, and three-cannula techniques. Either surgical cutdown or percutaneous insertion may be done using the modified or unmodified Seldinger technique. Clinicians must consider the need for sedation and analgesia during cannulation.

Considerations for ECMO including the correct way to begin the process, problems that may necessitate changing the circuit, and whether a second oxygenator is needed. If circuit gas embolism develops, which is an uncommon but life-threatening complication, the circuit may require emergency de-airing. Procedures unrelated to cannulation should be avoided during ECMO support. Possible complications include suction events, low circuit flow, and hypoxemia.

Conclusions.—ECMO can be life-saving for patients with severe ARDS but can also cause substantial patient harm. All of the aspects connected with the circuit, pump, oxygenator, and cannulas must be thoroughly understood, as well as the possibility of complications. A team approach is best and should include intensivists, cardiac anesthesiologists, surgeons, perfusionists, nurses, and other personnel as appropriate (Figs 2 and 7).

▶ I think intensivists need to read this article and understand it. There is a sea change happening in adult respiratory distress syndrome (ARDS) care and extracorporeal membrane oxygenation (ECMO) is it. With better intensive care unit organization and care as well as the optimal positive end-expiratory pressure/low tidal volume proven effective in the ARDS Net trial, the mortality for ARDS has steadily dropped from the original 66% in the Ashbaugh and Petty days to approximately 35% now. But we are at a plateau. No other ventilator strategies have proven additional efficacy. Proning may improve oxygenation but has not been proven to change survival.

But not every plateau creates a breakthrough. What is driving this move onward to ECMO? As the authors herein outline, there is now good evidence that ECMO is no longer just a technique for pediatrics. The CESAR study was thus a landmark.[1] I agree with the authors that the burning platform that forced many of us to jump to ECMO was H1N1. Suddenly, young, viable people were dying of ARDS despite every trick we tried. At the University of South Carolina/Palmetto Health Richland, we sent 2 of our 9 mortality patients to autopsy. The findings were stunning: The lungs had blood and diffuse alveolar damage. There was no normal lung and thus volume and pressure ventilator techniques had no chance to improve oxygenation.

The disease that H1N1 ARDS mimics most closely is, of course, *Hantavirus*-induced ARDS. It is no surprise that the University of New Mexico has a robust ECMO service.

Few of us likely know the vagaries of ECMO. These authors will teach us. Fig 2 has a very nice schematic of how ECMO is set up. Fig 7 shows the most common venovenous configuration. Of course, venoarterial configuration is also done. It depends on the institution and whether the goal is lung only support or heart lung support. Our young program here at Scott and White has an amazing 50% survival (personal communication, Kenton Zehr, MD). Some of these patients have been off the ventilator and ambulatory. Disruptive technology is real.

J. A. Barker, MD, CPE, FACP, FCCP, FAASM

Reference

1. Peek GJ, Mugford M, Tiruvoipati R, et al. Efficacy and economic assessment of conventional ventilatory support versus extracorporeal membrane oxygenation for severe adult respiratory failure (CESAR): a multicentre randomised controlled trial. *Lancet.* 2009;374:1351-1363.

Pharmacotherapy for Acute Respiratory Distress Syndrome

Shafeeq H, Lat I (St John's Univ, Jamaica, NY; Univ of Chicago Med Ctr, IL)
Pharmacotherapy 32:943-957, 2012

Acute lung injury (ALI) and acute respiratory distress syndrome (ARDS) represent a continuum of a clinical syndrome of respiratory failure due to refractory hypoxia. Acute respiratory distress syndrome is differentiated from ALI by a greater degree of hypoxemia and is associated with higher morbidity and mortality. The mortality for ARDS ranges from 22−41%, with survivors usually requiring long-term rehabilitation to regain normal physiologic function. Numerous pharmacologic therapies have been studied for prevention and treatment of ARDS; however, studies demonstrating clear clinical benefit for ARDS-related mortality and morbidity are limited. In this focused review, controversial pharmacologic therapies that have demonstrated, at minimum, a modest clinical benefit are discussed. Three pharmacologic treatment strategies are reviewed in detail: corticosteroids, fluid management, and neuromuscular blocking agents. Use of corticosteroids to attenuate inflammation remains controversial. Available evidence does not support early administration of corticosteroids. Additionally, administration after 14 days of disease onset is strongly discouraged. A liberal fluid strategy during the early phase of comorbid septic shock, balanced with a conservative fluid strategy in patients with ALI or ARDS during the postresuscitation phase, is the optimum approach for fluid management. Available evidence supports an early, short course of continuous-infusion cis-atracurium in patients presenting with severe ARDS. Evidence of safe and effective pharmacologic therapies for ARDS is limited, and clinicians must be knowledgeable about the areas of controversies to determine application to patient care.

▶ This is a useful review of medications and medication studies in acute respiratory distress syndrome (ARDS) studies. The new frontier, in my opinion, will be a retro approach: How can we block progression to ARDS and/or systemic inflammatory response syndrome in high-risk patients? Much effort was put into this in the 1970s and 1980s. However, care strategies appear to have plateaued after the ARDS Clinical Trials Network trial.

J. A. Barker, MD, CPE, FACP, FCCP, FAASM

The acute respiratory distress syndrome

Matthay MA, Ware LB, Zimmerman GA (UCSF; Vanderbilt Univ, Nashville, TN; Univ of Utah, Salt Lake City)
J Clin Invest 122:2731-2740, 2012

The acute respiratory distress syndrome (ARDS) is an important cause of acute respiratory failure that is often associated with multiple organ failure. Several clinical disorders can precipitate ARDS, including pneumonia, sepsis, aspiration of gastric contents, and major trauma. Physiologically, ARDS is characterized by increased permeability pulmonary edema, severe arterial hypoxemia, and impaired carbon dioxide excretion. Based on both experimental and clinical studies, progress has been made in understanding the mechanisms responsible for the pathogenesis and the resolution of lung injury, including the contribution of environmental and genetic factors. Improved survival has been achieved with the use of lung-protective ventilation. Future progress will depend on developing novel therapeutics that can facilitate and enhance lung repair.

▶ I wondered what a Journal of Clinical Investigation article on acute respiratory distress syndrome (ARDS) would be like, but this is actually a very good, thought-provoking read. Fig 3 in the original article outlines the current molecular mechanisms for capillary leak and progression to ARDS. Fig 5 in the original article shows the mechanisms of ventilator-associated lung injury (VALI) versus no VALI. The authors show attempts of therapy at different molecular sites as well as sites for possible future therapies. I am skeptical, but we have to understand the basics before amazing new therapies can be devised.

J. A. Barker, MD, CPE, FACP, FCCP, FAASM

The Berlin definition of ARDS: an expanded rationale, justification, and supplementary material

Ferguson ND, Fan E, Camporota L, et al (Univ of Toronto, Ontario, Canada; King's College London and Dept of Adult Critical Care, UK; et al)
Intensive Care Med 38:1573-1582, 2012

Purpose.—Our objective was to revise the definition of acute respiratory distress syndrome (ARDS) using a conceptual model incorporating reliability and validity, and a novel iterative approach with formal evaluation of the definition.

Methods.—The European Society of Intensive Care Medicine identified three chairs with broad expertise in ARDS who selected the participants and created the agenda. After 2 days of consensus discussions a draft definition was developed, which then underwent empiric evaluation followed by consensus revision.

Results.—The Berlin Definition of ARDS maintains a link to prior definitions with diagnostic criteria of timing, chest imaging, origin of edema, and

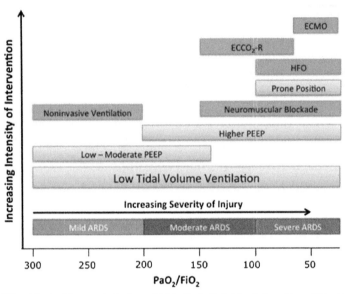

FIGURE.—Aligning Therapeutic Options with The Berlin Definition (adapted from [48] with permission). This figure depicts potential therapeutic options according to the severity of ARDS. Boxes in yellow represent therapies that in the opinion of the panel still require confirmation in prospective clinical trials. This figure is just a model based on currently available information. In the coming years, various aspects of the figure will likely change; proposed cutoffs may move, and some therapies may be found to not be useful, while others may be added. For interpretation of the references to color in this figure legend, the reader is referred to web version of this article. *Editor's Note:* Please refer to original journal article for full references. (With kind permission from Springer Science+Business Media: Ferguson ND, Fan E, Camporota L, et al. The Berlin definition of ARDS: an expanded rationale, justification, and supplementary material. *Intensive Care Med.* 2012;38:1573-1582, with permission from Springer and ESICM.)

hypoxemia. Patients may have ARDS if the onset is within 1 week of a known clinical insult or new/worsening respiratory symptoms. For the bilateral opacities on chest radiograph criterion, a reference set of chest radiographs has been developed to enhance inter-observer reliability. The pulmonary artery wedge pressure criterion for hydrostatic edema was removed, and illustrative vignettes were created to guide judgments about the primary cause of respiratory failure. If no risk factor for ARDS is apparent, however, objective evaluation (e.g., echocardiography) is required to help rule out hydrostatic edema. A minimum level of positive end-expiratory pressure and mutually exclusive PaO_2/FiO_2 thresholds were chosen for the different levels of ARDS severity (mild, moderate, severe) to better categorize patients with different outcomes and potential responses to therapy.

Conclusions.—This panel addressed some of the limitations of the prior ARDS definition by incorporating current data, physiologic concepts, and clinical trials results to develop the Berlin definition, which should facilitate case recognition and better match treatment options to severity in both research trials and clinical practice (Fig, Table 3).

▶ The Berlin definition is rapidly becoming the new way to classify acute respiratory distress syndrome (ARDS). It is actually more pragmatic than prior

TABLE 3.—The Berlin Definition of ARDS (with Permission From [22])

Acute Respiratory Distress Syndrome

	Mild	Moderate	Severe
Timing	Within 1 week of a known clinical insult or new/worsening respiratory symptoms		
Chest imaging[a]	Bilateral opacities—not fully explained by effusions, lobar/lung collapse, or nodules		
Origin of Edema	Respiratory failure not fully explained by cardiac failure or fluid overload; Need objective assessment (e.g., echocardiography) to exclude hydrostatic edema if no risk factor present		
Oxygenation[b]	$200 < PaO_2/FiO_2 \leq 300$ with PEEP or CPAP ≥ 5 cmH$_2$O[c]	$100 < PaO_2/TiO_2 \leq 200$ with PEEP ≥ 5 cmH$_2$O	$PaO_2/FiO_2 \leq 100$ with PEEP ≥ 5 cmH$_2$O

Editor's Note: Please refer to original journal article for full references.
ARDS acute respiratory distress syndrome, PaO_2 partial pressure of arterial oxygen, FiO_2 fraction of inspired oxygen, PEEP positive end-expiratory pressure, CPAP continuous positive airway pressure, N/A not applicable.
[a]Chest X-ray or CT scan.
[b]If altitude higher than 1000 m, correction factor should be made as follows: $PaO_2/FiO_2 \times$ (barometric pressure/760).
[c]This may be delivered non-invasively in the mild ARDS group.

definitions. These changes are overdue, quite honestly. We no longer routinely place pulmonary artery catheters, for example, and so new criteria and testing for cardiac function and volume status are needed. Many but not all practitioners used a 72-hour window from inciting event to syndrome. It is now defined as 7 days from the event. See Table 3 for the definition.

Usually redefinitions are aimed at improved precision for research design. However, the Berlin definition is actually useful in that it divides ARDS into mild, moderate, and severe categories. The Figure shows how this allows therapeutic planning in a meaningful way. For example, a patient at a small community hospital with level 3 ARDS should probably transfer to a center capable of extracorporeal membrane oxygenation. That same hospital would likely be quite satisfactory for patients with levels 1 or 2. I am sure there will be more to follow on this new ARDS definition.

J. A. Barker, MD, CPE, FACP, FCCP, FAASM

Trauma Issues

A model for predicting primary blast lung injury
MacFadden LN, Chan PC, Ho KH-H, et al (L-3 Communications/JAYCOR, San Diego, CA)
J Trauma Acute Care Surg 73:1121-1129, 2012

Background.—This article presents a model-based method for predicting primary blast injury. On the basis of the normalized work injury mechanism from previous work, this method presents a new model that accounts for the effects of blast orientation and species difference.

Methods.—The analysis used test data from a series of extensive experimental studies sponsored by the US Army Medical Research and Materiel

Command. In these studies, more than 1200 sheep were exposed to air blast in free-field and confined enclosures, and lung injuries were quantified as the percentage of surface area contused. Blast overpressure data were collected using blast test devices placed at matching locations to represent loadings to the thorax. Adopting the modified Lobdell model with further modifications specifically for blast and scaling, the thorax deformation histories for the left, chest, and right sides of the thorax were calculated for all sheep subjects. Using the calculated thorax velocities, effective normalized work was computed for each test subject representing the irreversible work performed on the lung tissues normalized by lung volume and ambient pressure.

Results.—Dose-response curves for four categories of injuries (trace, slight, moderate, and severe) were developed by performing log-logistic correlations of the computed normalized work with the injury outcomes, including the effect of multiple shots. A blast lethality correlation was also established.

Conclusion.—Validated by sheep data, the present work revalidates the previous understanding and findings of the blast lung injury mechanism and provides an anthropomorphic model for primary blast injury prediction that can be used for occupational and survivability analysis.

Level of Evidence.—Economic and decision analysis, level III.

▶ We must prepare for every form of disaster, and these researchers have created an excellent biomedical model for blast injury.

J. A. Barker, MD, CPE, FACP, FCCP, FAASM

Acute Respiratory Failure

A comparison of immunomodulation therapies in mechanically ventilated patients with Guillain Barré syndrome

Netto AB, Kulkarni GB, Taly AB, et al (Natl Inst of Mental Health and Neurosciences (NIMHANS), Bangalore, Karnataka, India)
J Clin Neurosci 19:1664-1667, 2012

A comparison of the effectiveness of immunomodulatory therapies in patients with Guillain Barré syndrome (GBS) who require mechanical ventilation (MV) is important for patient treatment and cost. We aimed to compare the effectiveness of three modes of intervention on the outcome of patients with GBS receiving MV: intravenous immunoglobulin (IVIgG); small volume plasmapheresis (SVP) and large volume plasmapheresis (LVP). Patients with GBS satisfying National Institute of Neurological and Communicative Disorders and Stroke 1990 criteria and requiring MV between 1997 between 2007 were analyzed. The primary outcome parameters evaluated were mortality, duration of MV, hospital stay and Hughes scale at discharge from hospital. Of the 173 (Male: Female, 118:55) patients who required MV during the study, 106 patients received single modality treatment (IVIgG 31, LVP 45, SVP 30) based on availability, affordability

TABLE 3.—Effect of Therapeutic Intervention on the Outcome of Patients with Guillain Barré Syndrome Receiving Mechanical Ventilation

Treatment	Deceased (%)	Hughes Scale >3	Hughes Scale ≤3	Hospital Stay (Days)	Duration of Ventilation (Days)
IVIgG alone (n = 31)	2 (6.7)	21 (70)	7 (23.3)	55.3 ± 38.3	33.3 ± 23.4
LVP alone (n = 45)	2 (4.4)	29 (64.4)	14 (31.1)	46.9 ± 39.2	29.9 ± 32.4
SVP alone (n = 30)	6 (21.4)	12 (42.8)	10 (35.7)	43.1 ± 31.9	26.2 ± 24.2
p value	NA*	0.31	0.31	0.44	0.61
No. patients included in analysis	10 (9.7)	62 (60.2)	31 (30.1)	106	106

LVP = large volume plasmapharesis, SVP = small volume plasmapharesis, IVIgG = intravenous immunoglobulin.
*NA, tests of significance not applicable due to the small sample (only two patients in each group). A total of 106 patients received single modality treatment; data on Hughes scale was not available on three patients.

and feasibility. Patients receiving IVIgG had a higher incidence of severe weakness and bulbar involvement. The mean duration of MV ($p = 0.61$), total hospital stay ($p = 0.44$) and Hughes scale at discharge ($p = 0.31$) did not differ among the three groups. Complications were similar in the three treatment groups except for hypoalbuminemia and anemia, which were more common in patients in the LVP group. In conclusion, the outcome of patients treated with these three immunomodulatory treatment modalities did not vary. The beneficial effects of SVP in our study warrant further randomized control trials especially in resource-constrained settings (Table 3).

▶ Guillain-Barré (GB) remains a serious and complex syndrome that we as intensivists see with regularity. Those patients with early bulbar involvement are lumped into the Miller Fischer variant. They have a higher rate of progression to acute respiratory failure in which they require mechanical ventilation. In addition, this subgroup of GB patients also has a relatively high rate of autonomic dysfunction.

This study from investigators in India looks at results from a different viewpoint: patients already on mechanical ventilatory support, and, thus, represents obviously severe patients. But this is probably reality for many if not most of us. Diagnosis is often delayed. From a practical point of view, it is much easier to administer intravenous immunoglobulin because many hospitals will not have the blood center support necessary to deliver plasma exchange.

Please review Table 3. There are no statistically significant changes in the 3 groups. However, the trend looks very good for small-volume plasma exchange. This would also be financially advantageous for many systems. Further study seems warranted.

J. A. Barker, MD, CPE, FACP, FCCP, FAASM

Airway Management

Complications and failure of airway management

Cook TM, Macdougall-Davis SR (Royal United Hosp, Bath, UK)
Br J Anaesth 109:i68-i85, 2012

Airway management complications causing temporary patient harm are common, but serious injury is rare. Because most airways are easy, most complications occur in easy airways: these complications can and do lead to harm and death. Because these events are rare, most of our learning comes from large litigation and critical incident databases that help identify patterns and areas where care can be improved: but both have limitations. The recent 4th National Audit Project of the Royal College of Anaesthetists and Difficult Airway Society provides important detailed information and our best estimates of the incidence of major airway complications. A significant proportion of airway complications occur in Intensive Care Units and Emergency Departments, and these more frequently cause patient harm/death and are associated with suboptimal care. Hypoxia is the commonest cause of airway-related deaths. Obesity markedly increases risk of airway complications. Pulmonary aspiration remains the leading cause of airway-related anaesthetic deaths, most cases having identifiable risk factors. Unrecognized oesophageal intubation is not of only historical interest and is entirely avoidable. All airway management techniques fail and prediction scores are rather poor, so many failures are unanticipated. Avoidance of airway complications requires institutional and individual preparedness, careful assessment, good planning and judgement, good communication and teamwork, knowledge and use of a range of techniques and devices, and a willingness to stop performing techniques when they are

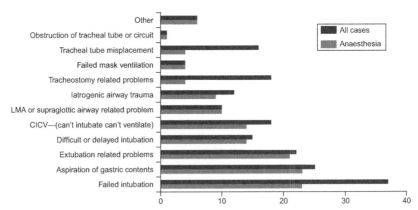

FIGURE 1.—Primary airway problem for all events and for anaesthesia events reported to NAP4. From Cook et al.,[2] with permission. *Editor's Note*: Please refer to original journal article for full references. (Reprinted from Cook TM, Macdougall-Davis SR. Complications and failure of airway management. *Br J Anaesth.* 2012;109:i68-i85, by permission of The Board of Management and Trustees of the British Journal of Anaesthesia, Oxford University Press.)

failing. Analysis of major airway complications identifies areas where practice is suboptimal; research to improve understanding, prevention, and management of such complications remains an anaesthetic priority (Fig 1).

▶ This is an excellent review of airway complications as characterized by type, frequency, and location of service. Interesting, isn't it, that an intensive care unit is thought equivalent to an emergency department as far as a high-risk location for an anesthesiologist?

Aspiration and esophageal intubation remain the most common complications. Particularly scary is the category CICV—ie, can't intubate, can't ventilate. The authors appropriately point out that each case should be planned as if it were a difficult airway. Fig 1 delineates the types of failures that are known to occur in the literature. There are many caveats in this article; for example, fiberoptic intubation has a failure rate of up to 11%.

J. A. Barker, MD, CPE, FACP, FCCP, FAASM

Ventilator-Associated Pneumonia

Clinical predictors of *Pseudomonas aeruginosa* or *Acinetobacter baumannii* bacteremia in patients admitted to the ED

Kang C-I, the Korean Network for Study on Infectious Diseases (KONSID) (Sungkyunkwan Univ School of Medicine, Seoul, Korea)
Am J Emerg Med 30:1169-1175, 2012

The identification of clinical characteristics that could identify patients at high risk for *Pseudomonas aeruginosa* or *Acinetobacter baumannii* bacteremia would aid clinicians in the appropriate management of these life-threatening conditions, especially in patients admitted to the emergency department (ED) with community-onset infections. To determine clinical risk factors for *P aeruginosa* or *A baumannii* bacteremia in patients with community-onset gram-negative bacteremia (GNB), a post hoc analysis of a nationwide bacteremia surveillance database including patients with microbiologically documented GNB was performed. Ninety-six patients with *P aeruginosa* or *A baumannii* bacteremia were compared with 1230 patients with *Escherichia coli* or *Klebsiella pneumoniae* bacteremia. A solid tumor or hematologic malignancy was more likely to be associated with *P aeruginosa* or *A baumannii* bacteremia, whereas concurrent neurologic disease was less frequently seen. In regards to the site of infection, pneumonia was more common in *P aeruginosa* or *A baumannii* bacteremia, whereas a urinary tract infection was less frequently seen. Factors associated with *P aeruginosa* or *A baumannii* bacteremia in multivariate analysis included pneumonia (odds ratio [OR], 3.60; 95% confidence interval [CI], 1.86-6.99), hematologic malignancy (OR, 2.71; 95% CI, 1.26-5.84), male sex (OR, 2.17; 95% CI, 1.31-3.58), solid tumor (OR, 1.89; 95% CI, 1.15-3.12), and health-care—associated infection (OR, 1.88; 95% CI, 1.48-2.41). Our data suggest that an initial empirical antimicrobial coverage of *P aeruginosa* or *A baumannii* bacteremia should be seriously considered in patients with pneumonia, a hematologic malignancy, solid tumor, or health-care—associated infection, when GNB is suspected, even in community-onset infections.

▶ These 2 gram-negative organisms are very important to recognize because they often have a more complex resistance pattern and thus require different antibiotics. These authors from Korea have nicely delineated the risk factors for *Pseudomonas aeruginosa* or *Acinetobacter baumannii*. I am guessing that these findings are universal to the United States as well (personal observation). So, consider broader coverage in male patients with hematologic malignancy, solid tumor, or healthcare associated pneumonia.

J. A. Barker, MD, CPE, FACP, FCCP, FAASM

Decreasing ventilator-associated pneumonia in the intensive care unit: A sustainable comprehensive quality improvement program
Heck K (Holland Hosp, MI)
Am J Infect Control 40:877-879, 2012

An intensive care unit implemented an oral care bundle to decrease ventilator-associated pneumonia (VAP). A retrospective analysis comparing like time periods revealed the VAP rate per 1,000 ventilator-days dropped significantly from 10.5 to 0 (*P* = .016). The oral care bundle remains in

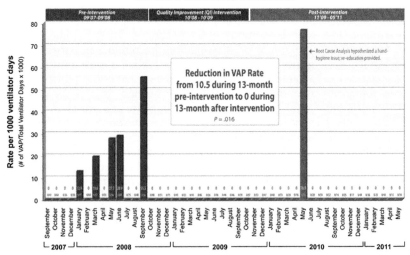

FIGURE 2.—Rate of ventilator-associated pneumonia (VAP) in the intensive care unit before and after initiation of the quality improvement initiative. (Reprinted from Heck K. Decreasing ventilator-associated pneumonia in the intensive care unit: a sustainable comprehensive quality improvement program. *Am J Infect Control.* 2012;40:877-879, with permission from the Association for Professionals in Infection Control and Epidemiology, Inc.)

place as of end of May 2011 and has proven to be a sustainable method for VAP prevention (Fig 2).

▶ Evidence-based practice and "bundles" really do work. Look at the wonderful results on this run chart from these investigators in the small town of Holland, Michigan (Fig 2).

And also note that one back-slide month occurred after the active intervention time. Unfortunately, quality improvement projects will always need reengineering or continued measurement to prevent erosion of improvement processes.

J. A. Barker, MD, CPE, FACP, FCCP, FAASM

Pulmonary Hypertension in the ICU

Aggressive Surgical Treatment of Acute Pulmonary Embolism With Circulatory Collapse

Takahashi H, Okada K, Matsumori M, et al (Kobe Univ Graduate School of Medicine, Japan)

Ann Thorac Surg 94:785-791, 2012

Background.—Acute high-risk pulmonary embolism is a life-threatening condition with high early mortality rates resulting from acute right ventricular failure and cardiogenic shock. We retrospectively analyzed the outcomes of surgical embolectomy among patients with circulatory collapse.

Methods.—Between July 2000 and September 2011, 24 consecutive patients (17 women and 7 men; mean age, 59.9 ± 17.2 years) underwent emergency surgical embolectomy to treat acute pulmonary embolism with circulatory collapse. Nineteen (79.2%) patients were in cardiogenic shock, and 16 (66.7%) patients received preoperative percutaneous cardiopulmonary support. Eleven (45.8%) patients were in cardiac arrest. The preoperative pulmonary artery obstruction index was 76.9% ± 16.4% (median, 88.9%; range, 44.4%−88.9%). The indications for surgical intervention were cardiogenic shock (n = 16 [66.7%]), failed medical therapy or catheter embolectomy (n = 4 [16.7%]), or contraindication for thrombolysis (n = 4 [16.7%]). Follow-up was 100% complete with a mean of 6.8 ± 3.9 years (median, 5.6 years).

Results.—The in-hospital mortality rate was 12.5% (n = 3). One patient underwent a repeated embolectomy on postoperative day 6. The postoperative course was complicated by cerebral infarction and by mediastinitis in 1 patient each. The 5-year cumulative survival rate was 87.5% ± 6.8%. Mean right ventricular pressure significantly decreased from 66.9 to 28.5 mm Hg among the survivors.

Conclusions.—Surgical pulmonary embolectomy is an excellent approach to treating acute pulmonary embolism with circulatory collapse. Providing immediate percutaneous cardiopulmonary support to patients with cardiogenic shock could help to resuscitate and stabilize cardiopulmonary function and allow for a good outcome of pulmonary embolectomy.

▶ Acute surgical embolectomy has not been standard therapy for acute massive or submassive pulmonary embolism. However, newer techniques coupled with cardiopulmonary bypass have markedly improved survival. These Japanese investigators confirm this marked improvement in survival in these very ill patients. Surgical embolectomy should now be inserted into treatment algorithms in centers that have high-level expertise such as described here.

J. A. Barker, MD, CPE, FACP, FCCP, FAASM

A Primary Pulmonary Artery Chondrosarcoma Manifesting as Acute Pulmonary Embolism
Schleger S, Weingartner JS, Costi M, et al (Hosp Bogenhausen, Munich, Germany)
Ann Thorac Surg 94:1731-1733, 2012

Primary cardiac malignancies are rare, and the majority are benign. Malignant tumors are often found to be sarcomas arising from structural cells such as muscle, connective tissue, and blood vessels. We report a case of a 62-year-old woman who presented with pulmonary embolism secondary to a primary pulmonary artery chondrosarcoma. Radical resection with curative intent was impossible, but partial resection and reconstruction of the pulmonary main stem was performed. The remaining tumor was treated with adjuvant chemotherapy. A positron emission

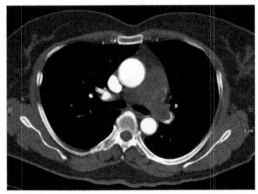

FIGURE 1.—A solid mass blocking the pulmonary bifurcation. (Reprinted from the Annals of Vascular Surgery. Schleger S, Weingartner JS, Costi M, et al. A primary pulmonary artery chondrosarcoma manifesting as acute pulmonary embolism. *Ann Thorac Surg.* 2012;94:1731-1733, Copyright 2012, with permission from Annals of Vascular Surgery, Inc.)

tomography—computed tomography scan 6 months postoperatively showed a nearly complete remission (Fig 1).

▶ I have seen 2 cases like this one in my career. It is so rare that I remember them! Both were initially called pulmonary emboli.

It is important for the pulmonologist to realize that primary pulmonary artery sarcoma is in the differential diagnosis for unusual large emboli (unilateral saddle embolism—does it happen?).

Fig 1 shows a typical computed tomography image. Magnetic resonance imaging/magnetic resonance angiography probably will show the sarcoma more clearly.

J. A. Barker, MD, CPE, FACP, FCCP, FAASM

World Health Organization Pulmonary Hypertension Group 2: Pulmonary hypertension due to left heart disease in the adult—a summary statement from the Pulmonary Hypertension Council of the International Society for Heart and Lung Transplantation
Fang JC, Demarco T, Givertz MM, et al (Univ Hosps Case Med Ctr, Cleveland, OH; Univ of California, San Francisco; Brigham and Women's Hosp, Boston, MA; et al)
J Heart Lung Transplant 31:913-933, 2012

Pulmonary hypertension associated with left heart disease is the most common form of pulmonary hypertension encountered in clinical practice today. Although frequently a target of therapy, its pathophysiology remains poorly understood and its treatment remains undefined. Pulmonary hypertension in the context of left heart disease is a marker of worse prognosis and disease severity, but whether its primary treatment is beneficial or harmful is unknown. An important step to the future study of this important clinical problem will be to standardize definitions across disciplines to facilitate an evidence base that is interpretable and applicable to clinical practice. In this current statement, we provide an extensive review and interpretation of the current available literature to guide current practice and future investigation. At the request of the Pulmonary Hypertension (PH) Council of the International Society for Heart and Lung Transplantation (ISHLT), a writing group was assembled and tasked to put forth this document as described above. The review process was facilitated through the peer review process of the *Journal of Heart and Lung Transplantation* and ultimately endorsed by the leadership of the ISHLT PH Council (Fig 1, Table 1).

▶ I think it behooves us as pulmonary/critical care physicians to understand and treat the most common cause of pulmonary hypertension (PH). This, of course, is type 2 or PH associated with left ventricular (LV) failure and/or diastolic dysfunction. Table 1 outlines the types of PH. Pulmonary arterial hypertension (PAH) or idiopathic pulmonary hypertension is much less common.

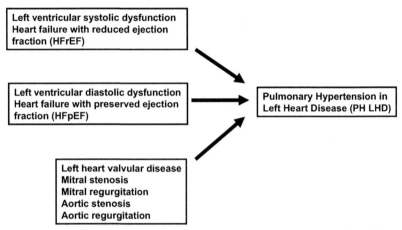

FIGURE 1.—World Health Organization Pulmonary Hypertension Group 2. (Reprinted from The Journal of Heart and Lung Transplantation. Fang JC, Demarco T, Givertz MM, et al. World Health Organization Pulmonary Hypertension Group 2: pulmonary hypertension due to left heart disease in the adult—A summary statement from the Pulmonary Hypertension Council of the International Society for Heart and Lung Transplantation. *J Heart Lung Transplant*. 2012;31:913-933, Copyright 2012, with permission from the International Society for Heart Transplantation.)

TABLE 1.—(A) World Health Organization Classification for Pulmonary Hypertension

Group	Description	Example
1	Pulmonary arterial hypertension	Idiopathic PAH
2	PH owing to left heart disease	Mitral stenosis
3	PH owing to lung diseases and/or hypoxemia	COPD
4	Chronic thromboembolic PH	Chronic pulmonary embolism
5	PH with unclear or multifactorial mechanisms	Histiocytosis X

COPD, Chronic obstructive pulmonary disease; PAH, pulmonary arterial hypertension; PH, pulmonary hypertension.

Fig 1 demonstrates a nice algorithm for separating LV failure likelihood from primary PAH (by echocardiogram). Part B of Fig 1 proceeds with the cardiac catheterization split of the 2 entities.

The remainder of the article discusses known and unknown areas of pathophysiology and also of pharmacologic therapy. The authors have done a wonderful job of making the complex seem understandable.

J. A. Barker, MD, CPE, FACP, FCCP, FAASM

Imaging and Monitoring in the ICU

Effect of Bedside Ultrasonography on the Certainty of Physician Clinical Decisionmaking for Septic Patients in the Emergency Department

Haydar SA, Moore ET, Higgins GL III, et al (Maine Med Ctr, Portland)
Ann Emerg Med 60:346-358, 2012

Study Objective.—Sepsis protocols promote aggressive patient management, including invasive procedures. After the provision of point-of-care ultrasonographic markers of volume status and cardiac function, we seek to evaluate changes in emergency physician clinical decisionmaking and physician assessments about the clinical utility of the point-of-care ultrasonographic data when caring for adult sepsis patients.

Methods.—For this prospective before-and-after study, patients with suspected sepsis received point-of-care ultrasonography to determine cardiac contractility, inferior vena cava diameter, and inferior vena cava collapsibility. Physician reports of treatment plans, presumed causes of observed vital sign abnormalities, and degree of certainty were compared before and after knowledge of point-of-care ultrasonographic findings. The clinical utility of point-of-care ultrasonographic data was also evaluated.

Results.—Seventy-four adult sepsis patients were enrolled: 27 (37%) sepsis, 30 (40%) severe sepsis, 16 (22%) septic shock, and 1 (1%) systemic inflammatory response syndrome. After receipt of point-of-care ultrasonographic data, physicians altered the presumed primary cause of vital sign abnormalities in 12 cases (17% [95% confidence interval {CI} 8% to 25%]) and procedural intervention plans in 20 cases (27% [95% CI 17% to 37%]). Overall treatment plans were changed in 39 cases (53% [95% CI 41% to 64%]). Certainty increased in 47 (71%) cases and decreased in 19 (29%). Measured on a 100-mm visual analog scale, the mean clinical utility score was 65 mm (SD 29; 95% CI 58 to 72), with usefulness reported in all cases.

Conclusions.—Emergency physicians found point-of-care ultrasonographic data about cardiac contractility, inferior vena cava diameter, and inferior vena cava collapsibility to be clinically useful in treating adult patients with sepsis. Increased certainty followed acquisition of point-of-care ultrasonographic data in most instances. Point-of-care ultrasonography appears to be a useful modality in evaluating and treating adult sepsis patients (Tables 4 and 5).

▶ This is a neat study and one that I believe forecasts the future. Because we have all stopped using pulmonary artery catheters, we need some technology to help us both confirm the type of shock and help us assess volume status. Although central venous pressure monitoring is currently recommended, it is invasive and also known to be relatively inaccurate in older patients with chronic diseases (which, after all, are our primary patient cohort, or so it seems). The certainty of both diagnosis and therapy was nicely enhanced after ultrasound, as evidenced

TABLE 4.—Mean Visual Analog Scale Scores for Physician Certainty Pre- and Postreceipt of Point-of-Care Ultrasonographic Data

Sepsis Severity (n)	Pre US Mean (SD)	Post US Mean (SD)	Certainty About Cause of Vital Sign Abnormalities Mean Difference Change (95% CI)	Effect Size, Cohen's d
SIRS (1)	86	90	-4.0	n/a
Sepsis (27)	71.2 (18.2)	76.9 (28.5)	-5.6 (-18.7 to 7.4)	-0.24
Severe sepsis (30)	74.9 (21.4)	87.6 (17.3)	-12.7 (-22.8 to -2.6)	-0.65
Septic shock (16)	73.3 (22.5)	82.8 (30.7)	-9.5 (-28.9 to 9.9)	-0.35
Certainty about planned interventions (intravenous fluid resuscitation, use of vasopressive medications, blood transfusions)				
SIRS (1)	88	92	-4.0	n/a
Sepsis (27)	78.3 (17.1)	78.6 (26.8)	-0.3 (-12.6 to 12.0)	-0.01
Severe sepsis (30)	76.8 (22.9)	86.7 (22.7)	-9.9 (-21.6 to 1.9)	-0.43
Septic shock (16)	77.3 (25.8)	79.5 (32.8)	-2.2 (-23.5 to 19.1)	-0.07
Certainty about interventions foreseen (central venous access, central venous pressure monitoring, mixed venous saturation monitoring, tracheal intubation)				
SIRS (1)	83	90	-7.0	n/a
Sepsis (27)	70.4 (26.5)	82.8 (18.6)	-12.3 (-24.8 to 0.16)	-0.54
Severe sepsis (30)	72.0 (25.9)	73.5 (26.9)	-1.5 (-15.1 to 12.2)	-0.06
Septic shock (16)	65.8 (32.8)	72.2 (33.9)	-6.4 (-30.5 to 17.7)	-0.19
Certainty about choosing correct series of interventions				
SIRS (1)	85	93	-8.0	n/a
Sepsis (27)	74.0 (19.6)	83.9 (15.3)	-9.9 (-19.5 to -0.30)	-0.56
Severe sepsis (30)	81.3 (13.5)	86.4 (11.8)	-5.1 (-11.7 to 1.4)	-0.40
Septic shock (16)	74.2 (24.1)	81.9 (30.4)	-7.8 (-27.5 to 12.0)	-0.28
Certainty about disposition				
SIRS (1)	85	82	-7.0	n/a
Sepsis (27)	70.7 (20.3)	78.7 (23.7)	-8.1 (-20.1 to 4.0)	-0.36
Severe sepsis (30)	74.9 (14.7)	82.8 (14.2)	-7.8 (-15.3 to -0.38)	-0.55
Septic shock (16)	77.9 (19.0)	83.3 (29.6)	-5.4 (-23.4 to 12.5)	-0.22

Editor's Note: Please refer to original journal article for full references.
US, Ultrasonography; SD, standard deviation.

TABLE 5.—Point-of-Care Ultrasonographic Measures by Sepsis Severity

POCUS Measure	SIRS, n = 1	Sepsis, n = 27	No. (%) Severe Sepsis, n = 30	Septic Shock, n = 16
IVC size				
<1.5	0	9 (33.3)	9 (30.0)	5 (33.3)
1.5−2.5	0	13 (48.1)	15 (50.0)	6 (40.0)
>2.5	0	3 (11.1)	3 (10.0)	2 (13.3)
Unable	1 (100)	2 (7.4)	3 (10.0)	2 (13.3)
IVC collapse				
Total collapse	0	7 (28.0)	8 (30.8)	4 (33.3)
>50%	0	7 (28.0)	11 (42.3)	2 (16.7)
<50%	0	11 (44.0)	6 (23.1)	6 (50.0)
No change	0	0	1 (3.8)	0
Unable	1 (100)	0	0	0
CVP				
0−5	0	9 (36.0)	9 (34.6)	3 (38.5)
5−10	0	6 (24.0)	10 (38.5)	2 (15.4)
11−15	0	9 (36.0)	6 (23.1)	4 (30.8)
16−20	0	1 (4.0)	1 (3.8)	2 (15.4)
Unable	1 (100)	0	0	0
Contractility				
Normal	1 (100)	23 (85.2)	25 (83.3)	11 (68.8)
Depressed	0	3 (11.1)	1 (3.3)	3 (18.8)
Severely depressed	0	1 (3.7)	4 (13.3)	1 (6.3)
Unable	0	0	0	1 (6.3)

IVC, Inferior vena cava; CVP, central venous pressure.

in Table 4. In addition, the physicians were largely successful at taking desired ultrasound measurements that aided them in both diagnosis and management.

This appeals to me: It is noninvasive. Information for important rule-outs is acquired (no tamponade, heart without severe drop in ejection fraction or abnormal wall motion). Volume status data can be acquired. Screening of gall bladder and other possible infection sites can also occur. A larger, multicenter study should follow this one.

J. A. Barker, MD, CPE, FACP, FCCP, FAASM

Accuracy of non-invasive measurement of haemoglobin concentration by pulse co-oximetry during steady-state and dynamic conditions in liver surgery

Vos JJ, Kalmar AF, Struys MMRF, et al (The Univ of Groningen, The Netherlands)

Br J Anaesth 109:522-528, 2012

Background.—The Masimo Radical 7 (Masimo Corp., Irvine, CA, USA) pulse co-oximeter® calculates haemoglobin concentration (SpHb) non-invasively using transcutaneous spectrophotometry. We compared SpHb with invasive satellite-lab haemoglobin monitoring (Hb$_{satlab}$) during major hepatic resections both under steady-state conditions and in a dynamic phase with fluid administration of crystalloid and colloid solutions.

Methods.—Thirty patients undergoing major hepatic resection were included and randomized to receive a fluid bolus of 15 ml kg^{-1} colloid ($n = 15$) or crystalloid ($n = 15$) solution over 30 min. SpHb was continuously measured on the index finger, and venous blood samples were analysed in both the steady-state phase (from induction until completion of parenchymal transection) and the dynamic phase (during fluid bolus).

Results.—Correlation was significant between SpHb and Hb$_{satlab}$ ($R^2 = 0.50$, $n = 543$). The modified Bland-Altman analysis for repeated measurements showed a bias (precision) of -0.27 (1.06) and -0.02 (1.07) g dl^{-1} for the steady-state and dynamic phases, respectively. SpHb accuracy increased when Hb$_{satlab}$ was <10 g dl^{-1}, with a bias (precision) of 0.41 (0.47) *vs* -0.26 (1.12) g dl^{-1} for values >10 g dl^{-1}, but accuracy decreased after colloid administration ($R^2 = 0.25$).

Conclusions.—SpHb correlated moderately with Hb$_{satlab}$ with a slight underestimation in both phases in patients undergoing major hepatic resection. Accuracy increased for lower Hb$_{satlab}$ values but decreased in the presence of colloid solution. Further improvements are necessary to improve device accuracy under these conditions, so that SpHb might become a sensitive screening device for clinically significant anaemia.

▶ This is a useful article. Most of the prior articles on this technology were industry sponsored. If hemoglobin concentration can be used reliably to monitor hemoglobin, blood draws can be saved and more rapid decision making is possible. The authors here conclude that the technology is reliable but appears to slightly underestimate levels. That probably is acceptable as long as trending curves are accurate.

J. A. Barker, MD, CPE, FACP, FCCP, FAASM

Decrease in central venous catheter placement due to use of ultrasound guidance for peripheral intravenous catheters

Au AK, Rotte MJ, Grzybowski RJ, et al (Thomas Jefferson Univ, Philadelphia, PA)
Am J Emerg Med 30:1950-1954, 2012

Study Objectives.—Obtaining intravenous (IV) access in the emergency department (ED) can be especially challenging, and physicians often resort to placement of central venous catheters (CVCs). Use of ultrasound-guided peripheral IV catheters (USGPIVs) can prevent many "unnecessary" CVCs, but the true impact of USGPIVs has never been quantified. This study set out to determine the reduction in CVCs by USGPIV placement.

Methods.—This was a prospective, observational study conducted in 2 urban EDs. Patients who were to undergo placement of a CVC due to inability to establish IV access by other methods were enrolled. Ultrasound-trained physicians then attempted USGPIV placement. Patients were followed up for up to 7 days to assess for CVC placement and related complications.

Results.—One hundred patients were enrolled and underwent USGPIV placement. Ultrasound-guided peripheral IV catheters were initially successfully placed in all patients but failed in 12 patients (12.0%; 95 confidence interval [CI], 7.0%-19.8%) before ED disposition, resulting in 4 central lines, 7 repeated USGPIVs, and 1 patient requiring no further intervention. Through the inpatient follow-up period, another 11 patients underwent CVC placement, resulting in a total of 15 CVCs (15.0%; 95 CI, 9.3%-23.3%) placed. Of the 15 patients who did receive a CVC, 1 patient developed a catheter related infection, resulting in a 6.7% (95 CI, 1.2%-29.8%) complication rate.

Conclusion.—Ultrasound prevented the need for CVC placement in 85% of patients with difficult IV access. This suggests that USGPIVs have the potential to reduce morbidity in this patient population.

▶ Ultrasound guidance can be useful for peripheral intravenous lines, peripheral intravenous central catheter (PICC) lines, and, of course, central lines. These investigators in Philadelphia show that central venous lines can be markedly decreased by using ultrasound-guided PICCs. Results were quite good here, although it should be noted that this is a less-ill patient cohort—some went home, most went to a floor bed, and 8% were admitted to the intensive care unit. Will PICCs replace central venous catheters? I doubt it, but we will see what time brings.

J. A. Barker, MD, CPE, FACP, FCCP, FAASM

A 61-year-old man with cough and abnormal chest x-ray

Lutwak N, Dill C (VA New York Harbor Healthcare Ctr; NYU School of Medicine)
Am J Emerg Med 30:387.e1-387.e3, 2012

We present a case of a 61-year-old male smoker presenting with complaints of nonproductive cough and flulike symptoms. The chest x-ray revealed an enlarged mediastinal silhouette and no evidence of pneumonia. A computerized axial tomography scan was done, which demonstrated a very large thoracic aortic aneurysm with evidence of a hyperattenuating crescent sign, indicative of impending rupture. The patient denied chest and abdominal pain. He went to the operating room and had repair of the aneurysm (Figs 1 and 2).

▶ This is very nice review of presentation and workup of a thoracic aortic aneurysm. This is a lethal yet relatively common disorder seen in our field. It is worthwhile to review the basics frequently. Figs 1 and 2 show the relatively subtle plain film finding, which is much more obvious on chest computed tomography.

J. A. Barker, MD, CPE, FACP, FCCP, FAASM

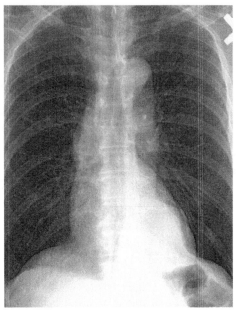

FIGURE 1.—Chest x-ray. (Reprinted from the American Journal of Emergency Medicine. Lutwak N, Dill C. A 61-year-old man with cough and abnormal chest x-ray. *Am J Emerg Med.* 2012;30:387.e1-387.e3, Copyright 2012, with permission from Elsevier.)

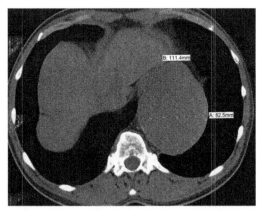

FIGURE 2.—Noncontrast CAT scan of thorax. (Reprinted from the American Journal of Emergency Medicine. Lutwak N, Dill C. A 61-year-old man with cough and abnormal chest x-ray. *Am J Emerg Med.* 2012;30:387.e1-387.e3, Copyright 2012, with permission from Elsevier.)

A National ICU Telemedicine Survey: Validation and Results

Lilly CM, Fisher KA, Ries M, et al (Univ of Massachusetts Med School, Worcester; Rush Univ Med Ctr, Chicago, IL; et al)
Chest 142:40-47, 2012

Background.—A recent ICU telemedicine research consensus conference identified the need for reliable methods of measuring structural features and processes of critical care delivery in the domains of organizational context and characteristics of ICU teams, ICUs, hospitals, and of the communities supported by an ICU.

Methods.—The American College of Chest Physicians Critical Care Institute developed and conducted a survey of ICU telemedicine practices. A 32-item survey was delivered electronically to leaders of 311 ICUs, and 11 domains were identified using principal components analysis. Survey reliability was judged by intraclass correlation among raters, and validity was measured for items for which independent assessment was available.

Results.—Complete survey information was obtained for 170 of 311 ICUs sent invitations. Analysis of a subset of surveys from 45 ICUs with complete data from more than one rater indicated that the survey reliability was in the excellent to nearly perfect range. Coefficients for measures of external validation ranged from 0.63 to 1.0. Analyses of the survey revealed substantial variation in the practice of ICU telemedicine, including ICU telemedicine center staffing patterns; qualifications of providers; case sign-out; ICU staffing models, leadership, and governance; intensivist review for new patients; adherence to best practices; use of quality and safety information; and ICU physician sign out for their patients.

Conclusions.—The American College of Chest Physicians ICU telemedicine survey is a reliable tool for measuring variation among ICUs with regard to staffing, structure, processes of care, and ICU telemedicine practices.

▶ Is remote or telemedicine intensive care unit practice still a novelty or is it becoming a standard practice? This survey from the American College of Chest Physicians helps to add to the body of literature evaluating it. The variation in practice is surprising because there is really only 1 primary vendor. I would guess the variability among intensive care unit practice in nontelemedicine locations is even more evident.

J. A. Barker, MD, CPE, FACP, FCCP, FAASM

A potentially hazardous complication during central venous catheterization: lost guidewire retained in the patient

Song Y, Messerlian AK, Matevosian R (Stanford Univ School of Medicine, CA; David Geffen School of Medicine at UCLA; et al)

J Clin Anesth 24:221-226, 2012

Guidewires are routinely used in the Seldinger technique during central venous catheter placement. A case in which a guidewire was unsuspectingly released and retained in a patient during the catheterization of the internal jugular vein is presented. Physicians from multiple services subsequently failed to detect the retained guidewire on several chest radiographs; however, the guidewire was incidentally discovered after a computed tomographic scan was obtained (Fig 1).

▶ It is maddening and saddening to see that patient safety issues remain largely unchanged even 30 years after my internship year. That year we saw numerous mishaps occur. It was, after all, soon after "House of God" was published. We were the heady young doctors out to save lives. The patients were already at high risk to die or have complications. So complications were part and parcel of work.... But we were wrong.

Now we can take a systems approach to try to avoid patient harm. (And, remember, it isn't the lonely resident's fault necessarily—although one of my

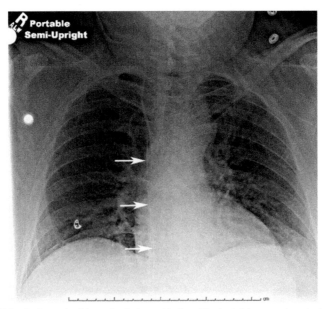

FIGURE 1.—Radiograph of the patient's chest with the guidewire (white arrows) retained in the right thorax. (Reprinted from Journal of Clinical Anesthesia, Song Y, Messerlian AK, Matevosian R. A potentially hazardous complication during central venous catheterization: lost guidewire retained in the patient. *J Clin Anesth.* 2012;24:221-226. Copyright 2012 with permission from Elsevier.)

colleagues lost 2 guidelines in 2 different patients.) Close supervision, checklists, redundancy, and systematic instrument counts as well as radiograph readings will counter the "Swiss cheese error" pointed out by the authors.

Multiple errors of omission and commission occurred to allow this x-ray to happen (Fig 1). Standardized work and redundancy can help us prevent this in our future patients. Fortunately for this patient, a good outcome occurred.

J. A. Barker, MD, CPE, FACP, FCCP, FAASM

Miscellaneous

Acquired Neuromuscular Weakness and Early Mobilization in the Intensive Care Unit

Lipshutz AKM, Gropper MA (Univ of California, San Francisco)
Anesthesiology 118:202-215, 2013

Survival from critical illness has improved in recent years, leading to increased attention to the sequelae of such illness. Neuromuscular weakness in the intensive care unit (ICU) is common, persistent, and has significant public health implications. The differential diagnosis of weakness in the ICU is extensive and includes critical illness neuromyopathy. Prolonged immobility and bedrest lead to catabolism and muscle atrophy, and are associated with critical illness neuromyopathy and ICU-acquired weakness. Early mobilization therapy has been advocated as a mechanism to prevent ICU-acquired weakness. Early mobilization is safe and feasible in most ICU patients, and improves outcomes. Implementation of early mobilization therapy requires changes in ICU culture, including decreased sedation and bedrest. Various technologies exist to increase compliance with early mobilization programs. Drugs targeting muscle pathways to decrease atrophy and muscle-wasting are in development. Additional research on early mobilization in the ICU is needed (Table 1).

▶ This is a must read for the modern intensivist. Table 1 gives a nice mnemonic for causes of muscle weakness. For example, I still see steroids excessively dosed

TABLE 1.—Mnemonic for Differential Diagnosis of Generalized Weakness in the ICU

M	Medications: steroids, neuromuscular blockers (pancuronium, vecuronium), zidovudine, amiodarone
U	Undiagnosed neuromuscular disorder: myasthenia, LEMS, inflammatory myopathies, mitochondrial myopathy, acid maltase deficiency
S	Spinal cord disease (ischemia, compression, trauma, vasculitis, demyelination)
C	Critical illness myopathy, polyneuropathy
L	Loss of muscle mass (cachectic myopathy, rhabdomyolysis)
E	Electrolyte disorders (hypokalemia, hypophosphatemia, hypermagnesemia)
S	Systemic illness (porphyria, AIDS, vasculitis, paraneoplastic, toxic)

Editor's Note: Please refer to original journal article for full references.
Reprinted with permission from Maramattom *et al.* and Wolters Kluwer Health.[19]
AIDS = acquired immunodeficiency syndrome; ICU = intensive care unit; LEMS = Lambert—Eaton myasthenic syndrome.

routinely. Few physicians seem to know that up to 50% of chronic obstructive pulmonary disease (COPD) patients admitted to an intensive care unit (ICU) will have demonstrable myopathy by the time they leave (by creatine phosphokinase, electromyogram, or muscle biopsy). Nor do most clinicians know that the current recommended dose of glucocorticoid for COPD exacerbation is now only 40 mg prednisone.

Similarly, there have been many times I have received or picked up ventilator patients labeled as "COPD" when they in fact had a paralyzed diaphragm, amyotrophic lateral sclerosis, or myasthenia gravis. Albuterol and prednisone make myasthenia worse!

Early mobilization is the new frontier in ICUs. It improves so many things: muscle function and mental awareness in addition to decreased skin breakdown. It also forces us to lower sedative medications. Yes, it may be difficult for staffing and there is some risk for dislodging tubes and lines. But these are surmountable problems.

This article covers 2 important facets of current ICU care. Read on!

J. A. Barker, MD, CPE, FACP, FCCP, FAASM

Adverse events are common on the intensive care unit: results from a structured record review
Nilsson L, Pihl A, Tågsjö M, et al (Linköping Univ, Sweden; Vrinnevi Hosp, Norrköping, Sweden; et al)
Acta Anaesthesiol Scand 56:959-965, 2012

Background.—Intensive care is advanced and highly technical, and it is essential that, despite this, patient care remains safe and of high quality. Adverse events (AEs) are supposed to be reported to internal quality control systems by health-care providers, but many are never reported. Patients on the intensive care unit (ICU) are at special risk for AEs. Our aim was to identify the incidence and characteristics of AEs in patients who died on the ICU during a 2-year period.

Methods.—A structured record review according to the Global Trigger Tool (GTT) was used to review charts from patients cared for at the ICU of a middle-sized Swedish hospital during 2007 and 2008 and who died during or immediately after ICU care. All identified AEs were scored according to severity and preventability.

Results.—We reviewed 128 records, and 41 different AEs were identified in 25 patients (19.5%). Health care-associated infections, hypoglycaemia, pressure sores and procedural complications were the most common harmful events. Twenty two (54%) of the AEs were classified as being avoidable. Two of the 41 AEs were reported as complications according to the Swedish Intensive Care Registry, and one AE had been reported in the internal AE-reporting system.

Conclusion.—Almost one fifth of the patients who died on the ICU were subjected to harmful events. GTT has the advantage of identifying more patient injuries caused by AEs than the traditional AE-reporting systems used on many ICUs.

▶ The IHI Global Trigger Tool is powerful when used. Our road ahead in intensive care units and hospitals is best done with a systems approach. The high number of adverse events (AEs) found here is emblematic of that need as we forge ahead. Fully 20% of patients in the sample group had significant AEs.

J. A. Barker, MD, CPE, FACP, FCCP, FAASM

A Historical Perspective on Sepsis
Ward PA, Bosmann M (Univ of Michigan Med School, Ann Arbor)
Am J Pathol 181:2-7, 2012

In North America, approximately 700,000 cases of sepsis occur each year, with mortality ranging between 30% and 50%. *The American Journal of Pathology* has featured numerous articles on the topic, revealing mechanistic insights gleaned from both experimental rodent models and human sepsis. Nonetheless, there remains urgent need to determine the basis for sepsis-related complications and how they can be avoided, as well as how they can be most effectively treated once recognized. This historical perspective reviews what we currently understand about the mechanisms of sepsis, as well as the barriers that remain in our treatment strategies (Fig).

▶ Why do some patients get septic with pneumonia and others only require oral outpatient antibiotics? What are the current mechanisms of sepsis—or at least the theory of the mechanism? These authors have cogently summarized current thought. It is nicely outlined in Figure 1. We will have to understand these mechanisms to modulate the inflammatory response to sepsis in the individual patient. Likewise, if we can understand the pathogenesis of sepsis, then there will be an opportunity to develop novel early pathway-blocking agents.

J. A. Barker, MD, CPE, FACP, FCCP, FAASM

SEPSIS

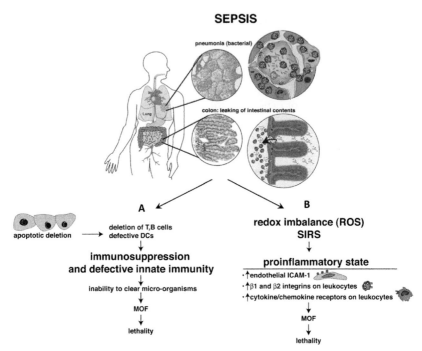

FIGURE.—Onset of sepsis beginning either as bacterial pneumonia or as peritonitis associated with extramural leaking of intestinal contents. **A:** Subsequent events include apoptotic deletion of T and B cells, defective DCs, and onset of immunosuppression, together with defective innate immunity. These events lead to loss of the ability to clear bacteria, resulting in development of multiorgan failure (MOF) and death. **B:** Development of sepsis can also lead to redox imbalance in a variety of cells (leukocytes) and organs due to buildup of reactive oxygen species (ROS). This is followed by an inflammatory response (SIRS), including a sustained immune response and other immune activation states in endothelial cells and leukocytes, ultimately associated with MOF and death. (Reprinted from the American Journal of Pathology. Ward PA, Bosmann M. A historical perspective on sepsis. *Am J Pathol*. 2012;181:2-7, Copyright 2012, with permission from American Society for Investigative Pathology.)

A 42-year-old woman with septic shock: an unexpected source

Sacks R, Kerr K (Univ of California, La Jolla)
J Emerg Med 42:275-278, 2012

Background.—Dog bites are the most common animal bite injuries occurring in the United States. Estimated infection rates range between 15% and 20%. Polymicrobial infections are most common. *Capnocytophaga canimorsus* (*C. canimorsus*) is a Gram-negative rod strongly associated with dog bites, and is known to cause life-threatening infection in humans.

Objectives.—1) Outline epidemiology of dog bites in the United States; 2) Identify host factors associated with infection, and common pathogens; 3) Discuss microbiology of *C. canimorsus*; 4) Discuss common clinical manifestations of *C. canimorsus* infection; 5) Outline treatment options.

Case Report.—A 42-year-old woman with a remote history of Hodgkin's lymphoma (treated with irradiation) and thyroid carcinoma, both of which were in remission, presented to the Emergency Department with fever, abdominal pain, and diarrhea. She was found to be in septic shock. She was aggressively resuscitated and administered broad-spectrum antibiotics. Blood cultures grew *C. canimorsus* in 2/4 bottles. The patient recalled being bitten by the family dog 48 h before her initial presentation. She made an uneventful recovery. She was felt to be "functionally hyposplenic" due to her prior irradiation.

Conclusions.—*C. canimorsus* is a rare pathogen strongly associated with dog bites. By eliciting a history of animal bite, clinicians may be able to alert the laboratory of suspected *C. canimorsus* infection. Prolonged laboratory incubation times may be necessary as the organism is fastidious. Predisposing conditions include, among others, prior splenectomy and alcoholism. The mortality rate from *C. canimorsus* sepsis is high, so treatment should be promptly initiated.

▶ I have a feeling that dog bites are pretty common. Immunosuppression is very common as well. Thus, it should be no surprise to any of us that a case such as this may occur. In particular, we should note the normal white blood cell count despite severe septic shock. It is always good to be reminded of the severity of asplenia, and this case certainly does that.

J. A. Barker, MD, CPE, FACP, FCCP, FAASM

A multicenter trial to compare blood culture with polymerase chain reaction in severe human sepsis
Bloos F, Hinder F, Becker K, et al (Univ Hosp Jena, Germany; Univ Hosp Münster, Germany; et al)
Intensive Care Med 36:241-247, 2010

Objective.—To assess the presence of microbial DNA in the blood by polymerase chain reaction (PCR) and its association with disease severity and markers of inflammation in severe sepsis and to compare the performance of PCR with blood culture (BC).

Design.—Prospective multicentric controlled observational study.

Setting.—Three surgical intensive care units in university centers and large teaching hospitals.

Patients.—One hundred forty-two patients with severe sepsis and 63 surgical controls.

Interventions.—Presence of microbial DNA was assessed by multiplex PCR upon enrollment, and each time a BC was obtained.

Measurements and Main Results.—Controls had both approximately 4% positive PCRs and BCs. In severe sepsis, 34.7% of PCRs were positive compared to 16.5% of BCs ($P < 0.001$). Consistently, 70.3% of BCs had a corresponding PCR result, while only 21.4% of PCR results were confirmed by BC. Compared to patients with negative PCRs at enrollment, those testing positive had higher organ dysfunction scores [SOFA, median (25th–75th percentile) 12 (7–15) vs. 9 (7–11); $P = 0.023$] and a trend toward higher mortality (PCR negative 25.3%; PCR positive 39.1%; $P = 0.115$).

Conclusions.—In septic patients, concordance between BC and PCR is moderate. However, PCR-based pathogen detection correlated with disease severity even if the BC remained negative, suggesting that presence of microbial DNA in the bloodstream is a significant event. The clinical utility to facilitate treatment decisions warrants investigation.

▶ I think this is an important article and probably signals the beginning of a change in practice for all of us. Patients with severe sepsis and septic shock do not always have positive blood cultures. In fact, most authorities quote only a 30% positive rate for blood cultures in septic shock. The polymerase chain reaction (PCR) results appear validated. Of interest, only 60% of the time were the blood cultures positive. Equally important were some apparent false negatives in the PCR group (positive blood cultures). Thus, at present both techniques would be needed for absolute best yield results.

Also reassuring are the negative results in nonseptic postoperative patients. These people are obviously quite inflamed yet not with active infection. It is important to see negative results for PCR in this group. Excessive sensitivity would render it a useless test.

J. A. Barker, MD, CPE, FACP, FCCP, FAASM

A systematic review and meta-analysis of clinical trials of thyroid hormone administration to brain dead potential organ donors
Macdonald PS, Aneman A, Bhonagiri D, et al (St Vincent's Hosp, Sydney, New South Wales, Australia; Liverpool Hosp, Sydney, New South Wales, Australia; et al)
Crit Care Med 40:1635-1644, 2012

Objectives.—To review all published clinical studies of thyroid hormone administration to brain-dead potential organ donors.

Methods.—A search of PubMed using multiple search terms retrieved 401 publications including 35 original reports describing administration of thyroid hormone to brain-dead potential organ donors. Detailed review of the 35 original reports led to identification of two additional publications not retrieved in the original search. The 37 original publications reported findings from 16 separate case series or retrospective audits and seven randomized controlled trials, four of which were placebo-controlled. Meta-analysis was restricted to the four placebo-controlled randomized controlled trials.

Results.—Whereas all case series and retrospective audits reported a beneficial effect of thyroid hormone administration, all seven randomized controlled trials reported no benefit of thyroid hormone administration either alone or in combination with other hormonal therapies. In four placebo-controlled trials including 209 donors, administration of thyroid hormone (n = 108) compared with placebo (n = 101) had no significant effect on donor cardiac index (pooled mean difference, 0.15 L/min/m^2; 95% confidence interval −0.18 to 0.48). The major limitation of the case series and retrospective audits was the lack of consideration of uncontrolled variables that confound interpretation of the results. A limitation of the randomized controlled trials was that the proportion of donors who were hemodynamically unstable or marginal in other ways was too small to exclude a benefit of thyroid hormone in this subgroup.

Conclusions.—The findings of this systematic review do not support a role for routine administration of thyroid hormone in the brain-dead potential organ donor. Existing recommendations regarding the use of thyroid hormone in marginal donors are based on low-level evidence.

▶ I found this article to be very useful. Thyroid hormone supplementation has become almost de rigueur in this small but very real population of critical care patients. It is paramount that we analyze common practice under the scrutiny of best available science.

Shout it from the treetops, "There is no indication for thyroid hormone in pre-donor brain dead patients."

J. A. Barker, MD, CPE, FACP, FCCP, FAASM

Recurrent Sepsis In a 69-Year-Old Woman

Konduru S, Koussa G, Naber M, et al (Albany Med Ctr, NY)
Chest 140:1091-1094, 2011

Background.—Quinine has been used as a herbal remedy for over 350 years and is used today to treat malaria and nocturnal leg cramps. However, the US Food and Drug Administration determined in 1994 that quinine's risk-to-benefit ratio in the treatment of leg cramps is unfavorable and banned all over-the-counter quinine products. Herbal products, tonic water, and bitter lemon still contain quinine and are available to consumers. In 2005 quinine was approved for the treatment of uncompleted malaria caused by *Plasmodium falciparum*, but prescribers still give patients quinine for the off-label treatment of nocturnal leg cramps. An American Academy of Neurology evidence-based review and a recent Cochrane systematic review of 23 trials have supported the effectiveness of quinine for reducing the number and intensity of muscle cramps, but patients should be informed of the possibility of serious adverse events. These include hypersensitivity reaction, aplastic or hemolytic anemia, thrombocytopenia, neutropenia, coagulopathy, hemolytic uremic

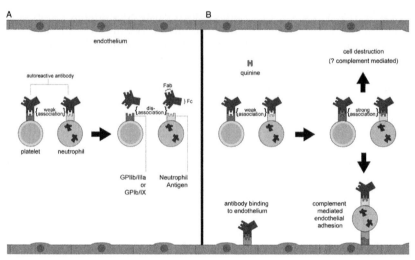

FIGURE 1.—A, Without quinine, the binding between autoreactive antibodies and the platelet or neutrophil receptor is weak and transient. B, When quinine is present, it facilitates favorable interactions between antibody and receptor, leading to sustained binding and stimulation of an autoimmune response resulting in cell destruction (possibly complement mediated), antibody binding to endothelium, and endothelial adhesion of neutrophils. These latter two events may lead to endothelial damage, with subsequent progression to a systemic inflammatory response and sepsis-like syndrome. Fab = antibody binding; Fc = antibody tail ; GP = glycoprotein. (Reprinted from Konduru S, Koussa G, Naber M, et al. Recurrent sepsis in a 69-year-old woman. *Chest.* 2011;140:1091-1094. © 2011 American College of Chest Physicians.

syndrome (HUS), and thrombotic thrombocytopenic purpura (TTP). Diagnosing quinine hypersensitivity is difficult because quinine use is often not disclosed in a medication history.

Case Report.—Woman, 69, had acute symptoms of fever, chills, nausea, vomiting, diarrhea, and dizziness lasting 4 hours. She was febrile, tachycardic, and hypotensive. She was managed with aggressive treatment of septic shock using fluid resuscitation, vasopressors, and broad-spectrum antibiotics. This was her third presentation to the hospital with similar symptoms in the past 2 years. Her medical history also included diabetes, hypertension, hyperlipidemia, asthma, gastroesophageal reflux disease, and peripheral neuropathy. She was taking irbesartan, atorvastatin, quinine, omeprazole, primidone, and desloratadine. Common elements in her three hospitalizations were pancytopenia and coagulopathy. She received antibiotics and vasopressors and underwent a thorough workup, the results of which were normal. Her first hospital visit was distinguished by the presence of microangiographic hemolytic anemia that required plasmapheresis and prolonged hemodialysis for acute renal failure. Her current laboratory results included profound leukopenia, mild thrombocytopenia, and anemia, and she demonstrated an elevated international normalized ratio and high liver transaminase and serum lactate dehydrogenase levels. She was admitted to the medical intensive care unit, and septic shock measures were continued. In 12 hours, her neutropenia resolved; in 24 hours, her fever and hypotension were gone. No causative microbiologic agent was identified. Quinine toxicity was highly suspected; quinine-dependent antibodies to neutrophils were detected, confirming the diagnosis. The patient was informed of her hypersensitivity to quinine and instructed to avoid its use.

Conclusions.—It is currently unknown why patients with quinine hypersensitivity develop a sepsis like syndrome, but endothelial dysfunction and capillary leak may contribute. This patient presented a life-threatening adverse event caused by quinine and required critical care support. Patients who come for treatment of such symptoms should be closely questioned about the medications they use, including complementary and alternative agents (Fig 1).

▶ A large percentage of patients use over-the-counter or herbal medications. In addition, quinine is available in many forms—medications, mixed drinks, and in herbal supplements.
The putative mechanism of endothelial damage is nicely outlined in Fig 1. I found this case particularly interesting. It outlines the importance of truly defining the type of shock one is dealing with. It is tempting to call this anaphylaxis but it does not fit with that (no urticaria, wheezing, etc). Instead the putative mechanism of noninfectious systematic inflammatory response syndrome as diagrammed in Fig 1 is the likely answer.

J. A. Barker, MD, CPE, FACP, FCCP, FAASM

Clinical characteristics and outcomes of obstetric patients admitted to the intensive care unit
Rios FG, Risso-Vázquez A, Alvarez J, et al (Hosp Nacional Profesor Alejandro Posadas, Buenos Aires, Argentina; Sanatorio Otamendi-Miroli, Buenos Aires, Argentina; Hospital Universitario Austral, Buenos Aires, Argentina)
Int J Gynecol Obstet 119:136-140, 2012

Objective.—To identify the reasons for admitting pregnant women to intensive care units (ICUs) in Buenos Aires, Argentina.
Methods.—The admission diagnoses of pregnant women hospitalized over 2 years at 4 ICUs were retrospectively studied.
Results.—During the studied period, 242 (3.9%) of the 6271 ICU patients were pregnant women, for an incidence of 8.1 per 1000 deliveries. The main reasons for admitting them at ICUs were hypertensive disorders, followed by postpartum hemorrhage and sepsis. More than a third (39.7%) was in a first pregnancy. The main nonobstetric reason for admission was pneumonia. The median pregnancy duration on admission was

36 weeks (range, 33—38 weeks) but it was less than 34 weeks for 66 (27.2%) of the women, 12.4% on whom required ventilation. Mortality was highest among those admitted for nonobstetric reasons (13.3% vs 0.5%; $P < 0.05$). The median stay for obstetric or nonobstetric conditions was 2 versus 5 days (range, 2—3 days vs 2—8 days) ($P < 0.001$).

Conclusion.—Postpartum hemorrhage and hypertensive disorders were the most common reasons for admitting pregnant women to an ICU, followed by sepsis. Nonobstetric causes of admission were associated with higher morbidity and mortality rates.

▶ Obstetric patients do make their way to adult intensive care units, although there is always significant angst among caregivers. The patients are usually young and healthy before the pregnancy. In addition, there are 2 lives at stake. Still, deaths do occur even with the best of care.

The worsening of prognosis with advancing age is useful to know. In addition, the nonobstetric disorders had markedly worse prognosis.

J. A. Barker, MD, CPE, FACP, FCCP, FAASM

Article Index

Chapter 1: Asthma, Allergy, and Cystic Fibrosis

Chapter 2: Chronic Obstructive Pulmonary Disease

Chapter 3: Lung Cancer

Chapter 4: Pleural, Interstitial Lung, and Pulmonary Vascular Disease

Chapter 5: Community-Acquired Pneumonia

Chapter 6: Lung Transplantation

Chapter 7: Sleep Disorders

Chapter 8: Critical Care Medicine

Author Index

A

Acosta-Pérez E, 2
Adamali HI, 117
Agbaje OF, 92
Agusti A, 54, 210
Aigner C, 180
Aitken ML, 197
Ak G, 120
Alarcão J, 174
Albert P, 54
Alex C, 198
Allen SJ, 232
Alpert HR, 73
Alvarez J, 265
Anagnostopoulos N, 69
Andersson M, 218
Andrews AL, 15
Aneman A, 262
Arcasoy SM, 187
Asadi L, 171
Ashraf H, 94
Au AK, 252
Aujesky D, 134
Aurora RN, 202
Austin ED, 136
Awad KM, 217

B

Bach PB, 74, 79
Bae S, 150
Bafadhel M, 43
Baldwin MR, 187
Banerjee SK, 190
Bannuru RR, 52
Barbé F, 214
Bargagli E, 116
Barlesi F, 88
Barnes M, 219
Barnet JH, 217
Barnett CF, 137
Barst RJ, 151
Basco WT Jr, 15
Bateman ED, 6, 9
Becker K, 261
Bellomi M, 96
Benza RL, 151
Berg S, 218
Bergethon K, 111
Bhonagiri D, 262
Bhorade S, 191
Bielsa S, 167
Biener L, 73

Bleecker ER, 6, 9
Blondon M, 134
Bloos F, 261
Blumenthal JA, 196
Boedeker E, 102
Bolster MB, 150
Bonser RS, 184
Bosmann M, 259
Brahmer JR, 105, 106
Brehm JM, 2
Breidthardt T, 162
Briel M, 165
Broffman M, 98
Brooks LJ, 229
Buatsi J, 132
Buikema AR, 12
Büller HR, 127
Burtin C, 194
Busse WW, 6
Buxton OM, 225

C

Cadirci O, 120
Caldeira D, 174
Camargos P, 3
Camporota L, 237
Campos-Rodríguez F, 207
Caporaso NE, 90
Carney RC, 196
Carratalà J, 167, 177
Castro-Rodriguez JA, 11
Catalán-Serra P, 207
Catalano PJ, 108
Celli BR, 37
Chan PC, 239
Chen Y-H, 155, 205
Chigbo C, 160
Choi P, 27
Chow LQM, 106
Chowdhuri S, 202
Christ-Crain M, 162, 165
Clancy JP, 24
Cole SR, 67
Colish J, 211
Collen J, 224
Connett JE, 34
Connolly GN, 73
Cook TM, 242
Correia LCL, 203
Corren J, 17
Costi M, 246
Crabtree TD, 123
Crawford-Achour E, 206

Crinò L, 88
Cronin A, 108

D

Dahl R, 8
Davies HE, 122
Demarco T, 247
DeSantis C, 103
Diderichsen F, 29
Dill C, 253
Dirksen A, 94
Dixon JB, 221
Donaldson GC, 41
Draper KA, 229
Drummond MB, 34
Duffy SW, 92

E

Eapen GA, 82
Edwards L, 54
Ehlken N, 139
Ehmann R, 102
Ellenbogen JM, 225
Elliott CG, 137
Elmayergi N, 211
Engel M, 8
Ettinger DS, 82
Eurich DT, 171

F

Fabre A, 117
Falguera M, 167
Fan E, 237
Fang JC, 247
Ferguson ND, 237
Finkelstein JA, 154
Fisher KA, 255
Flume PA, 25
Friedrich U, 102

G

Garcia G, 203
Garcia-Vidal C, 177
Gauthier M, 206
Givertz MM, 247
Goldhaber SZ, 50
Gonska T, 27
Gordon IO, 191

Printed and bound by CPI Group (UK) Ltd, Croydon, CR0 4YY

08/05/2025

01864755-0006